Board Review Series

Behavioral Science
3rd edition

Board Review Series

Behavioral Science

3rd edition

Barbara Fadem, Ph.D.
Professor
Department of Psychiatry
University of Medicine and Dentistry of New Jersey
New Jersey Medical School
Newark, New Jersey

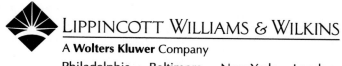

LIPPINCOTT WILLIAMS & WILKINS
A **Wolters Kluwer** Company
Philadelphia · Baltimore · New York · London
Buenos Aires · Hong Kong · Sydney · Tokyo

Editor: Elizabeth Nieginski
Development Editor: Emilie Linkins
Managing Editor: Marette D. Magargle-Smith
Marketing Manager: Jennifer Conrad

351 West Camden Street
Baltimore, Maryland 21201-2436 USA

227 East Washington Square
Philadelphia, PA 19106

Printed in the United States of America

Library of Congress Cataloging-in-Publication Data

Fadem, Barbara.
    Behavioral science / Barbara Fadem.—3rd ed.
      p. cm. — (Board review series)
    Includes index.
    ISBN 0-683-30681-2
    1. Psychiatry Outlines, syllabi, etc. 2. Psychology Outlines, syllabi, etc.
  3. Psychiatry Examinations, questions, etc. 4. Psychology Examinations,
questions, etc.
    I. Title. II. Series.
    [DNLM: 1. Behavioral Sciences Examination Questions. 2. Behavioral
Sciences Outlines. 3. Behavior Examination Questions. 4. Behavior
Outlines. WM 18.2 F144b 1999]
    RC457.2.F34 1999
    616.89'0076—DC21
    DNLM   999-20848
    for Library of Congress   CIP

To purchase additional copies of this book, call our customer service department at **(800) 638-3030** or fax orders to **(301) 824-7390**. International customers should call **(301) 714-2324**.

02 03
3 4 5 6 7 8 9 10

Dedication

I dedicate this book to Jonathan Fadem who has taught this teacher the true meaning of artistic passion, unwavering motivation, and physical courage.

Contents

Preface

The function and state of the mind are of significant importance to the physical health of an individual. The United States Medical Licensing Examination (USMLE) is closely attuned to the substantial power of the mind-body relationship and tests this area extensively on all three Steps of the examination. This review has been prepared as a learning tool to help students rapidly recall information that they have learned in the first two years of medical school in behavioral science, psychiatry, epidemiology and related courses.

The third edition of *BRS Behavioral Science* contains 9 sections divided into 26 chapters. All chapters start with a "Typical Board Question" (TBQ), which serves as an example for the way that the subject matter of that chapter is tested on the USMLE. Each chapter has been extensively updated to include the most current information. A total of at least 400 questions and answers with detailed explanations are presented after each chapter and in the Comprehensive Examination at the end of the book. Almost all of these questions have been written expressly for this third edition and reflect the new USMLE format utilizing clinical vignettes. Seventy-six tables are included in the book to provide essential information quickly.

Acknowledgments

The author wishes to thank Emilie Linkins, Julie Scardiglia, and Elizabeth Nieginski of Lippincott Williams and Wilkins for their encouragement, hard work, and practical assistance with the manuscript. The author also thanks Dr. Steven J. Schleifer, Chairman, and Dr. Steven S. Simring, Vice-Chairman for Education, both of the Department of Psychiatry of the New Jersey Medical School, for their enthusiasm, help, and support for this effort. Special thanks to Dr. Marian Passannante of the Department of Preventive Medicine and Community Health and Dr. Allan Siegel of the Department of Neurosciences for their generous contributions of time and knowledge and Todd Flannery for his help with the manuscript. Finally and as always, the author thanks with great affection and respect the caring, involved medical students with whom she has had the high honor of working over the years.

1

The Beginning of Life: Pregnancy through Preschool

Typical Board Question

A mother brings her 8-month-old child in to see the physician for a well-baby checkup. The mother appears concerned. She tells the doctor that the child recently saw an aunt whom he had not seen in 6 months. When the aunt approached him, the child cried, seemed fearful, and clung tightly to his mother. The doctor correctly tells the mother that this fearful, clinging behavior

(A) indicates that the child is developmentally delayed
(B) indicates that the child is emotionally disturbed
(C) indicates that the child has been abused by his aunt
(D) is more likely to occur in infants exposed to many different caregivers
(E) occurs in normal infants of this age when they are confronted with an unfamiliar person

(See "Answers and Explanations" at end of Chapter)

I. Pregnancy

A. Emotions

1. **Mood changes** are common during pregnancy and may be caused by **biological factors** (e.g., hormonal fluctuations) as well **as psychological factors** (e.g., concern over loss of physical attractiveness).

2. **Pseudocyesis (false pregnancy)**, the occurrence of many symptoms of pregnancy although conception has not taken place, may occur in women who have a **strong wish to be pregnant** or a **strong fear of pregnancy.**

3. Many pregnant women form a close emotional relationship with their unborn infant, thus beginning the **bonding** process prior to birth (See III A).

B. The marital relationship

1. Many obstetricians suggest cessation of sexual intercourse about 4 weeks prior to the expected date of delivery.

2. Reduction in sexual activity for any reason can put a strain on the mar-

riage. **Extramarital affairs** conducted by the husband, if they occur, are more likely to occur during the last 3 months of the wife's pregnancy.

II. Childbirth

A. Birth rate, infant mortality, and cesarean birth

1. About 4 million children are born each year in the United States.

2. **Infant mortality**
   a. In part because the United States **does not have socialized medicine** (health care for all citizens paid for by the government through taxes), the **infant mortality rate in the United States is high** compared with rates in other developed countries (see also Chapter 23).
   b. **Low socioeconomic status,** which is related in part to **ethnicity,** is associated with high infant mortality (Table 1-1).

3. **Cesarean birth**
   a. The number of **cesarean births** increased from the 1960s to the 1990s, partly because of physicians' fears of malpractice suits if an infant died or was injured during vaginal childbirth.
   b. Recently, however, the number of cesarean births (currently 21% of all births) has leveled off or even declined, partly in response to increasing evidence that women often undergo unnecessary surgical procedures.

B. Premature birth

1. Premature births are defined as those following a **gestation of less than 34 weeks** or in which the **birth weight is under 2500 g.**

2. Premature births, which are associated with low income, maternal illness or malnutrition, and young maternal age, occur in **6% of births to white women** and **13% of births to African-American women.**

3. Premature birth puts the child **at greater risk** for emotional, behavioral and learning problems, physical disability, and mental retardation.

C. Postpartum reactions

1. **Baby blues**
   a. Many women experience an emotional reaction called **"baby blues"** or **"postpartum blues"** lasting **up to 1 week** after childbirth.

Table 1-1. Ethnicity and Infant Mortality in the United States (1996)

Ethnic Group	Infant Deaths per 1000 Live Births
White, Asian American, and Mexican, Cuban, and other Hispanic American	5.1–6.1
Puerto Rican American	8.6
Native American (American Indian)	8.8
African-American	14.2
Overall	**7.2**

   b. This reaction results from psychological factors (e.g., the emotional stress of childbirth, the feelings of added responsibility), as well as physiological factors (e.g., **changes in hormone levels,** fatigue).

   c. Treatment involves support and practical help with the infant.

   2. Major depression and **brief psychotic disorder with postpartum onset** (postpartum psychosis) are reactions which are more serious than postpartum blues and which are treated with antidepressant and antipsychotic medications (Table 1-2) (and see Chapters 11 and 12).

III. Infancy: Birth to 15 Months

   A. Bonding of the parent to the infant

   1. Bonding between the caregiver and the infant is enhanced by **physical contact** between the two.

   2. Bonding **may be** adversely affected if:

   a. The child is of **low birth weight or ill,** leading to **separation from the mother** after delivery

   b. There are problems in the mother-father relationship

   3. Women who take **classes preparing them for childbirth** have shorter labors, fewer medical complications, less need for medication, and have closer initial interactions with their infants.

   B. Attachment of the infant to the parent

   1. The principal psychological task of infancy is the **formation of an intimate attachment** to the primary caregiver, usually the mother.

Table 1-2. Postpartum Maternal Reactions

Maternal Reaction	Incidence	Onset of Symptoms	Duration of Symptoms	Characteristics
Postpartum blues ("baby blues")	33%–50%	Within a few days after delivery	Up to 1 week after delivery	• Exaggerated emotionality and tearfulness • Interacting well with friends and family • Good grooming
Major depressive episode	5%–10%	Within 4 weeks after delivery	Up to 1 year without treatment; 3–6 weeks with treatment	• Feelings of hopelessness and helplessness • Lack of pleasure or interest in usual activities • Poor grooming
Brief psychotic disorder, postpartum onset ("postpartum psychosis")	0.1%–0.2%	Within 2–3 weeks after delivery	Up to 1 month	• Hallucinations, delusions, or other psychotic symptoms • Mother may harm infant

    2. Separation from the primary caregiver between 6–12 months of age leads to initial loud protests from the infant.

    3. With continued absence of the mother, the infant is at risk for **anaclitic depression,** in which he is **withdrawn** and **unresponsive** toward others.

        a. An infant may suffer from anaclitic depression even when he is living with his mother if the **mother is physically and emotionally distant and insensitive** to his needs.

        b. Depressed infants may exhibit **"failure to thrive"** which includes poor physical growth and poor health.

C. Studies of attachment

    1. Harry Harlow demonstrated that infant monkeys reared in relative isolation by **surrogate artificial mothers** do not develop normal mating, maternal, and social behaviors as adults.

        a. Males may be **more affected** than females by such isolation.

        b. Young monkeys raised in isolation for **less than 6 months** can be rehabilitated by playing with normal young monkeys.

    2. René Spitz documented that children without proper mothering (e.g., those in orphanages) show severe **developmental retardation,** poor health, and higher death rates (**"hospitalism"**) in spite of adequate physical care.

    3. Partly due to such findings, the "foster care" system was established for young children in the United States who do not have adequate home situations. "Foster families" are those who have been approved and funded by the state of residence to take care of a child in their homes.

D. Characteristics of the infant

    1. Reflexive behavior. At birth, the normal infant possesses simple reflexes such as the **startle** reflex (Moro reflex), the **palmar grasp** reflex, **Babinski's** reflex, and the **rooting** reflex. All of these reflexes disappear during the first year of life (Table 1-3).

    2. Motor, social, verbal, and cognitive development (Table 1-4)

        a. Although there is a reflexive smile present at birth, the **social smile** is one of the first markers of the infant's responsiveness to another individual.

Table 1-3. Reflexes Present at Birth and the Age at Which They Disappear

Reflex	Description	Age of disappearance
Palmar grasp	The child's fingers grasp objects placed in the palm	2 months
Rooting reflex	The child's head turns in the direction of a stroke on the cheek as though seeking a nipple	3 months
Startle (Moro) reflex	When the child is startled, the arms and legs extend	4 months
Babinski reflex	Dorsiflexion of the largest toe when the plantar surface of the child's foot is stroked	12 months
Tracking reflex	The child visually follows a human face	Continues

Table 1-4. Motor, Social, Verbal, and Cognitive Development of the Infant

Age	Skill Area		
	Motor	**Social**	**Verbal and Cognitive**
2–3 months	• Lifts head when lying on stomach	• Smiles in response to a human face (the "social smile")	• Coos or gurgles
5–6 months	• Turns over • Sits unassisted • Grasps with entire hand ("raking")	• Forms an attachment to primary caregiver • Recognizes familiar people	• Babbles (repeats single sounds over and over)
7–11 months	• Crawls on hands and knees • Pulls up to stand • Transfers toys to other hand • Picks up toys and food using "pincer" (thumb and forefinger) grasp	• Shows stranger anxiety • Plays social games such as peek-a-boo, waves "bye-bye"	• Imitates sounds • Uses gestures
11–15 months	• Walks unassisted	• Fears separation from primary caregiver (separation anxiety)	• Says first word • Understands words

> **b.** Crying and withdrawing in the presence of an unfamiliar person **(stranger anxiety) is normal** and begins at about 7 months of age.
>> **i.** This behavior indicates that the infant has developed a specific attachment to the mother and is able to distinguish her from a stranger.
>> **ii.** Infants exposed to many caregivers are less likely to show stranger anxiety than those exposed to few caregivers.

E. Theories of development

> **1. Chess and Thomas** showed that there are **endogenous differences** in the **temperaments** of infants which remain quite stable for the first 25 years of life. These differences include such characteristics as reactivity to stimuli, cyclic behavior patterns such as sleeping, responsiveness to people, mood, distractibility, and attention span.

> **2. Sigmund Freud** described development in terms of the parts of the body from which the most pleasure is derived at each stage of development (e.g., the "oral stage" occurs during the first year of life).

> **3. Erik Erikson** described development in terms of critical periods for the achievement of social goals; if a specific goal is not achieved at a specific age, the individual will never achieve the goal. For example, in Erikson's stage of **basic trust versus mistrust,** the child must learn to trust others during the first year of life or she will never be able to trust others.

> **4. Jean Piaget** described development in terms of learning capabilities of the child at each age.

5. Margaret Mahler described early development as a sequential process of separation of the child from the mother or primary caregiver.

IV. The Toddler Years: 15 Months to 2½ Years

A. Attachment
1. The **major theme** of the second year of life is to **separate from the mother** or primary caregiver, a process which is complete by about age 3.
2. There is **no evidence** that daily separation from working parents in a good day care setting has short- or long-term negative consequences for children.

B. Motor, social, verbal, and cognitive characteristics of the toddler (see Table 1-5)

V. The Preschool Child: 2½ to 6 Years

A. Attachment
1. After reaching 3 years of age a child should be able to spend a few hours away from the mother in the care of others (e.g., in day care).
2. A child who cannot do this after age 3 suffers from **separation anxiety disorder** (see Chapter 15).

B. Characteristics
1. The child's **vocabulary increases** rapidly (Table 1-5) and the child often finds humor in using "bathroom" profanity (e.g., saying "pee-pee").
2. The birth of a sibling is likely to occur in the preschool years and **sibling rivalry** may occur.
3. Sibling rivalry or other life stress, such as moving, may result in a child's use of **regression,** a defense mechanism in which the child temporarily behaves in a "babylike" way (e.g., he starts wetting the bed again).
4. The child can distinguish fantasy from reality (e.g., he knows that imaginary friends are not "real" people), although the line between them may still not be drawn sharply.
5. Other aspects of motor, social, verbal, and cognitive development of the preschool child can be found in Table 1-5.

C. Changes at 6 years of age: formation of the conscience
1. At the end of the preschool years (about age 6), the child's **conscience** (the **superego** of Freud) and **sense of morality** begin to be developed.
2. After age 6, the child can put himself in another person's place (**empathy**) and behave in a caring and sharing way toward others.
3. Morality and empathy increase further during the school-age years (see Chapter 2).

Table 1-5. Motor, Social, Verbal, and Cognitive Development of the Toddler and Preschool Child

Age	Skill Area		
	Motor	**Social**	**Verbal and cognitive**
18 months	• Throws a ball • Stacks 3 blocks • Climbs stairs one foot at a time • Scribbles on paper	• Moves away from and then returns to the mother for reassurance ("rapprochement")	• Uses about 10 individual words • Says own name
2 years	• Kicks a ball • Balances on one foot for one second • Stacks 6 blocks • Feeds self with fork and spoon	• Shows negativity (e.g., the favorite word is "no") • Plays alongside but not with another child ("parallel play": 2–4 years of age)	• Uses about 250 words • Speaks in 2-word sentences and uses pronouns (e.g., "me do") • Names body parts and objects
3 years	• Rides a tricycle • Undresses and partially dresses without help • Identifies some colors • Climbs stairs using alternate feet • Stacks 9 blocks • Cuts paper with scissors • Copies a circle ○	• Has a sense of self as male or female (gender identity) • Usually achieves bowel and bladder control [problems such as encopresis ("soiling") and enuresis ("bedwetting") cannot be diagnosed until 4 and 5 years of age, respectively] • Can spend part of the day with adults other than parents (e.g., in preschool setting)	• Uses about 900 words in speech • Understands about 3,500 words • Speaks in complete sentences (e.g., "I can do it myself")
4 years	• Catches a ball with arms • Dresses independently, using buttons and zippers • Grooms self (e.g., brushes teeth) • Hops on one foot • Copies a cross ✚	• Begins to play cooperatively with other children • Engages in role playing (e.g., "I'll be the mommy, you be the daddy") • May have imaginary companions • Has curiosity about sex differences, (e.g., plays "doctor" with other children) • Has nightmares and transient phobias (e.g., of "monsters")	• Shows good verbal self-expression (e.g., can tell detailed stories) • Comprehends and uses prepositions (e.g., under, above)
5 years	• Catches a ball with two hands • Draws a person in detail, (e.g., with arms, hair, eyes) • Skips using alternate feet • Copies a square □	• Has romantic feelings about the opposite sex parent (the "oedipal phase") at 4–5 years of age • Has overconcern about physical injury at 4–5 years of age	• Shows further improvement in verbal and cognitive skills
6 years	• Ties shoelaces • Rides a 2-wheeled bicycle • Prints letters • Copies a triangle △	• Begins to develop an internalized moral sense of right and wrong	• Begins to think logically (see Chapter 2) • Begins to read

Review Test

Directions: Each of the numbered items or incomplete statements in this section is followed by answers or by completions of the statement. Select the **one** lettered answer or completion that is **best** in each case.

1. An American couple would like to adopt a 10-month-old Russian child. However, they are concerned because the child has been in an orphanage ever since he was separated from his birth mother 2 months ago. Which of the following characteristics is the couple most likely to see in the child at this time?

(A) Loud crying and protests at the loss of his mother
(B) Increased responsiveness to adults
(C) Normal development of motor skills
(D) Depression
(E) Normal development of social skills

2. Although he previously slept in his own bed, after his parents separate, a 4-year-old boy insists on sleeping in his mother's bed every night. He continues to do well in nursery school and plays well with friends. The best description of this boy's behavior is

(A) separation anxiety disorder
(B) normal with regression
(C) delayed development
(D) lack of basic trust
(E) poor superego development

3. You conduct a well-child checkup on a normal 2-year-old girl. She is most likely to show which of the following skills or characteristics?

(A) Speaks in 2-word sentences
(B) Is completely toilet trained
(C) Can comfortably spend most of the day away from her mother
(D) Can ride a 2-wheeled bicycle
(E) Engages in cooperative play

4. You conduct a well-child checkup on a normal 4-year-old boy. He is most likely to show which of the following skills or characteristics?

(A) Identifies colors
(B) Reads a 3-word sentence
(C) Refuses to play with girls
(D) Ties shoelaces
(E) Has an internalized moral sense of right and wrong

5. A mother brings her normal 4-month-old child to the pediatrician for a well-baby examination. Which of the following developmental signposts can the doctor expect to be present in this infant?

(A) Stranger anxiety
(B) Social smile
(C) Rapprochement
(D) Core gender identity
(E) Phobias

6. The overall infant mortality rate in the United States in 1996 was approximately

(A) 1 per 1000 live births
(B) 3 per 1000 live births
(C) 7 per 1000 live births
(D) 21 per 1000 live births
(E) 40 per 1000 live births

7. The most important psychological task for a child between birth and 15 months is the development of

(A) the ability to think logically
(B) speech
(C) stranger anxiety
(D) a conscience
(E) an intimate attachment to the mother or primary caregiver

8. A 28-year-old woman and her husband are preparing for childbirth by taking a formal training program. Her physician can expect that when compared with women who do not take a formal training program, this woman will experience

(A) more medical complications
(B) longer labor
(C) closer initial interactions with her infant
(D) more need for medication during labor
(E) higher likelihood of postpartum emotional reactions

9. A new mother develops a sad mood 2 days following the birth of her child. Which of the following factors is most likely to contribute to the development of this condition?

(A) A positive childbirth experience
(B) Breastfeeding
(C) Feelings of decreased responsibility
(D) Changes in hormone levels
(E) Increased energy

10. A well-trained, highly qualified obstetrician has a busy practice. Which of the following is most likely to be true about postpartum reactions in this doctor's patients?

(A) Postpartum blues will occur in about 10% of patients
(B) Major depression will occur in about 25% of patients
(C) Postpartum psychosis will occur in about 8% of patients
(D) Postpartum psychosis will last about 1 year
(E) Postpartum blues will last up to one week

Questions 11–16

For each developmental milestone, select the age at which it commonly first appears.

11. Crawling on hands and knees

(A) 0–3 months
(B) 5–6 months
(C) 7–10 months
(D) 11–15 months
(E) 16–30 months

12. Sitting unassisted

(A) 0–3 months
(B) 5–6 months
(C) 7–10 months
(D) 11–15 months
(E) 16–30 months

13. Showing the rooting reflex

(A) 0–3 months
(B) 5–6 months
(C) 7–10 months
(D) 11–15 months
(E) 16–30 months

14. Using a "pincer" grasp

(A) 0–3 months
(B) 5–6 months
(C) 7–10 months
(D) 11–15 months
(E) 16–30 months

15. Using pronouns in speech

(A) 0–3 months
(B) 5–6 months
(C) 7–10 months
(D) 11–15 months
(E) 16–30 months

Answers and Explanations

TBQ-E. Stranger anxiety (the tendency to cry and cling to the mother in the presence of an unfamiliar person) develops in normal infants at 7–9 months of age. It does not indicate that the child is developmentally delayed, emotionally disturbed, or that the child has been abused, but rather that the child can now distinguish familiar from unfamiliar people. Stranger anxiety is seen less frequently in children exposed to many different caregivers.

1-D. This child is likely to show depression at this time. Loud protests occur initially when the mother leaves the child. With her continued absence of over 2 months and the child's placement in an orphanage, this child will suffer more serious consequences. These consequences include depression, decreased responsiveness to adults and deficits in the development of social and motor skills.

2-B. The best description of this boy's behavior is normal with regression (i.e., a defense mechanism involving acting like a child of a younger age). Because he continues to do well in nursery school and plays well with friends, this is not separation anxiety disorder. There is also no evidence of delayed development, lack of basic trust, or poor superego (conscience) development (see Chapter 6).

3-A. Two-year-old children speak in 2-word sentences (e.g., "Me go"). Toilet training or the ability to spend most of the day away from the mother does not usually occur until age 3. Children engage in cooperative play starting at about age 4 and can ride a 2-wheeled bicycle at about age 6.

4-A. Children can identify some colors by about age 3. The ability to tie shoelaces develops at about 6 years of age. Having an internalized moral sense of right and wrong (the superego), reading, and preference for playing with children of the same sex are characteristic of latency age children (7–11 years—See Chapter 2).

5-B. The social smile (smiling in response to seeing a human face) is one of the first developmental milestones to appear in the infant and is present by 1–2 months of age. Stranger anxiety (fear of unfamiliar people) appears at about 7 months of age and indicates that the infant has a specific attachment to the mother. Rapprochement (the tendency to run away from the mother and then run back for comfort and reassurance) appears at about 16 months of age. Core gender identity (the sense of self as male or female) is established between 2 and 3 years of age. Transient phobias (irrational fears) occur in normal children, appearing most commonly at 4–6 years of age.

6-C. In 1996, the overall infant mortality rate in the United States was about 7 per 1000 live births. This rate, which is closely associated with socioeconomic status, was about 14 per 1000 live births in African-American infants and about 6 per 1000 live births in white infants.

7-E. The most important psychological task of infancy is the development of an intimate attachment to the mother or primary caregiver. Stranger anxiety, which normally appears at about 7 months of age, demonstrates that the child has developed this attachment and can distinguish its mother from others. Speech, the ability to think logically, and the development of a conscience are skills which are developed over the first few years of life.

8-C. Women preparing for childbirth with a formal training program typically experience closer initial interactions with their infants, equal or lower likelihood of postpartum emotional reactions, shorter labors, fewer medical complications, and less need for medication during labor.

9-D. Changes in hormone levels, fatigue, physical and emotional stresses of childbirth and feelings of added responsibility contribute to the development of a sad mood in new mothers, otherwise known as the "baby blues." Breastfeeding usually is not a contributing factor in developing a sad mood after childbirth.

10-E. Postpartum psychosis is rare, occurring in less than 1% of new mothers and lasting up to one month after childbirth. Postpartum blues may occur in one third to one half of new mothers, and lasts up to one week. Intervention involves support and practical help with the child. Postpartum depression occurs in 5%–10% of new mothers and is treated primarily with antidepressant medication.

11-C. Crawling on hands and knees commonly begins between 7 and 10 months of age.

12-B. Infants can usually sit unassisted at about 6 months of age.

13-A. The rooting reflex is present at birth.

14-C. The thumb and forefinger "pincer" grasp begins at about 8 months of age. Prior to this, the child picks up objects using 4 fingers (no thumb) in a raking motion.

15-E. Children start using pronouns (e.g., "me") at about 2 years of age.

2

School Age, Adolescence, Special Issues of Development, and Adulthood

Typical Board Question

A 10-year-old girl with Down syndrome and an IQ of 60 is brought to the physician's office for a school physical. When the doctor interviews this girl, he is most likely to find that she

(A) has good self-esteem
(B) knows that she is handicapped
(C) communicates well with peers
(D) competes successfully with peers
(E) is socially outgoing

(See "Answers and Explanations" at end of Chapter)

I. Latency or School Age: 7–11 Years

A. Motor development. The normal grade school child, 7–11 years of age, engages in complex motor tasks (e.g., plays baseball, skips rope).

B. Social characteristics. The school age child:

1. Prefers to play with **children of the same sex**

2. Identifies with the parent of the same sex

3. Has relationships with **adults other than parents** (e.g., teachers, group leaders)

4. Demonstrates little interest in psychosexual issues

5. Has internalized a **moral sense of right and wrong (conscience)** and understands how to follow rules

C. Cognitive characteristics. The school age child:

1. Is **industrious** and organized (gathers collections of objects)

2. Has the capacity for **logical thought** and can determine that objects have more than one property (e.g., an object can be red and metal)

3. Understands the concept of **"conservation."** This concept involves the understanding that a **quantity of a substance remains the same** regardless of the size of the container it is in (e.g., two containers may contain the same amount of water even though one is a tall, thin tube and one is a short, wide bowl).

II. Adolescence: 11–20 Years

A. Early adolescence (11–14 years of age)

1. **Puberty** occurs in early adolescense and is marked by:
   a. The development of primary and **secondary sex characteristics** (Table 2-1) and increased skeletal growth
   b. **First menstruation** (menarche) in girls, which on average occurs at 11–12 years of age
   c. **First ejaculation** in boys, which on average occurs at 13–14 years of age
   d. **Cognitive maturation** and **formation of the personality**
   e. **Sex drives,** which are expressed through **physical activity** and **masturbation** (daily masturbation is normal).

2. Early adolescents show strong sensitivity to the opinions of peers but are generally obedient and unlikely to seriously challenge parental authority.

3. **Alterations in expected patterns of development** (e.g., acne, obesity, late breast development) may lead to psychological problems.

B. Middle adolescence (14–17 years of age)

1. **Characteristics**
   a. There is great interest in **gender roles, body image,** and **popularity.**
   b. Heterosexual **crushes** (love for an unattainable person such as a rock star) are common.
   c. **Homosexual experiences** may occur. Although parents may become alarmed, such practicing is part of normal development.
   d. Efforts to **develop an identity** by adopting current teen fashion in

Table 2-1. Tanner Stages of Sexual Development

Stage	Characteristics
1	Genitalia and associated structures are the same as in childhood; nipples, (papillae) are slightly elevated in girls
2	Scant, straight pubic hair, testes enlarge, scrotum develops texture; slight elevation of breast tissue in girls
3	Pubic hair increases over the pubis and becomes curly, penis increases in length and testes enlarge
4	Penis increases in width, glans develops, scrotal skin darkens; areola rises above the rest of the breast in girls
5	Male and female genitalia are like adult; pubic hair now is also on thighs, areola is no longer elevated above the breast in girls

clothing and music and preference for spending time with peers over family is normal, but may lead to conflict with parents.

2. Risk-taking behavior

a. Readiness to challenge parental rules and feelings of **omnipotence** may result in **risk taking behavior** (e.g., failure to use condoms, driving too fast, smoking).

b. Education with respect to **obvious short term benefits** rather than references to long term consequences of behavior are more likely to **decrease teenagers' unwanted behavior.**

—For example, **to discourage smoking,** telling teenagers that their teeth will stay white will be more helpful than telling them that they will avoid lung cancer in 30 years.

C. Late adolescence (17–20 years of age)

1. Development

a. Older adolescents develop **morals, ethics, self-control** and a realistic appraisal of their own abilities; they become concerned with humanitarian issues and world problems.

b. Some adolescents, but not all, develop the ability for abstract reasoning (Piaget's **stage of formal operations**).

2. In the effort to form one's own identity, an **identity crisis** commonly develops.

a. If the identity crisis is not handled effectively, the adolescent may suffer from **role confusion** in which he does not know where he belongs in the world.

b. With role confusion, the adolescent may display behavioral abnormalities with **criminality** or an **interest in cults.**

D. Teenage sexuality

1. In the United States, **first sexual intercourse** occurs on average at **16 years** of age; by 19 years of age, 80% of men and 70% of women have had sexual intercourse.

2. About 65% of teenagers **do not use contraceptives** for reasons which include the conviction that they will not get pregnant, lack of access to contraceptives, and lack of education about which methods are most effective.

3. Physicians may counsel minors (persons under 18 years of age) and provide them with contraceptives without parental knowledge or consent.

E. Teenage pregnancy

1. Teenage pregnancy is a social problem in the United States. Although the **birth rate and abortion rate** in American teenagers **are currently decreasing,** teenagers give birth to over 500,000 infants (12,000 of these infants are born to mothers under 15 years of age) and have about 400,000 abortions annually.

2. Abortion is legal in the United States. However, in about half of the states, minors must obtain parental consent for abortion.

3. Factors predisposing adolescent girls to pregnancy include depression, poor school achievement, and having divorced parents.

4. Pregnant teenagers are at high risk for **obstetric complications** because they are less likely to get prenatal care and because they are physically immature.

III. Special Issues in Child Development

A. **Illness and death in childhood and adolescence.** A child's reaction to illness and death is closely associated with the child's developmental stage.

1. During the **toddler years** (18 months to 2 ½ years) hospitalized children **fear separation** from the parent more than they fear bodily harm, pain, or death.

2. During the **preschool years** (2½ to 6 years) the child's greatest fear when hospitalized is of **bodily harm.**
   a. The preschool-age child does not fully understand the meaning of death.
   b. The child may expect that a dead friend, pet, or relative will **come back to life.**

3. **School-age children** (7–11 years of age) cope relatively well with hospitalization. Thus, this is the **best age to perform elective surgery.** Children of this age can understand the finality of death.

4. Ill **adolescents** may challenge the authority of doctors and nurses and resist being different than peers. Both of these factors can result in **noncompliance with medical advice.**

5. A child with an **ill sibling** or parent may respond by **acting badly** at school or home [use of the defense mechanism of "acting out" (see Chapter 6 II)].

B. **Adoption**

1. An **adoptive parent** is a person who voluntarily becomes the **legal parent** of a child who is not his or her genetic offspring.

2. Adopted children, particularly those adopted after infancy, may be at increased risk for behavioral problems in childhood and adolescence.

3. Children **should be told** by their parents that they are adopted **at the earliest age possible** to avoid the chance of others telling them first.

C. **Mental retardation**

1. **Etiology**
   a. The most common genetic cause of mental retardation is **Down syndrome;** the second is **Fragile X syndrome.**
   b. Other causes include metabolic factors affecting the mother or fetus, prenatal and postnatal **infection** and **maternal substance abuse;** many cases of mental retardation are of unknown etiology.

2. Mildly [intelligence quotient (IQ) of 50–69; see Chapter 8] and moderately (IQ of 35–49) mentally retarded children and adolescents commonly **know they are handicapped.** Because of this knowledge, they may become **frustrated and socially withdrawn** in part because of poor self-esteem due to difficulty in communicating and competing with peers.

3. The **Vineland Social Maturity Scale** can be used to evaluate social skills and skills for daily living in mentally retarded and other challenged individuals.

4. **Avoidance of pregnancy** in mentally retarded adults can become an issue particularly in residential social settings (e.g., summer camp). **Long-acting, reversible contraceptive methods** such as subcutaneous progesterone implants can be particularly useful for these individuals.

IV. Early Adulthood: 20–40 Years

A. Characteristics
1. At about **30 years of age,** there is a **period of reappraisal** of one's life.
2. The adult's **role in society is defined,** physical development peaks, and the adult becomes independent.

B. Responsibilities and relationships
1. The development of an **intimate (e.g., close, sexual) relationship with another person** occurs.
2. According to **Erikson,** this is the stage of **intimacy versus isolation;** if the individual does not develop the ability to sustain an intimate relationship by this stage of life, he or she suffers emotional isolation in the future.
3. By 30 years of age, most Americans are married and have children.
4. During their middle thirties, many women alter their lifestyles by returning to work or school or by **resuming their careers**.

V. Middle Adulthood: 40–65 Years

A. Characteristics. The person in middle adulthood possesses more **power** and **authority** than at other life stages.

B. Responsibilities. The individual either maintains a continued sense of productivity or develops a sense of emptiness (Erikson's stage of **generativity versus stagnation**).

C. Relationships
1. Seventy to eighty percent of men in their middle forties or early fifties exhibit a **midlife crisis.** This may lead to:
   a. A change in profession or lifestyle
   b. Infidelity, separation, or divorce
   c. Increased use of alcohol or drugs
   d. Depression
2. Midlife crisis is associated with an **awareness of one's own aging** and **death** and **severe or unexpected lifestyle changes** (e.g., death of a spouse, loss of a job, serious illness).

D. Climacterium is the change in physiologic function that occurs during midlife.

1. In **men,** although hormone levels do not change significantly, a decrease in muscle strength, endurance, and sexual performance (See Chapter 18) occurs in midlife.

2. In **women, menopause** occurs.

   a. The ovaries stop functioning, and menstruation stops in the **late forties** or **early fifties.**

   b. Absence of menstruation for one year defines **the end of menopause.** To avoid unwanted pregnancy, contraceptive measures should be used until at least **one year following the last missed menstrual period.**

   c. Most women experience menopause with relatively few physical or psychological problems.

   d. Vasomotor instability, called **hot flashes or flushes,** is a common **physical problem** seen in women in all countries and cultural groups. It may continue for years and can be relieved by estrogen replacement therapy.

Review Test

Directions: Each of the numbered items or incomplete statements in this section is followed by answers or by completions of the statement. Select the **one** lettered answer or completion that is **best** in each case.

1. A mother tells the physician that she is concerned about her son because he consistently engages in behavior which is dangerous and potentially life-threatening. The age of her son is most likely to be

(A) 11 years
(B) 13 years
(C) 15 years
(D) 18 years
(E) 20 years

2. A physician discovers that a 15-year-old patient is pregnant. Which of the following factors is likely to have contributed most to her risk of pregnancy?

(A) Living in a rural area
(B) Depressed mood
(C) Intact parental unit
(D) Achievement in school
(E) Education about contraceptive methods

3. A 50-year-old male patient comes in for an insurance physical. Which of the following developmental signposts is most likely to characterize this man?

(A) Decreased alcohol use
(B) Peak physical development
(C) Possession of power and authority
(D) Strong resistance to changes in social relationships
(E) Strong resistance to changes in work relationships

4. A woman has recently gone through menopause. Which of the following is most likely to characterize this transition?

(A) Sudden onset of symptoms
(B) Cessation of menstruation
(C) Severe depression
(D) Severe anxiety
(E) Occurrence in the fourth decade of life

5. Increase in penis width, development of the glans, and darkening of scrotal skin characterize Tanner stage

(A) 1
(B) 2
(C) 3
(D) 4
(E) 5

6. The adoptive parents of a newborn ask their physician when they should tell the child that she is adopted. The pediatrician correctly suggests that they tell her

(A) when she questions them about her background
(B) when she enters school
(C) as soon as possible
(D) at 4 years of age
(E) if she develops an illness that has a known genetic basis

7. A physician is conducting a school physical on a normal 10-year-old girl. When interviewing the child, the physician is most likely to find which of the following psychological characteristics?

(A) Lack of conscience formation
(B) Poor capacity for logical thought
(C) Identification with her father
(D) Relatively stronger importance of friends over family when compared to children of younger ages
(E) No preference with respect for the sex of playmates

8. A child's pet has recently died. The child believes that the pet will soon come back to life. This child is most likely to be age

(A) 4 years
(B) 6 years
(C) 7 years
(D) 9 years
(E) 11 years

9. A 5-year-old boy requires surgery to correct an inguinal hernia. When the child enters the hospital to have surgery, his greatest fear is likely to be

(A) separation from his mother
(B) the unknown environment
(C) the possibility that he will die during surgery
(D) unfamiliar people
(E) damage to his body

Answers and Explanations

TBQ-B. Mildly and moderately mentally retarded children are aware that they have a handicap. They often have low self-esteem and may become socially withdrawn. In part, these problems occur because they have difficulty communicating with and competing with peers.

1-C. The age of this woman's son is most likely to be 15 years. Middle adolescents (14–17 years) often challenge parental authority and have feelings of omnipotence (i.e., nothing bad will happen to them because they are all-powerful). Younger adolescents are unlikely to challenge parental rules and authority. Older adolescents (18–20 years) have developed self-control and a more realistic picture of their own abilities.

2-B. Teenagers who become pregnant frequently are depressed, come from homes where the parents are divorced, have problems in school, and may not know about effective contraceptive methods. Studies have not indicated that living in a rural area is related to teenage pregnancy.

3-C. While midlife is associated with the possession of power and authority, physical abilities decline. This time of life is also associated with a midlife crisis which may include increased alcohol and drug use as well as an increased likelihood of changes in social and work relationships.

4-B. Menopause is characterized by cessation of menstruation. Most women go through menopause gradually at about 50 years of age and with few psychological or physical problems.

5-D. Increase in penis width, development of the glans and darkening of scrotal skin characterize Tanner stage 4. Stage 1 is characterized by slight elevation of the papillae, and stage 2 by the presence of scant, straight pubic hair, testes enlargement, development of texture in scrotal skin, and slight elevation of breast tissue. In stage 3, pubic hair increases over the pubis and becomes curly, and the penis increases in length; in stage 5 male and female genitalia are much like those of the adult.

6-C. The best time to tell a child she is adopted is as soon as possible, usually when the child can first understand language. Waiting any longer than this will increase the probability that someone else will tell the child before the parents are able to.

7-D. When compared to younger ages, peers and non-familial adults become more important to the latency age child and the family becomes less important. Children 7–11 years of age have the capacity for logical thought, have a conscience, identify with the same-sex parent, and show a strong preference for playmates of their own sex.

8-A. Preschool children usually cannot comprehend the meaning of death and commonly believe that the dead person or pet will come back to life. Children over the age of 6 years commonly are aware of the finality of death.

9-E. The greatest fear of the preschool child is damage to his body. Children younger than age 3 are more fearful of separation from parents, an unknown environment and unfamiliar people. Fear of death is more prominent in older children who understand that death is not temporary.

3

Aging, Death, and Bereavement

Typical Board Question

An 80-year-old patient tells you that she is concerned because she forgets the addresses of people she has just met and takes longer than in the past to do the Sunday crossword puzzle. She enjoys family visits, lives comfortably on her own, and shops and cooks for herself. This patient

(A) is probably showing normal aging
(B) is probably suffering from Alzheimer's disease
(C) is probably suffering from depression
(D) is likely to develop an anxiety disorder
(E) should be advised not to live alone

(See "Answers and Explanations" at end of Chapter)

I. Aging

A. Demographics

1. By 2020, over 15% of the United States population will be more than 65 years of age.

2. The **fastest growing segment of the population** is people **over age 85.**

3. The average **life expectancy** in the United States is currently about **76 years;** however, this figure varies greatly by gender and race (Table 3-1).

4. Differences in life expectancies by gender and race have been decreasing over the past few years.

5. **Gerontology,** the study of aging, and **geriatrics,** the care of aging people, have become important new medical fields.

B. Somatic and neurologic changes

1. **Strength and physical health gradually decline**. This decline shows great variability, but commonly includes impaired vision, hearing, and immune responses; decreased muscle mass and strength; increased fat deposits; osteoporosis; decreased renal, pulmonary, and gastrointestinal func-

Table 3-1. Life Expectancy (in Years) at Birth in the United States by Sex and Race (1996 for African-American and White American; 1990 for Native American and Asian American)

	African-American	Native American	White American	Asian American
Men	66	71	74	82
Women	74	79	80	86

tion, reduced bladder control, and decreased responsiveness to changes in ambient temperature.

2. **Changes in the brain** occur with aging.

   a. These changes include **decreased weight, enlarged ventricles and sulci, and decreased cerebral blood flow.**

   b. **Senile plaques and neurofibrillary tangles** are present in the **normally aging brain** but **to a lesser extent than in dementia of the Alzheimer's type.**

C. **Cognitive changes**

1. Although learning speed may decrease, in the absence of brain disease, **intelligence remains approximately the same** throughout life.

2. **Slight memory problems** may occur in normal aging, (e.g., the patient may forget the name of a new acquaintance). However, these problems **do not interfere with the patient's functioning** and he is able to live independently.

D. **Psychological changes**

1. In late adulthood there is either a sense of ego integrity, (i.e., satisfaction, and pride in one's past accomplishments) or a sense of despair and worthlessness **(Erikson's stage of ego integrity versus despair).** Many elderly people achieve ego integrity.

2. **Psychopathology and related problems**

   a. **Depression** is the **most common psychiatric disorder** in the elderly. **Suicide is more common** in the elderly than in the general population.

      (1) Factors associated with depression in the elderly include loss of spouse, other family members, and friends; decreased social status; and decline of health.

      (2) **Depression may mimic and thus be misdiagnosed as Alzheimer's disease. This misdiagnosed disorder is referred to as pseudodementia** because it is associated with memory loss and cognitive problems (see Chapter 14)

      (3) Depression **can be treated successfully** with supportive psychotherapy in conjunction with pharmacotherapy or electroconvulsive therapy (see Chapter 15).

   b. **Sleep patterns change,** resulting in loss of sleep, poor sleep quality, or both (see Chapter 10).

   c. **Anxiety** and fearfulness may be associated with realistic fear-inducing situations (e.g., worries about developing a physical illness or falling and breaking a bone).

   d. **Alcohol-related disorders** are often unidentified but are present in 10%–15% of the geriatric population.

        e. Psychoactive agents may produce different effects in the elderly than in younger patients.

    E. Longevity has been associated with many factors, including:

        1. Family history of longevity

        2. Continuation of physical and occupational activity

        3. Advanced education

        4. Social support systems, including marriage

II. Stages of Dying And Death.

According to **Elizabeth Kübler-Ross,** the process of dying involves **five stages.** The stages usually occur in the following order, but also may be present simultaneously or occur in another order.

    A. Denial. The patient refuses to believe that she is dying ("The laboratory made an error").

    B. Anger. The patient may become angry at the physician and hospital staff ("It is your fault that I am dying. You should have checked on me weekly"). Physicians must learn not to take such comments personally (see also Chapter 21).

    C. Bargaining. The patient may try to strike a bargain with God or some higher being ("I will give half of my money to charity if I can get rid of this disease").

    D. Depression. The patient becomes preoccupied with death and may become emotionally detached ("I feel so distant from others and so hopeless").

    E. Acceptance. The patient is calm and accepts her fate ("I am ready to go now").

III. Bereavement (Normal Grief) Versus Depression (Abnormal Grief).

After the loss of a loved one, there is a normal grief reaction. This reaction also occurs with other losses, such as loss of a body part, or, for younger people, with a miscarriage or abortion. A normal grief reaction must be distinguished from depression, which is pathologic.

    A. Characteristics of normal grief (bereavement)

        1. Grief is characterized initially by **shock and denial.**

        2. In normal grief, the bereaved may experience an **illusion** (see also Table 11-1) that the deceased person is physically present.

        3. Normal grief generally **subsides after 1–2 years,** although some features may continue longer. Even after they have subsided, symptoms may return on holidays or special occasions (the **"anniversary reaction"**).

        4. The **mortality rate** is high for close relatives (especially **widowed men**) in the first year of bereavement.

    B. Comparison between normal and abnormal grief reactions can be found in Table 3-2.

Table 3-2. Comparison between Normal Grief Reactions and Abnormal Grief Reactions

Normal grief reaction (Bereavement)	Abnormal grief reaction (Depression)
Minor weight loss (e.g., 1–3 pounds)	Significant weight loss (e.g., > 8 pounds)
Minor sleep disturbances	Significant sleep disturbances
Some guilty feelings	Intense feelings of guilt and worthlessness
Illusions (thinking that one briefly sees the deceased person)	Hallucinations and delusions (hearing the dead person talking)
Attempts to return to work and social activities	Resumes few, if any, work or social activities
Cries and expresses sadness	Considers or attempts suicide
Severe symptoms resolve within 2 months	Severe symptoms persist for > 2 months
Moderate symptoms subside within 1 year	Moderate symptoms persist for > 1 year
Treatment includes increased calls and visits to the physician, supportive psychotherapy, and short-acting benzodiazepines for temporary problems with sleep	Treatment includes antidepressants, antipsychotics, or electroconvulsive therapy

(Adapted from Fadem B, Simring S: *High Yield Psychiatry.* Baltimore, Williams & Wilkins, 1998, p 31.)

C. Physician's response to death

1. The major **responsibility of the physician** is to give **support** to the dying patient and the patient's family.

2. Generally, physicians **make the patient completely aware** of the diagnosis and prognosis. However, a physician should follow the patient's lead as to how much he or she wants to know about the condition. With the patient's permission, the **physician may tell the family** the diagnosis and other details of the illness (see Chapter 23).

3. Physicians often feel a **sense of failure** at not preventing death. They may deal with this sense by becoming **emotionally detached** from the patient in order to deal with his imminent death. Such detachment can preclude helping the patient and family through this important transition.

Review Test

Directions: Each of the numbered items or incomplete statements in this section is followed by answers or by completions of the statement. Select the **one** lettered answer or completion that is **best** in each case.

1. A 70-year-old patient whose wife died 8 months ago reports that he sometimes wakes up an hour earlier than usual and often cries when he thinks about his wife. He also tells you that on one occasion he briefly followed a woman down the street who resembled his late wife. The patient also relates that he has rejoined his bowling team and enjoys visits with his grandchildren. For this patient, the best recommendation of the physician is

(A) medication for sleep
(B) antidepressant medication
(C) regular phone calls and visits to "check in" with the doctor
(D) psychotherapy
(E) a neuropsychological evaluation for Alzheimer's disease

2. A 70-year-old patient whose wife died 8 months ago appears unshaven and disheveled. He has lost 11 pounds, has persistent problems sleeping and has no interest in interacting with friends and family. For this patient, the best recommendation of the physician is

(A) medication for sleep
(B) antidepressant medication
(C) regular phone calls and visits to "check in" with the doctor
(D) psychotherapy
(E) a neuropsychological evaluation for Alzheimer's disease

3. An 80-year-old man is brought to a clinic by his wife who complains that he has become forgetful since he voluntarily gave up his driver's license one month previously. Which of the following statements best describes this patient?

(A) He probably has Alzheimer's disease
(B) He is probably suffering from depression
(C) He is at decreased risk of suicide when compared with a younger man in the same situation
(D) He cannot be treated effectively with psychoactive drugs
(E) He probably has a decreased intelligence quotient (IQ)

4. A terminally ill patient who uses a statement such as, "It is the doctor's fault that I became ill; she didn't do an electrocardiogram when I came for my last office visit," is most likely in which stage of dying, according to Elizabeth Kübler-Ross?

(A) Denial
(B) Anger
(C) Bargaining
(D) Depression
(E) Acceptance

5. A physician conducts a physical examination on an active, independent 75-year-old woman. Which of the following findings is most likely?

(A) Increased immune responses
(B) Increased muscle mass
(C) Decreased size of brain ventricles
(D) Decreased bladder control
(E) Severe memory problems

6. Ninety percent of the patients in a primary care physician's practice are over 65 years of age. When compared to the general population, these elderly patients are more likely to show which of the following psychological characteristics?

(A) Lower likelihood of suicide
(B) Less anxiety
(C) Lower intelligence
(D) Poorer sleep quality
(E) Less depression

7. The 78-year-old husband of a 70-year-old woman has just died. If this woman experiences normal bereavement, which of the following responses would be expected?

(A) Initial loss of appetite
(B) Feelings of worthlessness
(C) Threats of suicide
(D) Grief lasting 3–4 years after the death
(E) Feelings of hopelessness

8. A physician has just diagnosed a case of terminal pancreatic cancer in a 68-year-old man. Which of the following statements regarding the reactions and behavior of the physician is the most true?

(A) She should inform the family, but not the patient, about the serious nature of the illness.
(B) Her involvement with the patient's family should end when he dies.
(C) She should provide strong sedation for family members when the patient dies until the initial shock of his death wears off.
(D) She will feel that she has failed when the patient dies.
(E) She will feel closer and closer to the patient as his death approaches.

9. The average difference in life expectancy between white women and African-American men is approximately

(A) 3 years
(B) 6 years
(C) 10 years
(D) 14 years
(E) 20 years

Answers and Explanations

TBQ-A. This 80-year-old woman is probably showing normal aging, since she can function well living alone. Minor memory loss which does not interfere with normal functioning such as she describes is typically seen in normally aging people. There is no evidence that this patient is suffering from Alzheimer's disease, depression, or an anxiety disorder.

1-C. This patient whose wife died 8 months ago is showing a normal grief reaction. Although he sometimes wakes up an hour earlier than usual and cries when he thinks about his wife, he is showing efforts to return to his lifestyle by rejoining his bowling team and visiting with his family. The illusion of believing he sees and thus follows a woman who resembled his late wife is seen in a normal grief reaction. For a normal grief reaction, recommending regular phone calls and visits to "check in" with the doctor is the appropriate intervention. Sleep medication, antidepressants, psychotherapy, and a neuropsychological evaluation are not necessary for this patient.

2-B. This patient whose wife died 8 months ago demonstrates an abnormal grief reaction. He is showing signs of depression (i.e., poor grooming, significant weight loss, serious sleep problems, and no interest in interacting with friends and family) (see Chapter 12). For this patient, the physician should recommend antidepressant medication (see Chapter 15). Psychotherapy, while helpful, will be less useful than medication for this patient. His sleep will improve as the depression improves. There is no indication that this patient needs a neuropsychological evaluation for Alzheimer's disease.

3-B. Depression is commonly seen in elderly patients and memory problems are often seen in depression. Thus, depression in the elderly may mimic Alzheimer's disease (pseudodementia). The sudden onset of the condition with the concurrent loss of an important sign of youth and independence (the driver's license) indicate that the patient is likely to be suffering from depression rather than Alzheimer's disease. He can be treated effectively for depression with psychoactive drugs (i.e., antidepressants). This depressed patient is at increased risk of suicide when compared with a younger man in the same situation.

4-B. During the anger stage of dying, the patient is likely to blame the physician.

5-D. Of the listed findings, decreased bladder control is the most likely finding in the examination of an active, independent 75-year-old woman. In aging, immune responses and muscle mass decrease and brain ventricles increase in size. While mild memory problems may occur, severe memory problems do not occur in normal aging. Severe memory problems which interfere with normal function indicate the development of a dementia like Alzheimer's disease.

6-D. Sleep disturbances, such as decreased delta or slow wave sleep (see Chapter 10), commonly occur in the elderly. Suicide and depression are more common in the elderly than in the general population. Anxiety may arise easily due to fears of illness and injury. Intelligence does not decrease with age in normal people.

7-A. Initial loss of appetite is common in normal bereavement. Feelings of worthlessness or hopelessness, threats of suicide, and an extended period of grief characterize depression rather than normal bereavement.

8-D. Physicians often feel that they have failed when a patient dies. Rather than becoming closer, this physician may become emotionally detached from the patient in order to deal with his impending death. Heavy sedation is rarely indicated as treatment for the bereaved because it may interfere with the grieving process. Generally, physicians inform patients when they have a terminal illness and provide an important source of support for the family before and after the patient's death.

9-D. The difference in life expectancy between white women (80 years) and African-American men (66 years) is approximately 14 years. The difference in life expectancy by age and sex is currently decreasing.

4

Genetics, Anatomy, and Biochemistry of Behavior

Typical Board Question

A 28-year-old male patient is brought to the emergency room after a fight in which he attacked a man who cut into his line at the supermarket checkout. In the emergency room he remains assaultive and combative. The body fluids of this patient are most likely to show

(A) increased 3-methoxy-4-hydroxyphenylglycol (MHPG)
(B) decreased MHPG
(C) increased 5-hydroxyindoleacetic acid (5-HIAA)
(D) decreased 5-HIAA
(E) decreased homovanillic acid (HVA)

(See "Answers and Explanations" at end of Chapter)

I. Genetics

    A. There is a **genetic component** to the etiology of a variety of psychiatric disorders (e.g., schizophrenia, mood disorders, neuropsychiatric disorders, personality disorders, alcoholism), and personality traits.

    B. Studies for examining the genetics of behavior

        1. Pedigree studies use a **family tree** to show the occurrence of behavior disorders and traits within a family.

        2. Family risk studies compare how frequently a behavioral disorder or trait occurs in the relatives of the affected individual (**proband**) with how frequently it occurs in the general population.

        3. Twin studies

            a. Adoption studies using **monozygotic twins** (who are derived from a single fertilized ovum) or **dizygotic twins** (who are derived from two fertilized ova) reared in different homes, are used to differentiate the effects of genetic factors from environmental factors in the occurrence of psychiatric disorders.

      b. If there is a genetic component to the etiology, a disorder may be expected to have a higher **concordance rate** in monozygotic twins than in dizygotic twins (i.e., if concordant, the disorder occurs in both twins).

II. Neuroanatomy

—**The human nervous system** consists of the central nervous system (CNS) and the peripheral nervous system (PNS).

    A. The CNS contains the brain and spinal cord.

      1. The **cerebral cortex** of the brain can be divided

      —**Anatomically** into four lobes: frontal, temporal, parietal, and occipital

      —**By arrangement** of neuron layers or cryoarchitecture

      —**Functionally** into motor, sensory, and association areas

      2. The cerebral hemispheres

        a. The hemispheres are **connected** by the corpus callosum, anterior commissure, hippocampal commissure, and habenular commissure.

        b. The functions of the hemispheres are **lateralized.**

          (1) The **right,** or **nondominant hemisphere** is associated primarily with **perception;** it also is associated with **spatial relations, body image,** and musical and artistic ability.

          (2) The **left,** or **dominant, hemisphere** is associated with **language function** in about 96% of right-handed people and 70% of left-handed people.

        c. Sex differences in cerebral lateralization. Women may have a larger corpus callosum and anterior commissure and appear to have better interhemispheric communication than men. **Men** may have better-developed right hemispheres and appear to be better at spatial tasks than women.

      3. Brain lesions caused by accident, disease, or surgery are associated with particular neuropsychiatric effects (Table 4-1).

    B. The PNS contains all **sensory, motor,** and **autonomic** fibers outside of the CNS including the **spinal nerves, cranial nerves,** and **peripheral ganglia.**

      1. The PNS carries **sensory** information to the CNS, and carries **motor** information away from the CNS.

      2. The autonomic nervous system, which consists of **sympathetic** and **parasympathetic** divisions, innervates the internal organs.

      3. The autonomic nervous system coordinates emotions with visceral responses such as heart rate, blood pressure, and peptic acid secretion.

      4. Visceral responses occurring as a result of **psychological stress** are involved in the development and exacerbation of some **physical illnesses** (see Chapter 22).

Table 4-1. Neuropsychiatric Effects of Brain Lesions

Location of Lesion	Effects of Lesion on the Patient
Temporal lobes	• Impaired memory; psychomotor seizures • Inability to understand language [i.e. Wernicke's aphasia (left-side lesions)]
Limbic system Hippocampus	• Poor new learning • Implicated specifically in dementia of the Alzheimer type
Amygdala	• Changes in aggressive behavior, increased sexual behavior, hyperorality; (Klüver-Bucy syndrome) • Decreased fear response • Problems recognizing the meaningfulness of visual cues (visual agnosia)
Hypothalamus	• Hunger leading to obesity (ventromedial nucleus damage); loss of appetite leading to weight loss (lateral nucleus damage) • Effects on sexual activity and body temperature regulation
Frontal lobes	• Mood disorders [i.e., depression (especially left-side lesions)] • Problems with motivation, concentration, attention, orientation, and behavior • Inability to speak fluently, [i.e., Broca's aphasia (left-side lesions)]
Parietal lobes	• Impaired processing of visual-spatial information, [i.e., cannot copy a simple line drawing or a clock face correctly (right-sided lesions)] • Impaired processing of verbal information [i.e., cannot name fingers, cannot write (left-sided lesions)]
Occipital lobes	• Visual hallucinations and illusions • Inability to identify camouflaged objects • Blindness
Reticular system	• Changes in sleep-wake mechanisms
Basal ganglia	• Disorders of movement [i.e., Parkinson's disease (substantia nigra), Huntington's disease (caudate and putamen) and Tourette syndrome (caudate)]

Adapted from Fadem B, *High-Yield Behavioral Science*. Baltimore, Williams & Wilkins, 1996. Table 9-1, p. 32.

III. Neurotransmission

A. Synapses and neurotransmitters

1. Information in the nervous system is transferred across **synaptic cleft** (i.e., the space between the axon terminal of the presynaptic neuron and the dendrite of the postsynaptic neuron).

2. When the presynaptic neuron is stimulated, a **neurotransmitter** is released, travels across the synaptic cleft, and acts on receptors on the postsynaptic neuron.

—Neurotransmitters are **excitatory** if they increase the chances that a neuron will fire and **inhibitory** if they decrease these chances.

B. Presynaptic and postsynaptic receptors are proteins present in the membrane of the neuron that can recognize specific neurotransmitters.

1. The **changeability** of number or affinity of receptors for specific neurotransmitters (**neuronal plasticity**) can regulate the responsiveness of neurons.

2. **Second messengers.** When stimulated by neurotransmitters, postsynaptic receptors may alter the metabolism of neurons by the use of second messengers, which include **cyclic adenosine monophosphate (cAMP), lipids** (e.g., diacylglycerol), and **Ca^{2+}.**

C. **Classification of neurotransmitters. The biogenic amines** (monoamines), **amino acids,** and **peptides** are the three major classes of neurotransmitters.

D. **Regulation of neurotransmitter activity**

1. The concentration of neurotransmitters in the synaptic cleft is closely related to mood and behavior. A number of mechanisms affect this concentration.

2. After release by the presynaptic neuron, neurotransmitters are removed from the synaptic cleft by:

   a. **Reuptake** by the presynaptic neuron

   b. **Degradation** by enzymes such as **monoamine oxidase (MAO)**

3. Availability of specific neurotransmitters is associated with common psychiatric conditions (Table 4-2).

IV. Biogenic Amines

A. **Overview**

1. The **biogenic amines,** or **monoamines,** include catecholamines, indolamines, ethylamines, and quaternary amines.

2. The **monoamine theory of mood disorder** hypothesizes that **lowered monoamine activity results in depression.**

3. **Metabolites** of the monoamines are often measured in psychiatric research and diagnosis because they are more easily measured in body fluids than the actual monoamines (Table 4-3).

B. **Dopamine**

1. Dopamine, a catecholamine, is involved in the pathophysiology of **schizophrenia, Parkinson disease, mood disorders,** the conditioned fear response (see Chapter 7), and the "rewarding" nature of drugs of abuse (see Chapter 9).

Table 4-2. Psychiatric Conditions and Associated Neurotransmitter Activity

Psychiatric Condition	Neurotransmitter Activity Increased (↑) or Decreased (↓)
Depression	Norepinephrine (↓), serotonin (↓), dopamine (↓)
Mania	Dopamine (↑)
Schizophrenia	Dopamine (↑), Serotonin (↑)
Anxiety	γ-aminobutyric acid (GABA) (↓), serotonin (↓), norepinephrine (↑)
Dementia of the Alzheimer type	Acetylcholine (↓)

Adapted from Fadem B: *High-Yield Behavioral Science.* Baltimore, Williams & Wilkins, 1996, Table 9-2, p. 32.

Table 4-3. Metabolites of Monoamines and Associated Psychopathology

Neurotransmitter	Increased (↑) or Decreased (↓) Concentration of Metabolite in Blood Plasma, Cerebrospinal Fluid or Urine	Associated Psychopathology
Dopamine	(↑) HVA (homovanillic acid)	Schizophrenia and other conditions involving psychosis (see Chapters 9, 11 and 12)
	(↓) HVA	Parkinson's disease Patients treated with antipsychotic agents Depression
Norepinephrine	(↑) VMA (vanillylmandelic acid)	Adrenal medulla tumor (pheochromocytoma)
	(↓) MHPG (3-methoxy-4-hydroxyphenylglycol)	Severe depression and attempted suicide
Serotonin	(↓) 5-HIAA (5-hydroxyindoleacetic acid)	Severe depression and attempted suicide Aggressiveness and violence Impulsiveness Fire setting Tourette syndrome Alcohol abuse Bulimia

Adapted from Fadem B: *High-Yield Behavioral Science.* Baltimore, Williams & Wilkins, 1996, Table 9-3, p. 33.

    2. Synthesis. The amino acid tyrosine is converted to the precursor for dopamine by the enzyme **tyrosine hydroxylase.**

    3. Dopaminergic tracts

        a. The **nigrostriatal tract** is involved in the regulation of muscle tone and movement.

            (1) This tract **degenerates in Parkinson's disease.**

            (2) Treatment with antipsychotic drugs, which block postsynaptic dopamine receptors receiving input from the nigrostriatal tract, can result in parkinsonism-like symptoms.

        b. Dopamine acts on the **tuberoinfundibular tract** to inhibit the secretion of prolactin from the anterior pituitary.

            (1) Blockade of dopamine receptors by antipsychotic drugs prevents the inhibition of prolactin release and results in **elevated prolactin** levels.

            (2) This elevation in turn results in symptoms such as breast enlargement, galactorrhea, and sexual dysfunction.

        c. The **mesolimbic-mesocortical tract** may have a role in expression of **mood** since it projects into the limbic system, which is involved in emotional behavior.

  C. Norepinephrine, a catecholamine, plays a role in **mood, anxiety, arousal, learning,** and **memory.**

    1. Synthesis

a. Like dopaminergic neurons, noradrenergic neurons synthesize dopamine.

b. Dopamine β-hydroxylase, present in noradrenergic neurons, converts this dopamine to norepinephrine.

2. **Localization.** Most noradrenergic neurons (approximately 10,000 per hemisphere in the brain) are located in the **locus ceruleus.**

D. **Serotonin,** an indolamine, plays a role in **mood, sleep, sexuality,** and **impulse control;** elevation of serotonin is associated with **improved mood** and **sleep** but **decreased sexual function** (particularly delayed orgasm). Decreased serotonin is associated with poor impulse control, depression, and poor sleep.

1. **Synthesis.** The amino acid tryptophan is converted to serotonin [also known as **5-hydroxytryptamine (5-HT)**] by the enzyme tryptophan hydroxylase as well as by an amino acid decarboxylase.

2. **Localization.** Most serotonergic cell bodies in the brain are contained in the dorsal raphe nucleus.

3. **Antidepressants and serotonin**

   —Heterocyclic antidepressants, selective serotonin reuptake inhibitors, and MAO inhibitors ultimately increase the presence of serotonin and norepinephrine in the synaptic cleft.

   a. **Heterocyclics** block reuptake of serotonin and norepinephrine, and **selective serotonin reuptake inhibitors** such as fluoxetine [Prozac] selectively **block reuptake** of serotonin by the presynaptic neuron.

   b. **MAO inhibitors prevent** the **degradation** of serotonin and norepinephrine by MAO.

E. **Histamine**

1. Histamine, an **ethylamine,** is affected by psychoactive drugs.

2. Histamine receptor blockade with drugs such as antipsychotics and tricyclic antidepressants is associated with common side effects of these drugs such as **sedation** and **increased appetite** leading to weight gain.

F. **Acetylcholine (ACh),** a quaternary amine, is the transmitter used by **nerve-skeleton-muscle junctions.**

1. **Degeneration of cholinergic neurons** is associated with **dementia of the Alzheimer type, Down syndrome,** and **movement and sleep disorders.**

2. **Cholinergic neurons** synthesize ACh from acetyl coenzyme A and choline using **choline acetyltransferase.**

3. **Acetylcholinesterase** (AChE) breaks ACh down into choline and acetate.

4. Blocking the action of **AChE** with drugs such as tacrine [Cognex] and donepezil [Aricept] can delay the progression of dementia of the Alzheimer type but cannot reverse lost function.

5. **Blockade of muscarinic Ach receptors** with drugs such as antipsychotics and tricyclic antidepressants results in the classic "anticholinergic" adverse effects seen with use of these drugs, including dry mouth, blurred vision, urinary hesitancy, and constipation.

V. Amino Acid Neurotransmitters

—These neurotransmitters are involved in most synapses in the brain, and include γ-**aminobutyric acid (GABA), glycine,** and **glutamate.**

A. GABA

1. GABA is the principal inhibitory neurotransmitter in the CNS.

2. GABA is closely involved in the action of the antianxiety agents, benzodiazepines (e.g., diazepam [Valium]) and barbiturates (e.g., secobarbital [Seconal]).

    —Benzodiazepines and barbiturates increase the affinity of GABA for its binding site, allowing more chloride to enter the neuron. The chloride-laden neurons become hyperpolarized and inhibited, decreasing neuronal firing and ultimately decreasing anxiety.

B. **Glycine** is an inhibitory neurotransmitter which works on its own and as a regulator of glutamate activity.

C. **Glutamate** is an excitatory neurotransmitter and may be associated with **epilepsy, schizophrenia, neurodegenerative illnesses** and mechanisms of cell death.

VI. Neuropeptides

A. **Endogenous opioids**

1. **Enkephalins** and **endorphins** are opioids produced by the brain itself that decrease pain and anxiety and have a role in addiction and mood.

2. **Placebo effects** (see also Chapter 25) may be mediated by the endogenous opioid system. Prior treatment with an opiate receptor blocker such as naloxone may block the placebo effect.

B. **Other neuropeptides** have been implicated in the following conditions.

1. **Schizophrenia** [cholecystokinin (CCK) and neurotensin]

2. **Mood disorders** [somatostatin, substance P, vasopressin, oxytocin, and vasoactive intestinal peptide (VIP)]

3. **Huntington disease** (somatostatin and substance P)

4. **Dementia of the Alzheimer type** (somatostatin and VIP)

5. **Anxiety disorders** and **substance P** (CCK)

6. **Pain** and **aggression** (substance P)

Review Test

Directions: Each of the numbered items or incomplete statements in this section is followed by answers or by completions of the statement. Select the **one** lettered answer or completion that is **best** in each case.

1. Analysis of the blood plasma of a 45-year-old male patient shows an increased level of homovanillic acid (HVA). This patient is most likely to show which of the following conditions?

(A) Parkinson's disease
(B) Depression
(C) Bulimia
(D) Pheochromocytoma
(E) Schizophrenia

2. A very anxious patient is examined in the emergency room. If it could be measured, the γ-aminobutyric acid (GABA) activity in the brain of this patient would most likely be

(A) increased
(B) decreased
(C) unchanged
(D) higher than the activity of serotonin
(E) higher than the activity of norepinephrine

3. In a clinical experiment, a 48-year-old female patient with chronic pain who, in the past, has responded to placebos is given naloxone. Shortly thereafter the patient is given an inert substance which she believes is a painkiller. After the patient receives the inert substance, her pain is most likely to

(A) increase
(B) decrease
(C) be unchanged
(D) respond to lower doses of opiates than previously
(E) fail to respond to opiates in the future

4. Which of the following neuropeptides is most closely implicated in the psychopathology of pain?

(A) Cholecystokinin
(B) Vasopressin
(C) Substance P
(D) Somatostatin
(E) Vasoactive intestinal peptide

5. A 65-year-old female patient has had a stroke affecting the left hemisphere of her brain. Which of the following functions is most likely to be affected by the stroke?

(A) Perception
(B) Musical ability
(C) Spatial relations
(D) Language
(E) Artistic ability

6. Which of the following structures connects the two cerebral hemispheres?

(A) The basal ganglia
(B) The anterior commissure
(C) The reticular system
(D) The hippocampus
(E) The amygdala

7. A 23-year-old patient shows side effects such as sedation, increased appetite, and weight gain while being treated with antipsychotic medication. Of the following, the mechanism most closely associated with these effects is

(A) blockade of serotonin receptors
(B) blockade of dopamine receptors
(C) blockade of norepinephrine receptors
(D) blockade of histamine receptors
(E) decreased availability of serotonin

8. The autopsy of a 65-year-old man shows degeneration of cholinergic neurons in the hippocampus. In life, this man is most likely to have suffered from

(A) mania
(B) depression
(C) dementia of the Alzheimer type
(D) anxiety
(E) schizophrenia

9. The major neurotransmitter implicated in dementia of the Alzheimer type is

(A) serotonin
(B) norepinephrine
(C) dopamine
(D) γ-aminobutyric acid (GABA)
(E) acetylcholine (ACh)

10. The major neurotransmitter involved in the action of fluoxetine [Prozac] is

(A) serotonin
(B) norepinephrine
(C) dopamine
(D) γ-aminubutyric acid (GABA)
(E) acetylcholine (ACh)

11. The neurotransmitter metabolized to MHPG (3-methoxy-4-hydroxyphenylglycol) is

(A) serotonin
(B) norepinephrine
(C) dopamine
(D) γ-aminobutyric acid (GABA)
(E) acetylcholine (ACh)

12. The neurotransmitter metabolized to 5-HIAA (5-hydroxyindoleacetic acid) is

(A) serotonin
(B) norepinephrine
(C) dopamine
(D) γ-aminobutyric acid (GABA)
(E) acetylcholine (ACh)

13. A 25-year-old male patient sustains a serious head injury in an automobile accident. He had been aggressive and assaultive, but after the accident he is placid and cooperative. He also makes inappropriate suggestive comments to the nurses and masturbates a great deal. The area of the brain most likely to be affected in this patient is the

(A) right parietal lobe
(B) basal ganglia
(C) hippocampus
(D) reticular system
(E) amygdala
(F) left frontal lobe

14. A 35-year-old female patient reports that she has difficulty sleeping ever since she sustained a concussion in a subway accident. The area of the brain most likely to be affected in this patient is the

(A) right parietal lobe
(B) basal ganglia
(C) hippocampus
(D) reticular system
(E) amygdala
(F) left frontal lobe

15. When he attempts to reproduce a clock face drawn by the doctor, a 70-year-old man who has had a stroke crowds all twelve numbers into the one o'clock to six o'clock position, leaving the left side of the clock face blank. The area of the brain most likely to be affected in this patient is the

(A) right parietal lobe
(B) basal ganglia
(C) hippocampus
(D) reticular system
(E) amygdala
(F) left frontal lobe

16. An 80-year-old female patient has a tremor, difficulty walking, and problems initiating movement. The area of the brain most likely to be affected in this patient is the

(A) right parietal lobe
(B) basal ganglia
(C) hippocampus
(D) reticular system
(E) amygdala
(F) left frontal lobe

17. A 69-year-old former bank president cannot tell you the name of the current president and has difficulty identifying the woman sitting next to him (his wife). He began having memory problems 3 years ago. The area of the brain most likely to be affected in this patient is the

(A) right parietal lobe
(B) basal ganglia
(C) hippocampus
(D) reticular system
(E) amygdala
(F) left frontal lobe

18. A 45-year-old male patient becomes depressed following a head injury. The area of the brain most likely to be affected in this patient is the

(A) right parietal lobe
(B) basal ganglia
(C) hippocampus
(D) reticular system
(E) amygdala
(F) left frontal lobe

Answers and Explanations

TBQ-D. Assaultive, impulsive, aggressive behavior like that seen in this 28-year-old male patient is associated with decreased levels of serotonin in the brain. Levels of 5-HIAA (5-hydroxy-indoleacetic acid), the major metabolite of serotonin, have been shown to be decreased in the body fluids of violent, aggressive, impulsive individuals as well as depressed individuals. MHPG (3-methoxy-4-hydroxyphenylglycol), a metabolite of norepinephrine, is decreased in severe depression while homovanillic acid (HVA), a metabolite of dopamine, is decreased in Parkinson's disease and depression.

1-E. Increased body fluid level of homovanillic acid (HVA), a major metabolite of dopamine, is seen in schizophrenia. Decreased HVA is seen in Parkinson's disease, depression and in medicated schizophrenic patients. Increased vanillylmandelic acid (VMA), a metabolite of norepinephrine is seen in pheochromocytoma. Decreased body fluid level of 5-HIAA, a metabolite of serotonin, is seen in depression and in bulimia (see also answer to TBQ).

2-B. γ-Aminobutyric acid (GABA) is an inhibitory amino acid neurotransmitter in the CNS. Thus, the activity of GABA in the brain of this anxious patient is likely to be decreased. Other neurotransmitters are also involved in anxiety (see Table 4-2) There is no reason to believe that GABA activity is higher than the activity of serotonin or norepinephrine in this patient.

3-C. After receiving naloxone, a chronic pain patient receives placebo medication (a dose of an inert substance identified as a painkiller). Since the placebo response is based in part on activation of the endogenous opioid system, it will be blocked by naloxone, a substance which blocks descending pain inhibitory pathways, and her pain will be unchanged. This experiment will not necessarily affect her response to opiates in the future.

4-C. Substance P has been implicated in pain disorders. Cholecystokinin (CCK) is implicated in schizophrenia and anxiety disorders, vasopressin, somatostatin, and vasoactive intestinal peptide have been implicated in mood disorders. Somatostatin has been implicated also in Huntington's disease and dementia of the Alzheimer type.

5-D. Dominance for language in both right-handed and left-handed people is usually in the left hemisphere of the brain. Perception, musical ability, artistic ability, and spatial relations are functions of the right side of the brain.

6-B. The corpus callosum and the anterior and hippocampal commissures connect the two hemispheres of the brain. The basal ganglia, reticular system, hippocampus, and amygdala do not have this function.

7-D. Sedation, increased appetite, and weight gain are side effects of treatment with certain antipsychotic agents. The mechanism most closely associated with these side effects is blockade of histamine receptors since these antipsychotics are not specific for dopamine blockade. Blockade of dopamine receptors by these antipsychotic medications is associated with side effects such as parkinsonism-like symptoms and elevated prolactin levels.

8-C. Degeneration of cholinergic neurons in the brain is seen in dementia of the Alzheimer type, movement disorders, and Down syndrome.

9-E. Acetylcholine (ACh) is the major neurotransmitter implicated in dementia of the Alzheimer type.

10-A. Blockade of serotonin reuptake by presynaptic neurons is the primary action of the antidepressant fluoxetine.

11-B. Norepinephrine is metabolized to MHPG.

12-A. Serotonin is metabolized to 5-HIAA.

13-E. The patient is suffering from Klüver-Bucy syndrome, which includes hypersexuality and docility and is associated with damage to the amygdala.

14-D. Sleep-arousal mechanisms are affected by damage to the reticular system.

15-A. Damage to the right parietal lobe can result in impaired visual-spatial processing which can lead to problems copying simple drawings and left side neglect.

16-B. This patient is showing signs of Parkinson's disease which is associated with abnormalities of the basal ganglia.

17-C. This patient is probably suffering from dementia of the Alzheimer type. Of the listed brain areas the major one implicated in dementia of the Alzheimer type is the hippocampus.

18-F. Of the listed brain areas, depression is most likely to be associated with damage to the left frontal lobe.

5

Biological Assessment of Patients with Psychiatric Symptoms

Typical Board Question

A physician administers sodium lactate intravenously to a 28-year-old woman. Using this technique, the physician is trying to provoke and thus identify

(A) conversion disorder
(B) amnestic disorder
(C) malingering
(D) panic disorder
(E) major depression

(See "Answers and Explanations" at end of Chapter)

I. Overview

—Biological alterations and abnormalities can underlie psychiatric symptoms and influence their occurrence. A variety of studies are used clinically to identify such alterations and abnormalities in patients.

II. Measurement of Biogenic Amines and Psychotropic Drugs

A. Altered levels of biogenic amines and their metabolites occur in some psychiatric conditions (see Tables 4-2 and 4-3).

B. Plasma levels of some antipsychotic and antidepressant agents are measured to evaluate **patient compliance** or to determine whether **therapeutic blood levels** of the agent have been reached.

C. Laboratory tests are also used to monitor patients for complications of pharmacotherapy.

    1. Patients taking the antimanic agent carbamazepine [Tegretol] or the antipsychotic agent clozapine [Clozaril] must be observed for blood abnormalities such as agranulocytosis.

    2. Liver function tests are used in patients being treated with carbamazepine and valproic acid (an antimanic agent).

3. Thyroid function tests and renal panel should be used in patients who are being treated with the antimanic agent **lithium.**

 a. Patients taking lithium can develop **hypothyroidism** and, occasionally, hyperthyroidism.

 b. Lithium levels also should be monitored regularly because of the drug's **narrow therapeutic range.**

III. Dexamethasone Suppression Test (DST)

 A. In a normal patient with a normal hypothalamic-adrenal-pituitary axis, dexamethasone, a synthetic glucocorticoid, **suppresses the secretion of cortisol.** In contrast, approximately one half of patients with **major depressive disorder** have **a positive DST (i.e., this suppression is limited or absent).**

 B. There is some evidence that patients with a positive DST (indicating reduced suppression of cortisol) will respond well to treatment with antidepressant agents or to electroconvulsive therapy (see Chapter 16).

 C. The DST has limited clinical usefulness. Positive findings are **not specific;** nonsuppression is seen in conditions other than major depressive disorder. These disorders include: **schizophrenia, dementia,** pregnancy, anorexia nervosa, or severe weight loss and endocrine disorders. Nonsuppression is also seen with use, abuse, and withdrawal of alcohol and antianxiety agents.

IV. Tests of Endocrine Function

 A. Thyroid function tests are used to screen for **hypothyroidism and hyperthyroidism,** which can mimic depression and anxiety, respectively.

 B. Patients with depression may have other **endocrine irregularities** such as reduced response to a challenge with thyrotropin-releasing hormone, and abnormalities in growth hormone, melatonin, and gonadotropin.

 C. Reduced levels of gonadotropins are seen also in schizophrenia.

 D. Psychiatric symptoms are associated with endocrine disorders such as **Addison's disease** and **Cushing's disease.**

V. Neuroimaging and Electroencephalogram (EEG) Studies

—Structural brain abnormalities and EEG changes may correspond to specific psychiatric disorders (Table 5-1).

VI. Neuropsychological Tests

 A. Neuropsychological tests are designed to assess general intelligence, memory, reasoning, orientation, perceptuomotor performance, language function, attention, and concentration in patients with suspected neurologic problems, such as dementia and brain damage.

 B. Specific neuropsychological tests are described in Table 5-2.

VII. Other Tests

 A. Amobarbital sodium [Amytal] interview

 1. Intravenous (IV) administration of amobarbital sodium ("the Amytal interview") may be useful in determining whether organic pathology is re-

Table 5-1. Neuroimaging and Electroencephalography in the Biological Evaluation of the Psychiatric Patient

Specific test or measure	Uses and Characteristics
Computed tomography (CT)	• Identifies anatomically based brain changes (e.g., enlarged brain ventricles) in cognitive disorders such as dementia of the Alzheimer type as well as in schizophrenia
Nuclear magnetic resonance imaging (NMRI)	• Identifies demyelinating disease (e.g., multiple sclerosis). • Shows the biochemical condition of neural tissues as well as the anatomy without exposing the patient to ionizing radiation
Positron emission tomography (PET) or functional MRI (fMRI)	• Localizes areas of the brain that are physiologically active during specific tasks by characterizing and measuring metabolism of glucose in neural tissue
Electroencephalogram (EEG)	• Measures electrical activity in the cortex • Is useful in diagnosing epilepsy and in differentiating delirium (abnormal EEG) from dementia (often normal EEG) • Shows, in schizophrenic patients, decreased alpha waves, increased theta and delta waves, and epileptiform activity
Evoked EEG (evoked potentials)	• Measures electrical activity in the cortex in response to tactile, auditory, sound, or visual stimulation • Is used to evaluate vision and hearing loss in infants and brain responses in comatose and suspected brain dead patients

Table 5-2. Neuropsychological Diagnostic Tests Used in Psychiatry

Test	Uses and Characteristics
Halstead-Reitan battery	• Used to detect and localize brain lesions and determine their effects.
Luria-Nebraska neuropsychological battery	• Used to determine left or right cerebral dominance • Used to identify specific types of brain dysfunction, such as dyslexia
Bender Visual Motor Gestalt Test	• Used to evaluate visual and motor ability through the reproduction of designs

sponsible for symptomatology in patients who exhibit **malingering, dissociative disorder,** or **conversion disorder** (see Chapter 14).

2. Amobarbital sodium can **relax patients** with these disorders or other disorders involving high levels of anxiety and **mute psychotic states** (see Chapter 11), so that they can express themselves coherently during an interview.

B. Sodium lactate administration. IV administration of sodium lactate can **provoke a panic attack (see Chapter 13) in susceptible patients** and can thus help to identify individuals with panic disorder. Inhalation of carbon dioxide can produce the same effect.

C. Galvanic skin response **("lie detector" test)**

1. The electric resistance of skin (galvanic skin response) varies with the patient's psychological state.

2. Higher sweat gland activity, seen with sympathetic nervous system arousal (e.g., when lying), results in decreased skin resistance.

Review Test

Directions: Each of the numbered items or incomplete statements in this section is followed by answers or by completions of the statement. Select the **one** lettered answer or completion that is **best** in each case.

1. A 40-year-old woman reports that she has no appetite, sleeps poorly, and has lost interest in her normal activities. Which of the following is the most likely laboratory finding in this woman?

(A) Positive dexamethasone suppression test (DST)
(B) Normal growth hormone regulation
(C) Increased response to a challenge with thyrotropin-releasing hormone
(D) Normal melatonin levels
(E) Hyperthyroidism

2. A 34-year-old female patient develops agranulocytosis. This patient is most likely to be taking which of the following agents?

(A) Amobarbital sodium
(B) Clozapine
(C) Lithium
(D) Dexamethasone
(E) Sodium lactate

3. A 37-year-old male patient who has had a stroke cannot copy a design drawn by the examiner. The test that the examiner is most likely to be using to evaluate this patient is the

(A) Bender Visual Motor Gestalt Test
(B) Luria-Nebraska neuropsychological battery
(C) Halstead-Reitan battery
(D) dexamethasone suppression test
(E) electroencephalogram (EEG)

4. To determine which brain area is physiologically active when a 44-year-old male patient is translating a paragraph from Spanish to English, the most appropriate diagnostic technique is

(A) positron emission tomography (PET)
(B) computed tomography (CT)
(C) amobarbital sodium [Amytal] interview
(D) electroencephalogram (EEG)
(E) evoked EEG

5. To determine whether a 3-month-old infant is able to hear sounds, the most appropriate diagnostic technique is

(A) positron emission tomography (PET)
(B) computed tomography (CT)
(C) amobarbital sodium [Amytal] interview
(D) electroencephalogram (EEG)
(E) evoked EEG

6. A 27-year-old female patient shows a sudden loss of sensory function below the waist which cannot be medically explained. To determine whether psychological factors are responsible, the most appropriate diagnostic technique is

(A) positron emission tomography (PET)
(B) computed tomography (CT)
(C) amobarbital sodium [Amytal] interview
(D) electroencephalogram (EEG)
(E) evoked EEG

7. To identify anatomical changes in the brain of an 80-year-old female patient with dementia of the Alzheimer type, the most appropriate diagnostic technique is

(A) positron emission tomography (PET)
(B) computed tomography (CT)
(C) amobarbital sodium [Amytal] interview
(D) electroencephalogram (EEG)
(E) evoked EEG

8. To differentiate delirium from dementia in a 75-year-old male patient, the most appropriate diagnostic technique is

(A) positron emission tomography (PET)
(B) computed tomography (CT)
(C) amobarbital sodium [Amytal] interview
(D) electroencephalogram (EEG)
(E) evoked EEG

Answers and Explanations

TBQ-D. Intravenous administration of sodium lactate can help identify individuals with panic disorder since it can provoke a panic attack in such patients. Amobarbital sodium interviews may be useful in determining whether organic pathology is responsible for symptomatology in patients who exhibit malingering, amnestic, or conversion disorder (see Chapter 14). The dexamethasone suppression test can help in identifying major depression.

1-A. Poor appetite, poor sleep, and lack of interest in normal activities characterize patients suffering from major depression (see Chapter 12). In this depressed woman, the dexamethasone suppression test is likely to be positive. A positive result is seen when the synthetic glucocorticoid dexamethasone fails to suppress the secretion of cortisol as it would in a normal patient. Also, in depression there may be abnormal growth hormone regulation and melatonin levels and reduced response to a challenge with thyrotropin-releasing hormone. Hypothyroidism not uncommonly results in depression; hyperthyroidism is more commonly associated with the symptoms of anxiety.

2-B. Agranulocytosis (a disorder of the blood) is seen particularly in patients taking clozapine, an antipsychotic, or carbamazepine, an anticonvulsant which is used to treat bipolar disorder (see Chapter 12). Lithium, amobarbital sodium, dexamethasone, and sodium lactate are not specifically associated with agranulocytosis.

3-A. The Bender Visual Motor Gestalt Test is used to evaluate visual and motor ability by reproduction of designs. The Luria-Nebraska neuropsychological battery is used to determine cerebral dominance and to identify specific types of brain dysfunction, while the Halstead-Reitan battery is used to detect and localize brain lesions and determine their effects. The dexamethasone suppression test is used to predict which depressed patients will respond well to treatment with antidepressant agents or to electroconvulsive therapy. The electroencephalogram (EEG), which measures electrical activity in the cortex, is useful in diagnosing epilepsy and in differentiating delirium from dementia.

4-A. Positron emission tomography (PET) localizes physiologically active brain areas by measuring glucose metabolism. Thus, this test can be used to determine which brain area is being used during a specific task (e.g., translating a passage written in Spanish).

5-E. The auditory evoked EEG can be used to assess whether this child can hear. Evoked EEGs measure electrical activity in the cortex in response to sensory stimulation.

6-C. The sodium amobarbital (Amytal) interview is used to determine whether psychological factors are responsible for symptoms in this patient who shows a non-medically explained loss of sensory function (conversion disorder—see Chapter 14).

7-B. Computed tomography (CT) identifies organically based brain changes such as enlarged ventricles. Thus, although not diagnostic, this test can be used to identify anatomical changes in the brain such as enlarged ventricles of a patient with suspected dementia of the Alzheimer type.

8-D. Electroencephalogram (EEG) measures electrical activity in the cortex and can be useful in differentiating delirium (abnormal EEG) from dementia (usually normal EEG).

6

Psychoanalytic Theory

Typical Board Question

A doctor becomes very angry with a patient when the patient does not take his medication. The patient reminds the doctor of her rebellious son. This doctor's intense reaction to the patient's behavior is most likely to be a result of

(A) positive transference
(B) negative transference
(C) countertransference
(D) dislike of the patient
(E) anger at the patient

(See "Answers and Explanations" at end of Chapter)

I. Overview

—Psychoanalytic theory is based on Freud's concept that behavior is determined by forces derived from **unconscious mental processes. Psychoanalysis** and related therapies are psychotherapeutic treatments based on this concept (see Chapter 17).

II. Freud's Theories of the Mind

—To explain his ideas, Freud developed, early in his career, the topographic theory of the mind and, later in his career, the structural theory.

A. **Topographic theory of the mind.** In the topographic theory, the mind contains three levels: the unconscious, preconscious, and conscious.

1. The **unconscious mind** contains repressed thoughts and feelings which are not available to the conscious mind, and uses primary process thinking.

a. **Primary process** is a type of thinking associated with primitive drives, wish fulfillment, and pleasure seeking and has no logic or concept of time. Primary process thinking is seen in young children and psychotic adults.

b. **Dreams** represent gratification of unconscious instinctive impulses and wish fulfillment.

47

2. The **preconscious mind** contains memories that, while not immediately available, can be accessed easily.

3. The **conscious mind** contains thoughts that a person is currently aware of. It operates in close conjunction with the preconscious mind but does not have access to the unconscious mind. The conscious mind uses secondary process thinking (logical, mature, time-oriented) and can delay gratification.

B. **Structural theory of the mind.** In the structural theory, the mind contains three parts: the id, the ego, and the superego (Table 6-1).

II. Defense Mechanisms

A. **Definition.** Defense mechanisms are **unconscious mental techniques** used by the ego to keep conflicts out of the conscious mind, thus decreasing anxiety and maintaining a person's sense of safety, equilibrium, and self-esteem.

B. **Specific defense mechanisms (Table 6-2)**

1. Many defense mechanisms are **immature** (i.e., they are manifestations of childlike or disturbed behavior).

2. **Mature defense mechanisms** (e.g., altruism, humor, sublimation, and suppression) when used in moderation, directly help the patient or others.

3. **Repression,** pushing unacceptable emotions into the unconscious, is the **basic defense mechanism** on which all others are based.

Table 6-1. Freud's Structural Theory of the Mind

Structural component	Topographic level of operation	Age at which it develops	Characteristics
Id	Unconscious	Present at birth	• Contains instinctive sexual and aggressive drives • Controlled by primary process thinking • Not influenced by external reality
Ego	Unconscious, preconscious and conscious	Begins to develop immediately after birth	• Controls the expression of the id to adapt to the requirements of the external world primarily by the use of defense mechanisms • Enables one to sustain satisfying interpersonal relationships • Through reality testing (i.e., constantly evaluating what is valid and then adapting that to reality), enables one to maintain a sense of reality about the body and the external world
Superego	Unconscious, preconscious and conscious	Developed by about 6 years of age	• Associated with moral values and conscience • Controls the expression of the id

Table 6-2. Commonly Used Defense Mechanisms (listed alphabetically)

Defense mechanism	Explanation	Example
Acting out	• Avoiding personally unacceptable emotions by behaving in an attention-getting, often socially inappropriate manner	A depressed 14-year-old girl with no history of conduct disorder has sexual encounters with multiple partners after her parents divorce
Altruism	• Assisting others to avoid negative personal feelings (a relatively "mature" defense mechanism)	A man with a poor self-image, who is a social worker during the week, donates every other weekend to charity work
Denial	• Not believing aspects of reality that the person finds unbearable	An alcoholic insists that he is only a social drinker
Displacement	• Moving emotions from a personally intolerable situation to one that is personally tolerable	A surgeon attending with unacknowledged anger toward his mother is abrasive to the female residents on his service
Dissociation	• Mentally separating part of one's consciousness from real life events or mentally distancing oneself from others	A teenager has no memory of a car accident in which he was driving and his girlfriend was killed
Humor	• Expressing personally uncomfortable feelings without causing emotional discomfort (a relatively "mature" defense mechanism)	A man who is uncomfortable about his erectile problems makes jokes about Viagra (Sildenafil)
Identification (Identification with the Aggressor)	• Unconsciously patterning one's behavior after that of someone more powerful (can be either positive or negative)	A man who was terrorized by his gym teacher as a child, becomes a punitive, critical gym teacher
Intellectualization	• Using the mind's higher functions to avoid experiencing emotion	A sailor whose boat is about to sink calmly explains the technical aspects of the hull damage in great detail to the other crew members
Isolation of affect	• Failing to experience the feelings associated with a stressful life event, although logically understanding the significance of the event	Without showing any emotion, a woman tells her family the results of tests which indicate that her lung cancer has metastasized
Projection	• Attributing one's own personally unacceptable feelings to others • Associated with paranoid symptoms and prejudice	A man with unconscious homosexual impulses begins to believe that his boss is homosexual
Rationalization	• Distorting one's perception of an event so that its negative outcome seems reasonable	A man who loses an arm in an accident says the loss of his arm was good because it kept him from getting in trouble with the law
Reaction formation	• Adopting opposite attitudes to avoid personally unacceptable emotions; i.e. unconscious hypocrisy	A woman who unconsciously is resentful of the responsibilities of child rearing, over-

continued

Table 6-2. Commonly Used Defense Mechanisms (listed alphabetically)

Defense mechanism	Explanation	Example
		spends on expensive gifts and clothing for her children
Regression	• Reverting to behavior patterns like those seen in someone of a younger age	A 5-year-old child who was previously toilet-trained begins to wet the bed when his mother has a new baby
Splitting	• Categorizing people or situations into categories of either "fabulous" or "dreadful" because of intolerance of uncertainty • Seen in patients with borderline personality disorder	A patient tells the doctor that while all of the doctors in the group practice are wonderful, all of the nurses and office help are unfriendly and curt
Sublimation	• Expressing a personally unacceptable feeling (e.g., rage) in a socially acceptable way (a relatively "mature" defense mechanism)	A man who got into fights as a teenager, becomes a professional prize fighter
Suppression	• Deliberately pushing personally unacceptable emotions out of conscious awareness (the only defense mechanism that includes some aspect of consciousness)	A medical student taking a review course for the USMLE, mentally changes the subject when her mind wanders to the exam during a lecture
Undoing	• Believing that one can magically reverse past events caused by "incorrect" behavior by now adopting "correct" behavior	A woman who is terminally ill with AIDS caused by drug abuse, stops using drugs and alcohol and starts an exercise and healthful diet program

Adapted from Fadem B, Simring S: *High Yield Psychiatry.* Baltimore, Williams and Wilkins, 1998, p. 134.

III. Transference Reactions

A. **Definition**
—Transference and countertransference are **unconscious mental attitudes** based on important past personal relationships. These phenomena increase emotionality and may thus alter judgment and behavior in patients' relationships with their doctors (transference) and doctors' relationships with their patients (countertransference).

B. **Transference**

1. In **positive transference,** the patient has confidence in the doctor. If intense, the patient may over-idealize the doctor or develop sexual feelings toward the doctor.

2. In **negative transference,** the patient may become resentful or angry toward the doctor if the patient's desires and expectations are not realized. This may lead to noncompliance with medical advice.

C. In **countertransference,** feelings about a patient who reminds the doctor of a close friend or relative can interfere with the doctor's medical judgment.

Review Test

Directions: Each of the numbered items or incomplete statements in this section is followed by answers or by completions of the statement. Select the **one** lettered answer or completion that is **best** in each case.

1. A primary care physician notices that many of her patients use statements like "I can't stop smoking because I'll gain weight," or "when I'm sick, I only want to eat junk food." Statements like these

(A) produce conflict in the conscious mind
(B) are conscious mental techniques
(C) increase anxiety
(D) are examples of the use of defense mechanisms
(E) decrease patients' sense of self-esteem

2. Which of the following structures of the mind work on an unconscious level?

(A) The id only
(B) The id and the ego only
(C) The id, ego, and superego
(D) The ego and superego only
(E) Neither the id, ego, nor superego

3. Which of the following structures of the mind are developed in a normal 7-year-old child?

(A) The id only
(B) The id and the ego only
(C) The id, ego, and superego
(D) The ego and superego only
(E) Neither the id, ego, nor superego

4. A 34-year-old woman relates that she wakes up fully dressed at least twice a week but then is tired all day. She also frequently receives phone calls from men who say they met her in a bar but whom she does not remember meeting. The defense mechanism that this woman is using is

(A) denial
(B) sublimation
(C) dissociation
(D) regression
(E) intellectualization

5. A 35-year-old woman scheduled for surgery the next day insists that her mother stay overnight in the hospital with her. The defense mechanism that this patient is using is

(A) denial
(B) sublimation
(C) dissociation
(D) regression
(E) intellectualization

6. Which of the following defense mechanisms is classified as the most mature?

(A) Denial
(B) Sublimation
(C) Dissociation
(D) Regression
(E) Intellectualization

7. A patient whose father was often late for important family events storms out of the office when told that the doctor will be late because of an emergency. This patient's behavior is most likely to be a result of

(A) positive transference
(B) negative transference
(C) countertransference
(D) dislike of the doctor
(E) anger at the doctor

8. When having a manic episode, a 53-year-old patient with bipolar disorder shows primary process thinking. This type of thinking

(A) is logical
(B) is closely attuned to time
(C) is associated with reality
(D) is accessible to the conscious mind
(E) is associated with pleasure seeking

9. About 1 week after her final examination for a biochemistry course, a medical student's knowledge of the details of the Krebs cycle is most likely to reside in her

(A) unconscious mind
(B) preconscious mind
(C) conscious mind
(D) superego
(E) ego

10. A 15-year-old steals from family members and friends. When no one is watching, he also tortures the family cat. Which aspect of the mind is deficient in this teenager?

(A) The unconscious mind
(B) The preconscious mind
(C) The conscious mind
(D) The superego
(E) The ego

51

11. A man who has unacknowledged anger toward his wife kicks his dog. The defense mechanism that this man is using is

(A) Regression
(B) Acting out
(C) Denial
(D) Splitting
(E) Projection
(F) Dissociation
(G) Reaction formation
(H) Intellectualization
(I) Sublimation
(J) Displacement

12. A person who has unconscious violent feelings becomes a surgeon. The defense mechanism that this person is using is

(A) Regression
(B) Acting out
(C) Denial
(D) Splitting
(E) Projection
(F) Dissociation
(G) Reaction formation
(H) Intellectualization
(I) Sublimation
(J) Displacement

13. A husband who is unconsciously attracted to another woman accuses his wife of cheating. The defense mechanism that this man is using is

(A) Regression
(B) Acting out
(C) Denial
(D) Splitting
(E) Projection
(F) Dissociation
(G) Reaction formation
(H) Intellectualization
(I) Sublimation
(J) Displacement

14. A man who is unconsciously afraid of flying states his love of airplanes. The defense mechanism that this man is using is

((A) Regression
(B) Acting out
(C) Denial
(D) Splitting
(E) Projection
(F) Dissociation
(G) Reaction formation
(H) Intellectualization
(I) Sublimation
(J) Displacement

Answers and Explanations

TBQ-C. The doctor who becomes very angry at her patient for not taking his medication is showing a countertransference reaction. This excessive show of emotion is a result of reexperiencing feelings about her son's behavior in her relationship with the noncompliant patient. It is important for the doctor to identify this reaction because it can interfere with her medical judgement. In positive transference patients have a high level of confidence in the doctor. Patients may also over-idealize or develop sexual feelings toward the doctor. In negative transference, patients become resentful or angry toward the doctor if their desires and expectations are not realized. This may lead to noncompliance with medical advice. This doctor's reaction to the patient is unlikely to be related to dislike or fear of the patient.

1-D. Statements like "I can't stop smoking because I'll gain weight," or "when I'm sick, I only want to eat junk food" are examples of the defense mechanisms of rationalization and regression, respectively. In rationalization, a person distorts her perception of an event so that its negative outcome seems reasonable, (i.e., because she feels unable to stop smoking), this patient claims (and so she reasonably feels) that gaining weight is worse than smoking, a life-threatening habit. In regression, ill patients revert to behavior patterns like those seen in someone of a younger age, (i.e., eating junk food). Defense mechanisms such as these are unconscious mental techniques which decrease anxiety and help people to maintain a sense of equilibrium and self-esteem.

2-C. In Freud's structural theory, the mind is divided into the id, ego, and superego. The id operates completely on an unconscious level while the ego, and superego operate partly on an unconscious and partly on preconscious and conscious levels.

3-C. The id is present at birth, the ego begins to develop immediately after birth, and the superego is developed by about age 6 years.

4-C. This patient who relates that she wakes up fully dressed at least twice a week and receives phone calls from men whom she does not remember meeting is exhibiting dissociative identity disorder (multiple personality disorder). Dissociation, separating part of one's consciousness from real life events, is the defense mechanism used by individuals with this disorder. It is likely that this patient met the men who have her phone number but does not remember meeting them because at that time she was showing another personality (see also Chapter 14).

5-D. Regression, going back to a less mature way of behaving, is the defense mechanism used by this woman scheduled for surgery the next day who insists that her mother stay overnight in the hospital with her.

6-B. Sublimation, expressing an unacceptable emotion in a socially acceptable way, is classified as a mature defense mechanism. Denial, dissociation, regression, and intellectualization are all classified as less mature defense mechanisms.

7-B. The patient who becomes very angry at his doctor for being late is showing a negative transference reaction. This excessive show of emotion is a result of reexperiencing feelings about his father's lateness for important family events in his relationship with the doctor. In positive transference, a patient has confidence in and may idealize the doctor. In countertransference, a doctor's feelings about a patient who reminds her of a close friend or relative can interfere with her medical judgement. The patient's reaction to the doctor is unlikely to be related to dislike of or the doctor.

8-E. Primary process thinking is associated with pleasure seeking, disregards logic and reality, has no concept of time, and is not accessible to the conscious mind. Secondary process thinking is logical and is associated with reality.

9-B. Memory of the details of the Krebs cycle, while no longer in the forefront of the medical student's mind, can be recalled relatively easily one week after the examination. This memory therefore resides in the preconscious mind. The unconscious mind contains repressed thoughts and feelings, which are not available to the conscious mind. The conscious mind contains thoughts that a person is currently aware of. See Explanation 10 (below) for definitions of the ego and superego.

10-D. The superego is associated with moral values and conscience and controls impulses of the id. This teenager who steals from family members and friends and tortures the family cat is showing deficiencies in his superego. Children and adolescents under age 18 years who have poor superego development have conduct disorder (see Chapter 15). The id contains instinctive sexual and aggressive drives and is not influenced by external reality. The ego also controls the expression of the id, sustains satisfying interpersonal relationships and, through reality testing, maintains a sense of reality about the body and the external world.

11-J. In displacement, the man's personally unacceptable angry feelings toward his wife are taken out on his dog.

12-I. In sublimation, the surgeon reroutes his unconscious, unacceptable wish for committing a violent act to a socially acceptable route (cutting people during surgery).

13-E. Using projection, the husband attributes his unconscious, unacceptable sexual feelings toward another woman to his wife.

14-G. In reaction formation, the man denies his unconscious fear of flying and embraces the opposite idea by stating that he loves airplanes.

Chapter 8

7

Learning Theory

Typical Board Question

A 52-year-old woman has undergone three sessions of chemotherapy in a hospital. Before the fourth session, she becomes nauseated when she enters the hospital lobby. This patient's reaction is a result of the type of learning best described as

(A) operant conditioning
(B) classical conditioning
(C) modeling
(D) shaping
(E) biofeedback

(Answer in "Answers and Explanations" at end of Chapter)

I. Overview

    A. Learning is the acquisition of new behavior patterns.

    B. Methods of learning include **classical conditioning** and **operant conditioning.**

    C. Classical and operant conditioning are the basis of **behavioral treatment techniques,** such as systematic desensitization, aversive conditioning, flooding, biofeedback, token economy, and cognitive therapy (see Chapter 16).

II. Classical Conditioning

    A. Principles. In classical conditioning, a **natural, or reflexive response** (behavior) is elicited by a **learned stimulus** (a cue from an internal or external event).

    B. Elements of classical conditioning

        1. An **unconditioned stimulus** is something that automatically, without having to be learned, produces a response (e.g., the odor of food).

        2. An **unconditioned response** is a natural, reflexive behavior that does not have to be learned (e.g., salivation in response to the odor of food).

3. A **conditioned stimulus** is something that produces a response following learning (e.g., the sound of the lunch bell).

4. A **conditioned response** is a behavior that is learned by an association that is made between a conditioned stimulus and an unconditioned stimulus (e.g., salivation in response to the lunch bell).

C. **Response acquisition, extinction,** and **stimulus generalization**

1. In **acquisition,** the conditioned response (e.g., salivation in response to the lunch bell) is learned.

2. In **extinction,** the conditioned response decreases if the conditioned stimulus (e.g., the sound of the lunch bell) is never again paired with the unconditioned stimulus (e.g., the odor of food).

3. In **stimulus generalization,** a new stimulus (e.g., a fire bell) that resembles a conditioned stimulus (e.g., the lunch bell) causes a conditioned response (e.g., salivation).

D. **Aversive conditioning.** An unwanted behavior (e.g., setting fires) is paired with a painful, or aversive, stimulus (e.g., a painful electric shock). An association is created between the unwanted behavior (fire-setting) and the aversive stimulus (pain) and the fire-setting ceases.

E. **Learned helplessness**

1. An animal receives a series of painful electric shocks from which it is **unable to escape.**

2. By classical conditioning, the animal learns that there is an association between an aversive stimulus (e.g., painful electric shock) and the inability to escape.

3. Subsequently, the animal makes no attempt to escape when shocked or when faced with any new aversive stimulus; instead the animal becomes **hopeless and apathetic.**

4. Learned helplessness in animals may be a model system for **depression** (often characterized by hopelessness and apathy) in humans.

F. **Imprinting** is the tendency of organisms to make an association with and then follow the first thing they see after birth or hatching (in birds).

III. Operant Conditioning

A. **Principles**

1. Behavior is determined by its consequences for the individual. The consequence, or **reinforcement,** occurs immediately following a behavior.

2. In operant conditioning, a behavior that is **not part of the individual's natural repertoire** can be learned through reward or punishment.

B. **Features**

1. The likelihood that a **behavior** will occur is **increased by reinforcement** and **decreased by punishment.** (Table 7-1)

a. Types of reinforcement include:

Table 7-1. Features of Operant Conditioning

Example: A mother would like her 8-year-old son to stop hitting his 6-year-old brother. She can achieve this goal by using one of the following features of operant conditioning

Feature	Effect on Behavior	Example	Comments
Positive reinforcement	Behavior is increased by reward	Child increases his kind behavior toward his younger brother to get praise from his mother	• Reward or reinforcement (praise) increases desired behavior (kindness toward brother) • A reward can be praise or attention as well as a tangible reward like money
Negative reinforcement	Behavior is increased by avoidance or escape	Child increases his kind behavior toward his younger brother to avoid being scolded	• Active avoidance of an aversive stimulus (being scolded) increases desired behavior (kindness toward brother)
Punishment	Behavior is decreased by suppression	Child decreases his hitting behavior after his mother scolds him	• Delivery of an aversive stimulus (scolding) decreases unwanted behavior (hitting brother) rapidly but not permanently
Extinction	Behavior is eliminated by non-reinforcement	Child stops his hitting behavior when the behavior is ignored by his mother	• Extinction is more effective than punishment for long-term reduction in unwanted behavior • There may be an initial increase in hitting behavior before it disappears

> **(1) Positive reinforcement** (reward) is the introduction of a positive stimulus that results in an increase in the rate of behavior.
>
> **(2) Negative reinforcement** (escape) is the removal of an aversive stimulus that also results in an increase in the rate of behavior.

b. Punishment is the introduction of an aversive stimulus aimed at reducing the rate of an unwanted behavior.

2. Extinction in operant conditioning is the gradual disappearance of a learned behavior when reinforcement (reward) is withheld.

a. The pattern, or **schedule, of reinforcement** affects how quickly a behavior is learned and how quickly a behavior becomes extinguished when it is not rewarded (Table 7-2).

b. Resistance to extinction is the force which prevents the behavior from disappearing when a reward is withheld.

C. Shaping and modeling

1. Shaping involves rewarding closer and closer approximations of the wanted behavior until the correct behavior is achieved (e.g., a child learning to write).

2. Modeling is a type of observational learning (e.g., an individual behaves in a manner similar to that of someone she admires).

Table 7-2. Schedules of Reinforcement

Schedule	Reinforcement	Example	Effect on behavior
Continuous	Presented after every response	A teenager receives a candy bar each time she puts a dollar into a vending machine. One time she puts a dollar in and nothing comes out. She never buys candy from the machine again.	• Behavior (putting in a dollar to receive candy) is rapidly learned but disappears rapidly (has low resistance to extinction) when not reinforced (no candy comes out).
Fixed ratio	Presented after a designated number of responses	A man is paid $10 for every five hats he makes. He makes as many hats as he can during his shift.	• Fast response rate (many hats are made quickly)
Fixed interval	Presented after a designated amount of time	A student has an anatomy quiz every Friday. He studies for ten minutes on Wednesday nights, and for 2 hours on Thursday nights.	• The response rate (studying) increases toward end of each the interval (week). • When graphed, the response rate forms a scalloped curve.
Variable ratio	Presented after a random and unpredictable number of responses	After a slot machine pays off $5 for a single quarter, a woman plays $50 in quarters despite the fact that she receives no further payoffs.	• The behavior (playing the slot machine) continues (is highly resistant to extinction) despite the fact that it is only reinforced (winning money) after a large but variable number of responses
Variable interval	Presented after a random and unpredictable amount of time	After 5 minutes of fishing in a lake a man catches a large fish. He then spends 4 hours waiting for another bite.	• The behavior (fishing) continues (is highly resistant to extinction) despite the fact that it is only reinforced (a fish is caught) after varying certain time intervals

Review Test

Directions: Each of the numbered items or incomplete statements in this section is followed by answers or by completions of the statement. Select the one lettered answer or completion that is best.

Questions 1–3

For the past year, pizza has been sold from a white van outside a high school. The teenage students complain that they are often embarrassed because their stomachs begin to growl whenever they see any white vehicle, even on weekends. The principal then bans the van from selling pizza near the school and the students' stomachs stop growling at the sight of white vehicles.

1. For this scenario, which element represents the unconditioned response?

(A) Stomach growling in response to the white van
(B) Stomach growling in response to pizza
(C) The white van
(D) Pairing the white van with getting pizza
(E) pizza

2. For this scenario, which element represents the unconditioned stimulus?

(A) Stomach growling in response to the white van
(B) Stomach growling in response to pizza
(C) The white van
(D) Pairing the white van with getting pizza
(E) pizza

3. For this scenario, which element represents the conditioned stimulus?

(A) Stomach growling in response to the white van
(B) Stomach growling in response to pizza
(C) The white van
(D) Pairing the white van with getting pizza
(E) pizza

4. In the past, a child has on occasion received money for cleaning his room. Despite the fact that he has not received money for cleaning his room for the past month, the child's room cleaning behavior continues (is resistant to extinction). This behavior is most likely to have been learned using which of the following methods?

(A) Continuous reinforcement
(B) Fixed ratio reinforcement
(C) Fixed interval reinforcement
(D) Variable ratio reinforcement
(E) Punishment

5. A 7-year-old child who likes and looks up to her physician states that she wants to become a doctor when she grows up. This behavior by the child is an example of

(A) stimulus generalization
(B) modeling
(C) shaping
(D) imprinting
(E) learned helplessness

6. A 4-year-old child who has received beatings in the past from which he could not escape, appears unresponsive and no longer tries to escape new beatings. This behavior by the child is an example of

(A) stimulus generalization
(B) modeling
(C) shaping
(D) imprinting
(E) learned helplessness

7. A 2-year-old child is afraid of nurses in white uniforms. When his grandmother comes to visit him wearing a white jacket, he begins to cry. This behavior by the child is an example of

A) stimulus generalization
(B) modeling
(C) shaping
(D) imprinting
(E) learned helplessness

8. A father scolds his child when she hits the dog. The child stops hitting the dog. This change in the child's behavior is a result of

(A) punishment
(B) negative reinforcement
(C) positive reinforcement
(D) shaping
(E) classical conditioning

9. Although a father spanks his child when she hits the dog, the child continues to hit the dog. This child's hitting behavior is a result of

(A) punishment
(B) negative reinforcement
(C) positive reinforcement
(D) shaping
(E) classical conditioning

10. A patient with diabetes increases her time spent exercising in order to reduce the number of insulin injections she must receive. The increased exercising behavior is a result of

(A) punishment
(B) negative reinforcement
(C) positive reinforcement
(D) shaping
(E) classical conditioning

Questions 11–14

A child comes to the clinical laboratory to have a blood sample drawn for the first time and has a painful experience. The next time the child returns for this procedure, she begins to cry when she smells the odor of antiseptic in the clinic hallway. For each clinical scenario, select the definition that best describes it.

11. The painful blood withdrawal procedure at the child's initial visit can be called the

(A) unconditioned stimulus
(B) unconditioned response
(C) conditioned stimulus
(D) conditioned response

12. The antiseptic odor detected upon the child's return can be called the

(A) unconditioned stimulus
(B) unconditioned response
(C) conditioned stimulus
(D) conditioned response

13. The child's crying upon the smell of antiseptic can be called the

(A) unconditioned stimulus
(B) unconditioned response
(C) conditioned stimulus
(D) conditioned response

14. The child's crying when the blood sample is drawn can be called the

(A) unconditioned stimulus
(B) unconditioned response
(C) conditioned stimulus
(D) conditioned response

Answers and Explanations

TBQ-B. This common clinical phenomenon is an example of classical conditioning. In this example, a woman comes into the hospital for an intravenous (IV) chemotherapy treatment (unconditioned stimulus). The chemotherapy drug is toxic and she becomes nauseated after the treatment (unconditioned response). The following month, when she enters the hospital lobby (conditioned stimulus), she becomes nauseated (conditioned response). Thus, the hospital where the treatments took place (the conditioned stimulus) has become paired with chemotherapy (the unconditioned stimulus), which elicited nausea. Now, nausea (unconditioned response) can be elicited by entering the hospital lobby (conditioned stimulus). In operant conditioning, behavior is determined by its consequences. Modeling is a type of observational learning. Shaping involves rewarding closer and closer approximations of the wanted behavior until the correct behavior is achieved. Biofeedback is a treatment technique based on operant conditioning (see Chapter 17).

1-B. The unconditioned stimulus (the pizza) produces the unconditioned response (stomach growling in response to the pizza). The unconditioned response is reflexive and automatic and does not have to be learned.

2-E. The unconditioned stimulus (pizza) is the only element here which by itself will elicit a natural GI reflex (stomach growling).

3-C. The white van is an example of the conditioned stimulus. In this scenario, the conditioned or learned stimulus causes the same response as the unconditioned or unlearned stimulus only after it is paired with the pizza (stomach growling in response to pizza).

4-D. This child has received money at unpredictable times for cleaning his room. Behavior learned in this way (i.e., by variable ratio reinforcement), is very resistant to extinction and continues even when it is not rewarded. Behavior learned by fixed schedules of reinforcement (ratio or interval) are less resistant to extinction. Behavior learned by continuous reinforcement is least resistant to extinction. Punishment is aversive and is aimed at suppressing an undesirable behavior.

5-B. This behavior is an example of modeling; the child wants to become like the doctor she admires. In stimulus generalization, a new stimulus that resembles a conditioned stimulus causes a conditioned response. Shaping involves rewarding closer and closer approximations of the wanted behavior until the correct behavior is achieved. In learned helplessness, an association is made between an aversive stimulus and the inability to escape. Imprinting is the tendency of organisms to make an association with and then follow the first thing they see after birth or hatching.

6-E. In learned helplessness, an association is made between an aversive stimulus and the inability to escape. Subsequently, the person makes no attempt to escape but instead becomes hopeless and apathetic when faced with any new aversive stimulus. Learned helplessness may be a model system for the development of depression. Modeling is a type of observational learning. In stimulus generalization, a new stimulus that resembles a conditioned stimulus causes a conditioned response. Shaping involves rewarding closer and closer approximations of the wanted behavior until the correct behavior is achieved. Imprinting is the tendency of organisms to make an association with and then follow the first thing they see after birth or hatching.

7-A. Stimulus generalization occurs when a new conditioned stimulus (the grandmother's white jacket) that resembles the original conditioned stimulus (the nurse's white uniform) results in the conditioned response (crying when he sees his grandmother). Habit is a general term which refers to repetitive negative behavior, (i.e., smoking). Instrumental conditioning is another term for operant conditioning which can also be described as learning by trial and error. Extinction is the disappearance of a learned behavior when reinforcement is withheld.

8-A. Because the behavior (hitting the dog) decreased, the scolding that this child received is punishment. Both negative and positive reinforcement increase behavior. Shaping involves rewarding closer and closer approximations of the wanted behavior until the correct behavior is achieved. In classical conditioning, a natural, or reflexive response (behavior) is elicited by a learned stimulus (a cue from an internal or external event).

9-C. Because the behavior (hitting the dog) is increased, the scolding that this child received is positive reinforcement. Both negative and positive reinforcement increase behavior. The reward or reinforcement for this hitting behavior is most likely to be increased attention from the father. Punishment decreases behavior. Shaping involves rewarding closer and closer approximations of the wanted behavior until the correct behavior is achieved. In classical conditioning, a natural, or reflexive response (behavior) is elicited by a learned stimulus (a cue from an internal or external event).

10-B. Because the behavior (exercise) is increased to avoid something negative (insulin injections), this is an example of negative reinforcement. Both negative and positive reinforcement increase behavior. Punishment decreases behavior. Shaping involves rewarding closer and closer approximations of the wanted behavior until the correct behavior is achieved. In classical conditioning, a natural, or reflexive response (behavior) is elicited by a learned stimulus (a cue from an internal or external event).

11-A. The painful blood withdrawal procedure is the unconditioned stimulus.

12-C. The antiseptic odor in the clinic has become associated with the painful procedure and elicits the same response. It is therefore the conditioned stimulus.

13-D. The conditioned response, which is crying in response to the smell of the antiseptic, has been learned.

14-B. Because crying in response to the pain of an injection is automatic and does not have to be learned, it is the unconditioned response.

8

Clinical Assessment of Intelligence, Personality, and Achievement

Typical Board Question

A child in the fifth grade is functioning mentally at the level of a child in the first grade. What category of intellectual function best describes this child?

(A) Severely retarded
(B) Moderately retarded
(C) Mildly retarded
(D) Borderline
(E) Normal

(See "Answers and Explanations" at end of Chapter)

I. Overview of Psychological Tests

A. Types of tests

1. Psychological tests are used to assess intelligence, achievement, personality, and psychopathology.
2. These tests are classified by functional area and by whether information is gathered objectively or projectively.

B. Objective versus projective tests

1. An objective test is based on questions that are **easily scored** and statistically analyzed.
2. A projective test requires the subject to **interpret the questions**. Responses are assumed to be based on the subject's motivational state and defense mechanisms.

C. Individual versus group testing

1. Tests administered to one individual at a time allow careful observation and evaluation of that particular person; a **test battery** looks at functioning of an individual in a number of different functional areas.

2. Tests given to a group of people simultaneously have the advantages of efficient administration, grading and statistical analysis.

II. Intelligence Tests

A. Intelligence and mental age

1. Intelligence is defined as the ability to understand abstract concepts; reason; assimilate, recall, analyze, and organize information; and meet the special needs of new situations.

2. **Mental age (MA),** as defined by Alfred Binet, reflects a person's level of intellectual functioning. **Chronological age (CA)** is the person's actual age in years.

B. Intelligence quotient (IQ)

1. IQ is the ratio of MA to CA times 100: **MA/CA × 100 = IQ.** An IQ of **100** means that the person's mental and chronological ages are equivalent.

2. The highest CA used to determine IQ is 15 years.

3. IQ is determined to a large extent by genetics. However, **poor nutrition** and illness during development can negatively affect IQ.

4. IQ is relatively stable throughout life. In the absence of brain pathology, an individual's **IQ is essentially the same in old age as in childhood.**

5. The results of IQ tests are influenced by a person's cultural background and emotional response to testing situations.

C. Normal intelligence

1. As stated above, an IQ of 100 means that the MA and CA are approximately the same. **Normal, or average, IQ is in the range of 90–109.**

2. The standard deviation (see Chapter 26) in IQ scores is 15. A person with an IQ that is more than two standard deviations below the mean (IQ < 70) is usually considered mentally retarded (see Chapter 2). DSM-IV **classifications of mental retardation** (the overlap or gap in categories is related to differences in testing instruments) are:

   a. Mild (IQ 50–70)

   b. Moderate (IQ 35–55)

   c. Severe (IQ 20–40)

   d. Profound (IQ <20)

3. A score between **71 and 84** indicates **borderline** intellectual functioning.

4. A person with an IQ more than two standard deviations above the mean (IQ >130) has very superior intelligence.

D. Wechsler intelligence tests

1. The Wechsler Adult Intelligence Scale-Revised (WAIS-R) is the most commonly used IQ test.

2. The WAIS-R has 11 subtests: 6 verbal and 5 performance. The subtests evaluate general information, comprehension, similarities, arithmetic, vocabulary, picture assembly, picture completion, block design, object assembly, digit span, and digit symbol.

3. The Wechsler Intelligence Scale for Children-Revised **(WISC-R)** is used to test intelligence in children **6–16½** years of age.

4. The Wechsler Preschool and Primary Scale of Intelligence **(WPPSI)** is used to test intelligence in children **4–6½** years of age.

E. Related tests
—The **Vineland Social Maturity Scale** is used to evaluate skills for daily living in mentally retarded (see Chapter 2) and other challenged people (e.g., those with impaired vision or hearing).

III. Achievement Tests

A. Uses

1. Achievement tests evaluate how well an individual has mastered **specific subject areas** such as reading and mathematics.

2. These tests are used for evaluation and career counseling in schools and industry.

B. Specific achievement tests

1. The Wide-Range Achievement Test **(WRAT),** which is often used clinically, evaluates arithmetic, reading, and spelling skills.

2. Achievement tests often used by school systems include the California, Iowa, Stanford, and Peabody Achievement Tests.

IV. Personality Tests

A. Personality tests are used to evaluate psychopathology and personality characteristics.

B. Commonly used personality tests are described in Table 8-1.

V. Psychiatric Evaluation of the Patient with Emotional Symptoms

A. Psychiatric history
—The patient's psychiatric history is taken as part of the medical history. The psychiatric history includes questions about mental illness, drug and alcohol use, sexual activity, current living situation, and sources of stress.

B. The mental status examination and related instruments

1. The mental status examination evaluates an individual's current state of mental functioning (Table 8-2).

2. The **Folstein Mini-Mental State Examination** is commonly used at the bedside to follow improvement or deterioration in function (Table 8-3).

3. Objective rating scales of depression that are commonly used include the Hamilton, Raskin, and Zung scales.

4. Terms used to describe psychophysiologic symptoms and mood in patients with psychiatric illness are listed in Table 8-4.

Table 8-1. Personality Tests

Name of test	Uses	Characteristics	Examples
Minnesota Multiphasic Personality Inventory MMPI-2	• The most commonly used objective personality test • Useful for primary care physicians because no training is required for administration and scoring	• Objective test • Patients answer 566 true (T) or false (F) questions about themselves • Clinical scales include depression, paranoia, schizophrenia and hypochondriasis • Validity scales identify trying to look ill ("faking bad") or trying to look well ("faking good")	"I avoid most social situations" (T or F) "I often feel jealous" (T or F) "I like being active" (T or F)
Rorschach Test	• The most commonly used projective personality test • Used to identify thought disorders and defense mechanisms	• Projective test • Patients are asked to interpret 10 bilaterally symmetrical ink blot designs, eg. "Describe what you see in this figure"	
Thematic Apperception Test (TAT)	• Stories are used to evaluate unconscious emotions and conflicts	• Projective test • Patients are asked to create verbal scenarios based on 30 drawings depicting ambiguous situations, (eg., "Using this picture, make up a story that has a beginning, a middle, and an end")	
Sentence Completion Test (SCT)	• Used to identify worries and problems using verbal associations	• Projective test • Patients complete sentences started by the examiner	"My mother . . ." "I wish . . ." "Most people. . . . ."

(Original source of Rorshach illustration: Kleinmuntz B: *Essentials of abnormal psychology.* New York, Harper & Row, 1974. Original source of TAT illustration: Phares EJ, Clinical psychology: Concepts, methods, and profession, 2nd edition. Homewood, IL , Dorsey, 1984. Both from Krebs D and Blackman R: *Psychology; A First Encounter.* Harcourt, Brace, Jovanovich, 1988, p. 632. Used by permission of the publisher.)

Table 8-2. Variables Evaluated on the Mental Status Examination

Variable	Patient example
General presentation: Appearance Behavior Attitude toward the interviewer	A 40-year-old male patient looks older than his age, is well-groomed and seems defensive when asked about his experiences with drugs in the past
Sensorium and cognition: Level of consciousness Orientation, memory, attention Cognitive, spatial and abstraction abilities	A 55-year-old female patient has a Glasgow coma scale score of 15 (see Table 8-4) is oriented to person, place and time, is attentive and shows normal memory (cognitive ability), understanding of three dimensional space (spatial ability) and can tell you how an apple and an orange are alike (abstraction ability)
Speech: Volume, speed, articulation Language deficiencies	A 24-year-old male patient speaks too quickly and has a poor vocabulary
Mood and affect: Described (mood) and demonstrated (affect) emotions Match of emotions with current events	A 35-year-old male patient describes feeling "low" and shows less external expression of mood than expected (depressed with a restricted affect)
Thought: Form or process of thought Thought content (e.g., delusion)	A 40-year-old female patient tells you that the Mafia is after her (delusion)
Perception: Illusion Hallucination	A 12-year-old girl tells you that the clothes in her closet look like a person is in there (illusion). She then describes hearing voices (hallucination)
Judgment and insight	A 38-year-old woman tells you that she would open a stamped letter found on the sidewalk to see if it contained money. She also says that she knows this would be dishonest (normal, insightful response)
Reliability	A 55-year-old patient correctly provides the details of his previous illnesses (a reliable patient)
Control of aggressive and sexual impulses	A 35-year-old man tells you that he often overreacts emotionally although there is little provocation (poor impulse control)

Table 8-3. Folstein Mini-Mental State Examination

Skill evaluated	Sample instructions to the patient	Maximum score*
Orientation	Tell me where you are and what day it is	10
Language	Name the object that I am holding	8
Attention and calculation	Subtract 7 from 100 and then continue to subtract 7s	5
Registration	Repeat the names of these three objects	3
Recall	After 5 minutes, recall the names of these three objects	3
Construction	Copy this design	1

*Maximum total score=30; total score <25 suggests cognitive problems; total score <20 suggests significant impairment. (Adapted from Fadem B, Simring S: *High-Yield Psychiatry.* Baltimore, Williams & Wilkins, 1998, p 9.)

Table 8-4. Psychophysiologic States

Mood
Euphoric mood: strong feelings of elation
Expansive mood: feelings of self-importance and generosity
Irritable mood: easily annoyed and quick to anger
Euthymic mood: normal mood, with no significant depression or elevation of mood
Dysphoric mood: subjectively unpleasant feeling
Anhedonic mood: inability to feel pleasure
Labile mood (mood swings): alternations between euphoric and dysphoric moods

Affect
Restricted affect: decreased display of emotional responses
Blunted affect: strongly decreased display of emotional responses
Flat affect: complete lack of emotional responses
Labile affect: sudden alterations in emotional responses not related to environmental events

Fear and Anxiety
Fear: fright caused by real danger
Anxiety: fright caused by imagined danger
Free floating anxiety: fright not associated with any specific cause

Consciousness and Attention
Normal: alert, can follow commands, normal verbal responses (Glasgow Coma Scale score of 15)
Clouding of consciousness: inability to respond normally to external events
Somnolence: abnormal sleepiness
Stupor: little or no response to environmental stimuli
Coma: total unconsciousness (Glasgow Coma Scale score of 3)

Review Test

Directions: Each of the numbered items or incomplete statements in this section is followed by answers or by completions of the statement. Select the **one** lettered answer or completion that is **best** in each case.

1. A child is tested and found to have a mental age of 12 years. The child's chronological age is 10 years. What is the IQ of this child?

(A) 40
(B) 60
(C) 80
(D) 100
(E) 120

2. A child is tested and is found to have an IQ of 90. What category of intellectual function best describes this child?

(A) Severely retarded
(B) Moderately retarded
(C) Mildly retarded
(D) Borderline
(E) Normal

3. A 29-year-old woman tells the doctor that she often hears the voice of Abraham Lincoln speaking directly to her. This woman is showing a disorder of

(A) perception
(B) insight
(C) judgment
(D) mood
(E) affect

4. A 6-year-old child has an IQ of 50. The mental ability of this child is equivalent to that of a child aged

(A) 2 years
(B) 3 years
(C) 4 years
(D) 5 years
(E) 7 years

5. A doctor is evaluating a 20-year-old female patient. Which of the following characteristics of the patient is best evaluated using the Minnesota Multiphasic Personality Inventory (MMPI)?

(A) Skills for daily living
(B) Hypochondriasis
(C) Knowledge of general information
(D) Reading comprehension
(E) Intelligence

6. A 67-year-old male stroke patient has scored 18 on the Folstein Mini-Mental State Examination. From this score, what can the doctor conclude about this patient?

(A) He has a lower than normal IQ.
(B) He cannot read.
(C) He is cognitively impaired.
(D) He is "faking bad."
(E) He is normal.

7. You examine a severely depressed 75-year-old woman. She relates to you that she feels so low that she cannot enjoy anything in her life and that even winning the state lottery would not make her feel any better. The best description of this patient's mood is:

(A) anhedonic
(B) dysphoric
(C) euthymic
(D) labile
(E) euphoric

8. For evaluating the self-care skills of a 22-year-old woman with an IQ of 60 for placement in a group home, what is the most appropriate test?

(A) Thematic Apperception Test (TAT)
(B) Minnesota Multiphasic Personality Inventory (MMPI)
(C) Wechsler Intelligence Scale for Children-Revised (WISC-R)
(D) Rorschach Test
(E) Vineland Social Maturity Scale
(F) Wide Range Achievement Test (WRAT)
(G) Folstein Mini-Mental State Examination
(H) Glasgow Coma Scale

9. For determining, using bilaterally symmetrical ink blots, which defense mechanisms are used by a 25-year-old woman, what is the most appropriate test?

(A) Thematic Apperception Test (TAT)
(B) Minnesota Multiphasic Personality Inventory (MMPI)
(C) Wechsler Intelligence Scale for Children-Revised (WISC-R)
(D) Rorschach Test
(E) Vineland Social Maturity Scale
(F) Wide Range Achievement Test (WRAT)
(G) Folstein Mini-Mental State Examination
(H) Glasgow Coma Scale

10. For evaluating, by a primary care physician, depression in a 54-year-old male patient, what is the most appropriate test?

(A) Thematic Apperception Test (TAT)
(B) Minnesota Multiphasic Personality Inventory (MMPI)
(C) Wechsler Intelligence Scale for Children-Revised (WISC-R)
(D) Rorschach Test
(E) Vineland Social Maturity Scale
(F) Wide Range Achievement Test (WRAT)
(G) Folstein Mini-Mental State Examination
(H) Glasgow Coma Scale

11. For following, using a bedside test, deterioration or improvement in function in a 75-year-old patient with suspected dementia, what is the most appropriate test?

(A) Thematic Apperception Test (TAT)
(B) Minnesota Multiphasic Personality Inventory (MMPI)
(C) Wechsler Intelligence Scale for Children-Revised (WISC-R)
(D) Rorschach Test
(E) Vineland Social Maturity Scale
(F) Wide Range Achievement Test (WRAT)
(G) Folstein Mini-Mental State Examination
(H) Glasgow Coma Scale

Answers and Explanations

TBQ-C. In the United States, a child in the fifth grade is approximately 10 years of age while a child in the first grade is approximately 6 years of age. Thus, the IQ of this child is 6 years (mental age) over 10 years (chronological age) = 60 (IQ). Individuals with IQs of 60 are classified as mildly mentally retarded.

1-E. Using the formula 12 years (mental age) over 10 years (chronological age) × 100, the IQ of this child is 120.

2-E. An individual with an IQ of 90 is classified as having normal intellectual function (IQ 90–109).

3-A. This 29-year-old woman who believes that she hears the voice of Abraham Lincoln is showing an auditory hallucination which is a disorder of perception. Disorders of judgment and insight and of mood and affect are other categories of disorders.

4-B. The mental ability of a 6-year-old child with an IQ of 50 is 3 years. This is calculated using the IQ formula: IQ = MA/CA × 100, i.e. 50 = x/6 × 100: x=3.

5-B. Clinical scales of the Minnesota Multiphasic Personality Inventory (MMPI) evaluate hypochondriasis as well as depression, paranoia, and schizophrenia. Intelligence, including general information and reading comprehension, can be tested using the Wechsler Adult Intelligence Scale-Revised (WAIS-R).

6-C. The Folstein Mini-Mental State Examination is used to evaluate a person's current state of mental functioning. The total maximum score on this exam is 30. A total score <25 suggests some cognitive problems while a total score <20 indicates significant impairment. Therefore, with a score of 18, you can conclude that this 67-year-old male stroke patient is cognitively impaired. This test does not evaluate IQ, reading skills, or whether the patient is making believe he is in worse condition than he appears (i.e., "faking bad").

7-A. This severely depressed 75-year-old woman is showing anhedonia, the inability to feel pleasure, a characteristic of severe depression. Euphoric mood is an elated mood while euthymic mood is a normal mood, with no significant depression or elevation. Dysphoric mood is a subjectively unpleasant feeling. Labile moods (mood swings) are alterations between euphoric and dysthymic moods.

8-E. The Vineland Social Maturity Scale is the most appropriate test for evaluating the self-care skills of a 22-year-old woman with an IQ of 60 for placement in a group home.

9-D. The Rorschach Test, which utilizes bilaterally symmetrical ink blots, is the most appropriate test to determine which defense mechanisms are used by a 25-year-old woman.

10-B. The Minnesota Multiphasic Personality Inventory (MMPI) is the most appropriate test for use by a primary care physician to evaluate depression in a 54-year-old male patient since it is an objective test and no special training is required for administration and scoring.

11-G. The Folstein Mini-Mental State Examination is the most appropriate test to be used at the bedside to follow deterioration or improvement in function in patients with suspected neurological problems such as dementia.

9

Substance Abuse

Typical Board Question

Three days after admission to the hospital for a fractured hip due to a fall, a 63-year-old woman begins to show an intense hand tremor and tachycardia. She tells you that she has started to see spiders crawling on the walls and that she can feel them crawling on her arms. Of the following, what is the most likely cause of this picture?

(A) Alcohol use
(B) Alcohol withdrawal
(C) Heroin use
(D) Heroin withdrawal
(E) Amphetamine withdrawal

See "Answers and Explanations" at end of Chapter

I. Substance Abuse, Dependence, Withdrawal, Tolerance, and Demographics

A. Definitions

1. Substance **abuse** is a pattern of abnormal substance use that leads to impairment of occupational, physical, or social functioning.

2. Substance **dependence** is substance abuse plus withdrawal symptoms, tolerance, or a pattern of repetitive use.

   a. **Withdrawal** is the development of physical or psychological symptoms after the reduction or cessation of intake of a substance.

   b. **Tolerance** is the need for increased amounts of the substance to achieve the same positive psychological effect.

   c. **Cross-tolerance** is the development of tolerance to one substance as the result of using another substance.

B. Epidemiology and Demographics

1. Caffeine, alcohol, nicotine, marijuana and, to a lesser extent, cocaine, amphetamines, and heroin, are the most commonly used and abused substances in the United States (Table 9-1).

Table 9-1. Epidemiology of Commonly Used Psychoactive Substances

Substance	Percentage of Population that Used Substance		Comments
	In Last Year	**In Lifetime**	
Caffeine	75%	80%	• Used more commonly than any other psychoactive substance
Alcohol	50%	85%	• 10%–13% lifetime prevalence of abuse or dependence • The male:female ratio of abusers is at least 2:1 • Higher rate of use occurs in Native Americans and Eskimos, the 21–34-year-old age group, and residents of the Northeastern states • The lowest rate of use occurs in Utah because the Mormon religion prohibits alcohol use
Nicotine	30%	55%	• Use has increased in women (female smokers outnumber male smokers), adolescents, and African-American adults • In adolescents, use among African-Americans is lower than in whites
Marijuana	10%	33%	• Used more commonly than any other illegal psychoactive drug • Use has increased recently in the 12–25-year-old age group
Cocaine	3%	12%	• Used primarily by people in lower socioeconomic groups in its inexpensive crack form • Used by people in higher socioeconomic groups in its expensive, pure form • Use has declined after peaking in 1985
Amphetamine	1.3%	7%	• Higher rate of use in professionals, people who work late at night (e.g., musicians, students), and 18- to 25-year-olds
Heroin	0.2%	1.3%	• Higher rate of use among people living in large cities • The male:female ratio of users is 3:1

2. The use of illegal substances is more common among young adults **(18–25 years of age)** and is three times **more common in males.**

3. **Classes of abused substances** include stimulants, sedatives, opioids, and hallucinogens.

II. Stimulants

A. Overview

1. **Stimulants** are central nervous system activators that include caffeine, nicotine, amphetamines and cocaine.

2. The effects of use and withdrawal of these substances can be found in **Table 9-2.**

Table 9-2. Effects of Use and Withdrawal of Stimulant Drugs

Substances	Effects of Use	Effects of Withdrawal
	Psychological	
Caffeine Nicotine	• Increased alertness & attention span • Mild improvement in mood • Agitation and insomnia	• Lethargy • Mild depression of mood
	Physical	
	• Decreased appetite • Increased blood pressure and heart rate (tachycardia) • Increased gastrointestinal activity	• Increased appetite with slight weight gain • Fatigue • Headache
	Psychological	
Amphetamines Cocaine	• Significant elevation of mood (lasting only 1 hour with cocaine) • Increased attention span • Aggressiveness, impaired judgment • Psychotic symptoms (e.g., paranoid delusions with amphetamines and formication with cocaine)	• Significant depression of mood • Strong psychological craving (peaking a few days after the last dose) • Irritability
	Physical	
	• Loss of appetite and weight • Agitation and insomnia • Pupil dilation • Increased energy • Tachycardia & other cardiovascular effects which can be life-threatening • Seizures (particularly with cocaine) • Hypersexuality	• Hunger (particularly with amphetamines) • Pupil constriction • Fatigue

B. Caffeine is found in coffee (125 mg/cup), tea (65 mg/cup), cola (40 mg/cup), nonprescription stimulants, and diet agents.

C. Nicotine is a toxic substance present in tobacco. Cigarette smoking decreases life expectancy more than the use of any other substance.

D. Amphetamines are used clinically and are also drugs of abuse.

    1. They are medically indicated in the treatment of attention-deficit hyperactivity disorder **(ADHD)** (see Chapter 14) and **narcolepsy** (see Chapter 10). They are sometimes used to treat **depression** in the elderly and terminally ill, and depression and obesity in patients who do not respond to other treatments (see Chapter 12).

    2. The most common clinically used amphetamines are **dextroamphetamine** (Dexedrine), **methamphetamine** (Desoxyn), and a related compound, **methylphenidate** (Ritalin).

    3. **"Speed"**, **"ice"** (methamphetamine), and **"ecstasy"** [methylene dioxymethamphetamine (MDMA)] are street names for amphetamine compounds.

E. Cocaine

    1. **"Crack"** and **"freebase"** are smokable forms of **cocaine;** in pure form cocaine is sniffed into the nostrils **("snorted").**

    2. **Hyperactivity** and **growth retardation** are seen in **newborns** of mothers who used cocaine during pregnancy.

    3. Tactile hallucinations of bugs crawling on the skin (formication) is seen with use of cocaine ("cocaine bugs").

F. Neurotransmitter associations

    1. Stimulant drugs work primarily by **increasing** the availability of **dopamine (DA).**

    2. Amphetamine use causes the **release of DA. Cocaine blocks the reuptake of DA.**

      —Both the release of DA and the block of DA reuptake result in increased availability of this neurotransmitter in the synapse.

    3. Increased availability of DA in the synapse is apparently involved in the euphoric effects of stimulants and opiates (the "reward" system of the brain). As in **schizophrenia** (see Chapter 11), increased DA availability may also result in **psychotic symptoms.**

III. Sedatives

A. Overview

    1. Sedatives are **central nervous system depressants** that include alcohol, barbiturates, and benzodiazepines.

    2. Sedative agents work primarily by **increasing** the activity of the inhibitory neurotransmitter γ-aminobutyric acid **(GABA).**

    3. Hospitalization of patients for withdrawal from sedatives is prudent; the withdrawal syndrome may include seizures and cardiovascular symptoms that could be life-threatening. The effects of use and withdrawal of sedatives can be found in **Table 9-3.**

B. Alcohol

    1. Acute associated problems

Table 9-3. Effects of Use and Withdrawal of Sedative Drugs

Substances	Effects of use	Effects of withdrawal
	Psychological	
Alcohol Benzodiazepines Barbiturates	• Mild elevation of mood • Decreased anxiety • Somnolence • Behavioral disinhibition	• Mild depression of mood • Increased anxiety • Insomnia • Psychotic symptoms (e.g., delusions and formication) • Disorientation
	Physical	
	• Sedation • Poor coordination • Respiratory depression	• Tremor • Seizures • Cardiovascular symptoms, such as tachycardia and hypertension

      a. Traffic accidents, homicide, suicide, and **rape,** are correlated with the concurrent use of alcohol.

      b. Child physical and **sexual abuse,** spouse abuse, and elder abuse are also associated with alcohol use.

  2. Chronic problems

      a. Thiamine deficiency resulting in **Wernicke** and **Korsakoff syndromes** (see Chapter 14) is associated with long term use of alcohol.

      b. Liver dysfunction, gastrointestinal problems (e.g., ulcers), and reduced life expectancy are also seen in heavy users of alcohol.

      c. Fetal alcohol syndrome (including facial abnormalities, reduced height and weight, and mental retardation) is seen in the offspring of women who drink during pregnancy.

      d. A childhood history of problems such as **attention-deficit hyperactivity disorder** and **conduct disorder** correlate with alcoholism in the adult.

  3. Intoxication

      a. Legal intoxication is defined as **0.08%–0.15% blood alcohol concentration,** depending on individual state laws.

      b. Coma occurs at a blood alcohol concentration of 0.40%–0.50% in nonalcoholics.

  4. Delirium tremens ("the DTs")

      a. Alcohol withdrawal delirium (also called delirium tremens or **"the DTs"**) may occur during the first week of withdrawal from alcohol (most commonly on the third day of hospitalization). It usually occurs in patients who have been drinking heavily for at least **5 years.**

      b. Delirium tremens is **life threatening;** the mortality rate is about 20%.

C. Barbiturates

  1. Barbiturates are used medically as **sleeping pills,** sedatives, antianxiety agents (tranquilizers), anticonvulsants, and anesthetics.

  2. Frequently used and abused barbiturates include amobarbital, pentobarbital, and secobarbital.

  3. Barbiturates cause respiratory depression and have a **low safety margin;** they are the drugs most commonly taken to **commit suicide.**

D. Benzodiazepines

  1. Benzodiazepines are used medically as **tranquilizers,** sedatives, muscle relaxants, anticonvulsants, and anesthetics, and **to treat alcohol withdrawal** (particularly long-acting agents like chlordiazepoxide and diazepam. (See Chapter 16).

  2. Benzodiazepines have a **high safety margin** unless taken with another sedative, such as alcohol.

IV. Opioids

A. Overview

  1. Narcotics or opioid drugs include **agents used medically as analgesics** (e.g., morphine) as well as as drugs of abuse (e.g., heroin). The effects of use and withdrawal of some opioids can be found in **Table 9-4.**

Table 9-4. Effects of Use and Withdrawal of Opioid Drugs

Substance	Effects of use	Effects of withdrawal
	Psychological	
Heroin, Methadone Other Opioids	• Elevation of mood • Relaxation • Somnolence	• Depression of mood • Anxiety • Insomnia
	Physical	
	• Sedation • Analgesia • Respiratory depression (overdose may be fatal) • Constipation • Pupil constriction	• Sweating and fever • Rhinorrhea (running nose) • Piloerection (goose bumps) • Yawning • Stomach cramps and diarrhea • Pupil dilation

  2. When compared to medically used opioids like morphine and methadone, **abused opioids** such as heroin are more potent, cross the blood-brain barrier more quickly, have a faster onset of action and have **more euphoric action.**

  3. In contrast to barbiturate withdrawal, which may be fatal, **death from withdrawal of opioids is rare** unless a serious physical illness is present.

B. Methadone

  1. Methadone and l-alpha-acetylmethodol acetate (LAMM) are **synthetic opioids** used to treat heroin addiction (see Table 9-8); both also cause physical dependence and tolerance.

  2. These legal opioids can be substituted for illegal opioids, such as heroin, to prevent withdrawal symptoms.

  3. **Advantages** over heroin
      a. Methadone and LAMM are dispensed by **federal health authorities.**
      b. They **can be taken orally.** The intravenous method of drug use employed by many heroin addicts may involve sharing contaminated needles, thus contributing to AIDS and hepatitis B infection.
      c. They have a **longer duration of action.**
      d. They cause **less euphoria and drowsiness,** allowing people on maintenance regimens to keep their jobs and avoid the criminal activity that is necessary to maintain a costly heroin habit.

V. Hallucinogens

A. Overview

  1. Hallucinogens include lysergic acid diethylamide (LSD), phencyclidine (PCP, "angel dust"), cannabis (tetrahydrocannabinol, marijuana, hashish), psilocybin (from mushrooms) and mescaline (from cactus).

  2. **Hallucinogens** promote altered states of consciousness.

  3. Increased availability of **serotonin** is associated with the effects of some of these agents (e.g., LSD). The effects of use and withdrawal of hallucinogens can be found in **Table 9-5.**

Table 9-5. Effects of Use and Withdrawal of Hallucinogenic Drugs

Substances	Effects of use	Effects of withdrawal
	Psychological	
Cannabis (marijuana, hashish) Lysergic acid diethylamide (LSD) Phencyclidine (PCP, "angel dust") Psilocybin Mescaline	• Altered perceptual states (auditory and visual hallucinations, alterations of body image, distortions of time and space) • Elevation of mood • Impairment of memory (may be long-term) • Reduced attention span • "Bad trips" (panic reactions that may include psychotic symptoms) • "Flashbacks" (a reexperience of the sensations associated with use in the absence of the drug even months after the last dose)	• Few if any psychological withdrawal symptoms
	Physical	
	• Impairment of complex motor activity • Cardiovascular symptoms • Sweating • Tremor	• Few if any physical withdrawal symptoms

B. Marijuana

   1. Tetrahydrocannabinol **(THC)** is the primary active compound found in marijuana.

   2. In low doses, marijuana **increases appetite** and relaxation and causes conjunctival reddening.

   3. Chronic users experience **lung problems** associated with smoking and a decrease in motivation **("the amotivational syndrome")** characterized by lack of desire to work and increased apathy.

   4. Although illegal in the United States, at least two states permit limited medical use to treat glaucoma and cancer-related nausea and vomiting.

C. LSD and PCP

   1. **LSD is ingested** and **PCP is smoked** in a marijuana or other cigarette.

   2. While LSD and PCP both cause altered perception, in contrast to LSD, **episodes of violent behavior** occur with **PCP use.**

   3. Emergency department findings for **PCP** include hyperthermia and **nystagmus** (vertical or horizontal abnormal eye movements).

   4. Consumption of more than 20 mg of PCP may cause convulsions, coma, and death.

VI. Clinical Features of Substance Abuse

    A. **Laboratory findings** can often confirm substance use **(Table 9-6).**

    B. **Emergency department (ED) findings.** Changes in the pupil of the eye and presence or absence of psychotic symptoms can quickly narrow the search for the substance responsible for patients' symptoms in the ED **(Table 9-7).**

VII. Treatment

    A. **Treatment of substance abuse** ranges from abstinence and peer support groups to drugs that block withdrawal symptoms **(Table 9-8).**

    B. **Dual diagnosis** or medically ill-chemically addicted (MICA) patients require treatment for both substance abuse and the comorbid psychiatric illness (e.g., major depression), often on a special unit in the hospital.

Table 9-6. Laboratory Findings for Selected Drugs of Abuse

Class of Substance	Elevated levels in body fluids (e.g., blood, urine)	Length of time after use that substance can be detected
Stimulants	• Cotinine (nicotine metabolite)	1–2 days
	• Amphetamine	1–2 days
	• Benzoylecgonine (cocaine metabolite)	1–3 days in occasional users; 7–12 days in heavy users
Sedatives	• Alcohol	Hours
	• Gamma-glutamyltransferase (GGT)	Hours
	• Specific barbiturate or benzodiazepine or its metabolites	7 days or less
Opiates	• Opiate other than methadone	0.5–1.5 hours
	• Methadone	2–3 days
Hallucinogens	• Cannabinoid metabolites	7–28 days
	• Serum glutamic-oxaloacetic transaminase (SGOT) level and creatinine phosphokinase (CPK) (with PCP use)	More than 7 days

PCP=phencyclidine

Table 9-7. Quick Emergency Department Identification of the Abused Substance

Emergency Department Observation	Seen with Use of	Seen with Withdrawal from
Pupil dilation	• Cocaine • Amphetamines • LSD	• Heroin • Methadone • Alcohol
Pupil constriction	• Heroin • Methadone	• Cocaine • Amphetamines
Psychotic symptoms (i.e., hallucinations and delusions)	• Cocaine • Amphetamines • Alcohol • Hallucinogens	• Alcohol • Benzodiazepines • Barbiturates

LSD=lysergic acid diethylamide

Table 9-8. Treatment of Substance Use and Abuse

Substance	Most effective treatment	Other treatments
Alcohol	Alcoholics Anonymous (AA) and other voluntary peer support groups (12-step programs)	• Disulfiram [Antabuse]to prevent use (causes a toxic reaction when alcohol is ingested) • Benzodiazepines for withdrawal symptoms • Thiamine (Vitamin B1) for immediate emergency room treatment
Benzodiazepines and barbiturates	Hospitalization and gradual reduction in dosage of the abused drug by substituting long-acting barbiturates (such as phenobarbital) for the more commonly abused short-acting types	• Replacement with nonaddictive antianxiety agent (i.e., buspirone [Buspar]) or sleep agent (i.e., zolpidem [Ambien])
Caffeine	Elimination from the diet and replacement with decaffeinated beverages	• Analgesics to control headache due to withdrawal
Heroin	Methadone or l-alpha-acetylmethodol acetate (LAMM) maintenance program	• Narcotics anonymous (NA) or other 12-step program • Naloxone (blocks opiate receptors) to precipitate withdrawal and to maintain abstinence • Clonidine for withdrawal symptoms
Marijuana	Abstinence	• Education
Nicotine	Peer support group (80% of abstainers relapse within 2 years and only 66% relapse when members of a peer support group; 45% of all smokers eventually stop smoking)	• Nicotine transdermal patch or chewing gum • Antidepressants (particularly bupropion [Zyban])

Review Test

Directions: Each of the numbered items or incomplete statements in this section is followed by answers or by completions of the statement. Select the **one** lettered answer or completion that is **best** in each case.

1. A 29-year-old man comes to the emergency department complaining of stomach cramps and diarrhea. He is sweating, has a fever, runny nose, and goose bumps on his skin. His pupils are dilated and he yawns frequently. Of the following, what is the most likely cause of this picture is

(A) Alcohol use
(B) Alcohol withdrawal
(C) Heroin use
(D) Heroin withdrawal
(E) Amphetamine withdrawal

2. After 20 years of smoking, a 45-year-old female patient has decided to quit. Of the following, what physical effect is most likely to be seen as a result of this patient's withdrawal from nicotine?

(A) Weight gain
(B) Euphoria
(C) Excitability
(D) Delirium tremens
(E) Long-term abstinence

3. Which of the following drugs is the one most frequently abused in the United States?

(A) Marijuana
(B) Cocaine
(C) Speed
(D) Lysergic acid diethylamide (LSD)
(E) Heroin

4. A 20-year-old female patient tells the doctor that she has little interest in going back to school or in getting a job. She also reports that she often craves snack food and has gained over 10 pounds in the last 4 months. What substance is this patient is most likely to be using?

(A) Phencyclidine (PCP)
(B) Lysergic acid diethylamide (LSD)
(C) Marijuana
(D) Cocaine
(E) Heroin

5. A 22-year-old student tells the doctor that he has been using "speed" nightly. Which of the following complaints is the patient most likely to report?

(A) Increased fatigue
(B) Decreased pain threshold
(C) Increased appetite
(D) Decreased body weight
(E) Decreased libido

6. A patient has been abusing heroin for the past year. Which of the following is most likely to characterize this patient?

(A) 16 years of age
(B) Female gender
(C) Small town resident
(D) Anxious mood when using the drug
(E) Elevated mood when using the drug

7. A person who uses illegal drugs is most likely to be in what age range?

(A) 10–15 years
(B) 15–18 years
(C) 18–25 years
(D) 25–35 years
(E) 35–45 years

8. A 35-year-old patient who has abused drugs in the past is brought to the emergency department with life-threatening cardiovascular symptoms. The drug that this patient is most likely to be withdrawing from is

(A) phencyclidine (PCP)
(B) lysergic acid diethylamide (LSD)
(C) heroin
(D) secobarbital
(E) marijuana

9. Amnestic disorder (Korsakoff syndrome) is associated with long-term use of which substance?

(A) Amphetamines
(B) Alcohol
(C) Barbiturates
(D) Cocaine
(E) Lysergic acid diethylamide (LSD)

10. A doctor discovers that his 28-year-old patient is abusing cocaine. Which of the following can he expect to see in this patient?

(A) Severe physical signs of withdrawal
(B) Little psychological craving in withdrawal
(C) Euphoria lasting 3–4 days
(D) Hallucinations
(E) Sedation with use

11. A 20-year-old man who has been drinking 8 cups of coffee a day for the past week comes in for a physical examination. At this time, this man is most likely to show

(A) tachycardia
(B) decreased peristalsis
(C) weight gain
(D) fatigue
(E) headache

12. A 40-year-old female patient who has been taking a benzodiazepine in moderate doses over the past five years, decides to stop taking the drug. When you see her two days after her last dose, she is most likely to show

(A) hypersomnia
(B) tremor
(C) lethargy
(D) respiratory depression
(E) sedation

13. A 24-year-old patient is experiencing intense hunger as well as tiredness and headache. He is most likely to be withdrawing from which of the following substances?

(A) Alcohol
(B) Amphetamines
(C) Benzodiazepines
(D) Phencyclidine (PCP)
(E) Heroin

14. In the United States, the group in which smoking currently shows the largest increase are

(A) teenaged males
(B) middle-aged males
(C) teenaged females
(D) middle-aged females
(E) elderly females

15. What is the major mechanism of action of cocaine on neurotransmitter systems in the brain?

(A) Blocks reuptake of dopamine
(B) Blocks release of dopamine
(C) Blocks reuptake of serotonin
(D) Blocks release of serotonin
(E) Blocks release of norepinephrine

16. A 32-year-old woman presents in the emergency department. She is euphoric, is speaking rapidly in an excited fashion, and her pupils are dilated. One hour later, she is in a very low mood and shows little response to your presence. Use of which substance is most likely to be responsible for these symptoms?

(A) Alcohol
(B) Secobarbital
(C) Cocaine
(D) Methylphenidate
(E) Caffeine
(F) Diazepam
(G) Heroin
(H) Marijuana
(I) Nicotine
(J) Phencyclidine (PCP)

17. A 32-year-old man is brought to a New York City hospital. He appears sedated, but shows an elevated mood. A blood test reveals the presence of HIV. What substance is most likely to be responsible for these symptoms?

(A) Alcohol
(B) Secobarbital
(C) Cocaine
(D) Methylphenidate
(E) Caffeine
(F) Diazepam
(G) Heroin
(H) Marijuana
(I) Nicotine
(J) Phencyclidine (PCP)

Answers and Explanations

TBQ-B. The most likely cause of tremor, tachycardia, and visual and tactile hallucinations (e.g., formication—the feeling of insects crawling on the skin) in this patient is alcohol withdrawal, since use of alcohol during the past few days of hospitalization is unlikely. Her fractured hip may have been sustained in a fall while intoxicated. Heroin use and heroin and amphetetamine withdrawal generally are not associated with psychotic symptoms.

1-D. The most likely cause of this patient's symptoms of sweating, stomach cramps, diarrhea, fever, runny nose, goose bumps, yawning, and dilated pupils is heroin withdrawal. While alcohol withdrawal may be associated with pupil dilation, alcohol use and withdrawal and amphetamine withdrawal are less likely to cause this constellation of symptoms.

2-A. Weight gain commonly occurs following nicotine withdrawal. Mild depression of mood and lethargy are also seen. Long term abstinence is uncommon in smokers; 80% of smokers who quit relapse within two years. Delirium tremens occurs with withdrawal from alcohol.

3-A. Marijuana is the most frequently abused illegal drug in the United States. In the population, 33% have used marijuana, 12% have used cocaine, 1.3% have used heroin and a smaller percentage have used phencyclidine (PCP) or lysergic acid diethylamide (LSD) at some time during their lives.

4-C. The amotivational syndrome and increased appetite, particularly for snack foods, are characteristic of chronic users of marijuana. Cocaine, heroin, phencyclidine (PCP), and lysergic acid diethylamide (LSD) may cause work-related problems, but are less likely to increase appetite.

5-D. Like other stimulant drugs, amphetamines like "speed" reduce appetite; use can thus result in decreased body weight. Amphetamines also decrease fatigue, increase pain threshold, and increase libido.

6-E. Heroin abusers show an elevated, relaxed mood. Abusers are most likely to be male, 26–34 years of age and live in large cities.

7-C. Illegal drug use is most common in people from 18–25 years of age.

8-D. This 35-year-old patient is most likely to be withdrawing from is secobarbital, a barbiturate. Barbiturate withdrawal is associated with life-threatening cardiovascular symptoms. There are few physical withdrawal symptoms associated with marijuana, phencyclidine (PCP), or lysergic acid diethylamide (LSD), and those associated with heroin are uncomfortable but rarely physically dangerous.

9-B. Ananestic disorder (Korsakoffs syndrome) (see Chapter 14) is associated with long-term use of alcohol.

10-D. Hallucinations and other symptoms of psychosis are seen with use of cocaine. The intense euphoria produced by cocaine lasts only up to 1 hour. Severe psychological craving for the drug peaks 2–4 days after the last dose, although there may be few physiologic signs of withdrawal. Cocaine intoxication is characterized by agitation and irritability.

11-A. Tachycardia, increased peristalsis, increased energy, and decreased appetite are physical effects of stimulants like caffeine. Headache may result from withdrawal, not use of stimulant drugs.

12-B. Withdrawal from benzodiazepines is associated with tremor, insomnia, and anxiety. Respiratory depression and sedation are associated with use of, not withdrawal from sedative drugs.

13-B. Tiredness and headache are seen with withdrawal from stimulants. While increased appetite can be seen in withdrawal from all stimulants, intense hunger is most commonly seen with withdrawal from amphetamines.

14-C. In the United States, the group in which smoking currently shows the largest increase are teenaged females.

15-A. The major mechanism of action of cocaine is to block reuptake of dopamine, thereby increasing its availability in the synapse. Increased availability of dopamine is involved in the "reward" system of the brain and the euphoric effects of stimulants.

16-C. The fact that this patient has gone from euphoric and agitated to depressed and unresponsive in only one hour and the finding of dilated pupils, indicate that she has used cocaine.

17-G. The presence of HIV as well as signs of sedation and euphoria indicate that this patient is an intravenous heroin abuser.

10

Normal Sleep and Sleep Disorders

Typical Board Question

A 22-year-old student in the middle of finals week tells her doctor that for the last 2 weeks she has been studying late into the night and has started to have trouble falling asleep. What is the doctor's most appropriate recommendation?

(A) Exercise before bedtime
(B) A large meal before bedtime
(C) A glass of milk before bedtime
(D) A fixed wake-up and bedtime schedule
(E) A short-acting benzodiazepine at bedtime

(See "Answers and Explanations" at end of Chapter)

I. Normal Sleep

A. Awake state. Beta and alpha waves characterize the electroencephalogram (EEG) of the awake individual (Table 10-1) .

1. **Beta waves** over the frontal lobes are commonly seen with **active mental concentration.**

2. **Alpha waves** over the occipital and parietal lobes are seen when a person **relaxes** with closed eyes.

B. Sleep state. During sleep, brain waves show distinctive changes (see Table 10-1).

1. Sleep is divided into **REM** (rapid eye movement) sleep and **non-REM** sleep. Non-REM sleep consists of **stages 1, 2, 3, and 4.**

2. Mapping the transitions from one stage of sleep to another during the night produces a structure known as **sleep architecture** (Figure 10-1).

   a. Sleep architecture changes with age. The elderly often have poor sleep quality because **aging** is associated with **reduced REM sleep, delta sleep (stage 3–4 or slow-wave) and total sleep time** and increased **nighttime awakenings (Table 10-2).**

   b. **Sedative agents,** such as barbiturates and, to a lesser extent, ben-

Table 10-1. Characteristics of the Awake State and of Sleep Stages

Sleep Stage	Associated EEG Pattern	% Sleep Time in Young Adults	Characteristics
Awake	Beta	–	Active mental concentration
	Alpha	–	Relaxed with eyes closed
Stage 1	Theta	5%	Lightest stage of sleep characterized by peacefulness, slowed pulse and respiration, decreased blood pressure, and episodic body movements
Stage 2	Sleep spindle and K-complex	45%	Largest percentage of sleep time
Stages 3 and 4	Delta (slow-wave sleep)	25% (decreases with age)	Deepest, most relaxed stage of sleep; sleep disorders, such as night terrors, sleepwalking (somnambulism), and bed-wetting (enuresis) may occur
Rapid eye movement (REM) sleep	"Sawtooth", beta, alpha, and theta	25% (decreases with age)	Dreaming; penile and clitoral erection; increased pulse, respiration and blood pressure; absence of skeletal muscle movement

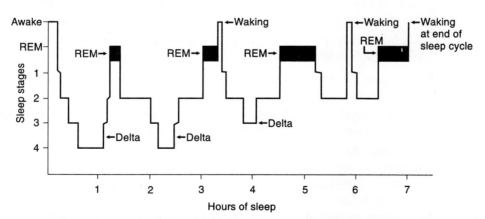

Figure 10-1. Sleep architecture in young adults. *REM* = rapid eye movement (Adapted from Wedding: *Behavior & Medicine.* St. Louis, Mosby Year Book, 1995, p. 416)

Table 10-2. Characteristics of Sleep in Depression and Aging

Sleep measure	Normal young adult patients	Depressed young adult patients	Normal elderly patients
Percentage REM	about 25%	> 25%	< 25%
REM latency	about 90 minutes	< 90 minutes	—
REM pattern	increased REM toward morning	decreased REM toward morning	—
Percentage delta	about 25%	< 25%	< 25%
Nighttime awakenings	≤ 3 per night	> 3 per night	> 3 per night

REM=rapid eye movement

zodiazepines, are associated also with **reduced REM sleep and delta sleep.**

   c. Most **delta sleep** occurs during the **first half of the sleep cycle.**

   d. **Longest REM periods** occur during the **second half of the sleep cycle.**

3. **During REM sleep, high levels of brain activity** occur.

   a. Average time to the first REM period after falling asleep **(REM latency) is 90 minutes.**

   b. REM periods of 10–40 minutes each occur about **every 90 minutes** throughout the night.

   c. A person who is deprived of REM sleep one night (e.g., because of inadequate sleep or repeated awakenings) has increased REM sleep the next night **(REM rebound).**

   d. Extended REM deprivation or total sleep deprivation may also result in the transient display of psychopathology, usually **anxiety** or psychotic symptoms.

   e. **REM** is the stage of sleep most commonly seen **just before awakening.**

C. **Neurotransmitters** are involved in the production of sleep.

   1. **Increased** levels of **acetylcholine (Ach) increase both total sleep time and REM sleep.** Acetylcholine levels, total sleep time and REM sleep decrease in normal aging as well as in Alzheimer's disease.

   2. **Increased** levels of **dopamine decrease total sleep time.** Treatment with antipsychotics, which block dopamine receptors, may improve sleep in patients with psychotic symptoms.

   3. **Increased** levels of **norepinephrine decrease both total sleep time and REM sleep.**

   4. **Increased** levels of **serotonin increase both total sleep time and delta sleep.** Damage to the dorsal raphe nuclei, which produce serotonin, decreases both of these measures.

II. Classification of Sleep Disorders

—The Diagnostic and Statistical Manual of Mental Disorders, 4th edition (DSM-IV), classifies sleep disorders in two major categories.

A. **Dyssomnias** are characterized by problems in the timing, quality, or amount of sleep. They include insomnia, hypersomnia, narcolepsy, breathing-related sleep disorder (sleep apnea), and circadian rhythm sleep disorder.

B. **Parasomnias** are characterized by abnormalities in physiology or in behavior associated with sleep. They include sleepwalking, sleep terror disorder, and nightmare disorders (see Table 10-3).

C. Insomnia, breathing-related sleep disorder, and narcolepsy are described below.

D. Other sleep disorders are described in **Table 10-3.**

III. Insomnia

A. Insomnia is **difficulty falling asleep or staying asleep** that occurs 3 times per week **for at least 1 month** and leads to sleepiness during the day

Table 10-3. Other Sleep Disorders and Their Characteristics

Sleep Disorder	Characteristics
Sleep terror disorder	• Repetitive experiences of fright in which a person (usually a child) screams in fear during sleep • The person cannot be awakened and has no memory of having a dream • Occurs during delta (slow-wave) sleep • Onset in adolescence may indicate temporal lobe epilepsy
Nightmare disorder	• Repetitive, frightening dreams that cause nighttime awakenings • The person usually can recall the nightmare • Occurs during REM sleep
Sleepwalking disorder	• Repetitive walking around during sleep • No memory of the episode • Begins in childhood (usually 4–8 years of age) • Occurs during delta (slow-wave) sleep
Circadian rhythm sleep disorder	• Delayed sleep phase type involves falling asleep and waking later than wanted • Jet lag type lasts 2–7 days after a change in time zones • Shift work type (e.g., in physician training) can result in physician error
Nocturnal myoclonus	• Repetitive, abrupt muscular contractions in the legs from toes to hips • Causes nighttime awakenings • More common in the elderly
Restless leg syndrome	• Uncomfortable sensation in the legs necessitating frequent motion • Causes difficulty falling asleep and nighttime awakenings • More common in middle age
Kleine-Levin syndrome	• Recurrent periods of hypersomnia and hyperphagia (overeating), each lasting 1–3 weeks • Rare, more common in adolescence; first attack usually at age 10–21 years
Sleep drunkenness	• Difficulty awakening fully after adequate sleep • Rare, must be differentiated from substance abuse or other sleep disorder • Associated with genetic factors
Menstrual-associated syndrome	• Hypersomnia and hyperphagia occurring only in the premenstrual period

or causes problems fulfilling social or occupational obligations. It is present in 30% of the population.

B. **Psychological causes** of insomnia include the affective and anxiety disorders.

1. **Major depressive disorder**

a. Characteristics of the **sleep pattern** in depression
1) Normal sleep onset
2) Repeated nighttime awakenings
3) **Waking too early** in the morning (terminal insomnia) is the most common sleep characteristic of depressed patients.

b. Characteristics of the **sleep stages** in depression (see Table 10-2).
(1) **Short REM latency** (appearance of REM within minutes of falling asleep)
(2) **Increased REM early in the sleep cycle** and decreased REM later in the sleep cycle (i.e., in the early morning hours) may lead to waking too early in the morning.
(3) Long first REM period and **increased total REM**
(4) **Reduced delta** sleep

2. **Bipolar disorder. Manic or hypomanic** patients have trouble falling asleep and **need less sleep.**

3. **Anxious** patients often have trouble falling asleep.

C. **Physical causes** of insomnia

1. **Use of central nervous system (CNS) stimulants** (e.g., caffeine) is the most common cause of insomnia.

2. **Withdrawal of drugs with sedating action** (e.g., alcohol, benzodiazepines, opiates) can result in wakefulness.

3. **Medical conditions** causing pain also result in insomnia, as do endocrine and metabolic disorders.

IV. Breathing-related Sleep Disorder (Sleep Apnea)

A. Patients with sleep apnea **stop breathing** for brief intervals. Low oxygen or high carbon dioxide level in the blood **awakens the patient repeatedly** during the night, resulting in **daytime sleepiness.**

1. In patients with **central sleep apnea** (more common in the elderly), little or no respiratory effort occurs, resulting in less air reaching the lungs.

2. In patients with **obstructive sleep** apnea, respiratory effort occurs, but an airway obstruction prevents air from reaching the lungs. Obstructive sleep apnea occurs most often in people 40–60 years of age, and is more common in men (8:1 male-to-female ratio) and in the obese (pickwickian syndrome). **Patients often snore.**

B. Sleep apnea occurs in **1%–10% of the population** and is related to depression, headaches, and **pulmonary hypertension.** It also may result in **sudden death** during sleep in the elderly and in infants.

V. Narcolepsy

A. Patients with narcolepsy have **sleep attacks** (i.e., fall asleep suddenly during the day) despite having a normal amount of sleep at night.

B. Narcolepsy is also characterized by

1. **Hypnagogic or hypnopompic hallucinations.** These are strange perceptual experiences which occur just as the patient falls asleep or wakes up, respectively, and occur in 20%–40% of patients.

2. **Short REM latency.**

3. **Cataplexy.** This is a sudden physical collapse caused by the loss of all muscle tone after a strong emotional stimulus, and occurs in 70% of patients.

4. **Sleep paralysis.** This is the inability to move the body for a few seconds after waking, and occurs in 30%–50% of patients.

C. Narcolepsy is uncommon, occurring most frequently in **adolescents and young adults.** There may be a **genetic component.**

VI. Treatment of Sleep Disorders

—The treatment of insomnia, breathing-related sleep disorder, and narcolepsy are described in Table 10-4.

Table 10-4. Treatment of the Major Sleep Disorders

Disorder	Treatment (in order of highest to lowest utility)
Insomnia	• Avoidance of caffeine, especially before bedtime • Development of a series of behaviors associated with bedtime (i.e., "a sleep ritual" or "sleep hygiene") • A fixed sleeping and waking schedule • Daily exercise (but not just before sleep) • Relaxation techniques • Psychoactive agents (i.e., limited use of benzodiazepines to establish an effective sleep pattern and antidepressants or antipsychotics if appropriate)
Breathing-related sleep disorder (obstructive sleep apnea)	• Weight loss • Continuous positive airway pressure (CPAP)—a device applied to the face at night to gently move air into the lungs • Uvulopalatoplasty • Tracheostomy (as a last resort)
Narcolepsy	• Stimulant drugs (e.g., methylphenidate [Ritalin]; if cataplexy is present, antidepressants may be added) • Timed daytime naps

Review Test

Directions: Each of the numbered items or incomplete statements in this section is followed by answers or by completions of the statement. Select the **one** lettered answer or completion that is **best** in each case.

1. A 45-year-old female patient reports that over the last 3 months she has lost her appetite and interest in her usual activities, and often feels hopeless and helpless. Which of the following would be most likely to characterize the sleep of this patient?

(A) Increased slow-wave sleep
(B) Lengthened REM latency
(C) Reduced percentage of REM sleep
(D) Shift in REM from the last part to the first part of the sleep cycle
(E) Short first REM period

2. During a sleep study a physician discovers that a patient shows too little REM sleep during the night. In order to increase REM sleep the physician should give the patient a medication that increases circulating levels of

(A) serotonin
(B) norepinephrine
(C) acetylcholine
(D) dopamine
(E) histamine

3. During a sleep study a male patient's electroencephalograph (EEG) shows primarily sawtooth waves. Which of the following is most likely to characterize this patient at this time?

(A) Penile erection
(B) Movement of skeletal muscles
(C) Decreased blood pressure
(D) Decreased brain oxygen use
(E) Decreased pulse

4. During a sleep study a female patient's electroencephalogram (EEG) shows primarily delta waves. Which of the following is most likely to characterize this patient at this time?

(A) Clitoral erection
(B) Paralysis of skeletal muscles
(C) Sleepwalking (somnambulism)
(D) Nightmares
(E) Increased brain oxygen use

5. An 85-year-old patient reports that he sleeps poorly. Sleep in this patient is most likely to be characterized by increased

(A) total sleep time
(B) REM sleep
(C) nighttime awakenings
(D) stage 3 sleep
(E) stage 4 sleep

6. A woman reports that most nights during the last year she has lain awake in bed for more than 2 hours before she falls asleep. The next day, she is tired and forgetful and often makes mistakes at work. Of the following, the most effective long-term treatment for this woman is

(A) continuous positive airway pressure (CPAP)
(B) an antipsychotic agent
(C) a sedative agent
(D) a stimulant agent
(E) development of a "sleep ritual"

Questions 7 and 8

A 22-year-old medical student who goes to sleep at 11:00 pm and wakes at 7:00 am falls asleep in lab every day. He tells the doctor that he sees strange images as he is falling asleep and sometimes just as he wakes up. He has had a few minor car accidents that occurred because he fell asleep while driving.

7. Of the following the most effective treatment for this student is

(A) continuous positive airway pressure (CPAP)
(B) an antipsychotic agent
(C) a sedative agent
(D) a stimulant agent
(E) development of a "sleep ritual"

8. Which of the following is this student most likely to experience?

(A) Long REM latency
(B) Auditory hallucinations
(C) Tactile hallucinations
(D) Delusions
(E) Cataplexy

Questions 9 and 10

A patient reports that he is sleepy all day despite having 8 hours of sleep each night. His wife reports that his loud snoring keeps her awake.

9. Of the following, the best treatment for this patient is

(A) continuous positive airway pressure (CPAP)
(B) an antipsychotic agent
(C) a sedative agent
(D) a stimulant agent
(E) development of a "sleep ritual"

10. Of the following, this patient is most likely to be

(A) depressed
(B) age 25 years
(C) overweight
(D) using a stimulant drug
(E) withdrawing from a sedative drug

11. Sawtooth waves are most characteristic of what sleep stage?

(A) Stage 1
(B) Stage 2
(C) Stages 3 and 4
(D) REM sleep

12. Sleep spindles and K-complexes are most characteristic of what sleep stage?

(A) Stage 1
(B) Stage 2
(C) Stages 3 and 4
(D) REM sleep

13. Theta waves are most characteristic of what sleep stage?

(A) Stage 1
(B) Stage 2
(C) Stages 3 and 4
(D) REM sleep

14. What sleep stage takes up the largest percentage of sleep time in young adults?

(A) Stage 1
(B) Stage 2
(C) Stages 3 and 4
(D) REM sleep

15. Bedwetting is characteristic of what sleep stage?

(A) Stage 1
(B) Stage 2
(C) Stages 3 and 4
(D) REM sleep

16. A 5-year-old child often screams during the night. His parents cannot awaken him and he has no memory of these experiences in the morning. Which of the following sleep disorders best matches this picture?

(A) Kleine-Levin syndrome
(B) Nightmare disorder
(C) Sleep terror disorder
(D) Sleep drunkenness
(E) Circadian rhythm sleep disorder
(F) Nocturnal myoclonus
(G) Restless leg syndrome

17. Another 5-year-old child often screams during the night. Although he seems upset, he relates to his parents the details of his frightening dreams. Which of the following sleep disorders best matches this picture?

(A) Kleine-Levin syndrome
(B) Nightmare disorder
(C) Sleep terror disorder
(D) Sleep drunkenness
(E) Circadian rhythm sleep disorder
(F) Nocturnal myoclonus
(G) Restless leg syndrome

18. The mother of a 13-year-old boy reports that he has "bouts" of overeating and of oversleeping each lasting about 2 weeks. Which of the following sleep disorders best matches this picture?

(A) Kleine-Levin syndrome
(B) Nightmare disorder
(C) Sleep terror disorder
(D) Sleep drunkenness
(E) Circadian rhythm sleep disorder
(F) Nocturnal myoclonus
(G) Restless leg syndrome

Answers and Explanations

TBQ-D. The most appropriate intervention for this 22-year-old student who is having temporary problems with sleep during finals week is to recommend a fixed wake-up and bedtime schedule. Benzodiazepines are not appropriate because of their high abuse potential and possibility of causing daytime sedation in this student during examinations. These agents also decrease sleep quality by reducing REM and delta sleep. Exercise should be done early in the day; if done before bedtime it can be stimulating and cause wakefulness. A large meal before bedtime is more likely to interfere with sleep than to help sleep. While many lay people believe that milk helps induce sleep, this effect has never been proven scientifically.

1-D. This woman is likely to be suffering from a major depressive episode (see Chapter 12). Major depression is associated with a shift in REM from the last to the first part of the sleep cycle, reduced slow wave sleep, shortened REM latency, greater percentage of REM, and long first REM period.

2-C. Acetylcholine (ACh) is involved in both increasing REM sleep and increasing total sleep time. Increased levels of dopamine decrease total sleep time. Increased levels of norepinephrine decrease both total sleep time and REM sleep while increased levels of serotonin increase both total sleep time and delta (slow-wave) sleep.

3-A. Sawtooth waves characterize REM sleep which also is associated with penile erection; dreaming; increased pulse, respiration, and blood pressure; and paralysis of skeletal muscles.

4-C. Delta waves characterize sleep stages 3 and 4 (slow-wave sleep) which also is associated with somnambulism, night terrors, episodic body movements, and enuresis. Delta sleep is the deepest, most relaxed stage of sleep. Clitoral erection, paralysis of skeletal muscles, nightmares, and increased brain oxygen use occur during REM sleep.

5-C. Sleep in the elderly is characterized by increased nighttime awakenings, decreased REM sleep, decreased delta sleep (stages 3 and 4), and decreased total sleep time.

6-E. The most effective long-term treatment for this woman with insomnia is the development of a series of behaviors associated with bedtime (i.e., a "sleep ritual"). By the process of classical conditioning (see Chapter 7) the sleep ritual then becomes associated with going to sleep. Sleep rituals can include things like taking a warm bath, pulling down the blinds and listening to soothing music. Continuous positive airway pressure is used to treat sleep apnea, stimulant drugs are used to treat narcolepsy, and antipsychotics are used to treat psychotic symptoms. Sedative drugs have a high abuse potential and, because they tend to reduce REM and delta sleep, their use may result in sleep of poorer quality.

7-D, 8-E. This medical student who falls asleep in lab every day despite a normal amount of sleep at night is probably suffering from narcolepsy. Of the listed choices, the most effective treatment for narcolepsy is the administration of stimulant drugs such as dextroamphetamine. Sedative drugs are not particularly useful for narcolepsy. In narcolepsy, short REM latency, sleep paralysis, and cataplexy occur. The student's strange perceptual experiences as he is falling asleep and waking up are hypnogogic and hypnopompic hallucinations.

9-A , 10-C. This man who snores and reports that he is sleepy all day despite having 8 hours of sleep each night is probably suffering from obstructive sleep apnea. Of the listed choices, the best treatment for this patient is continuous positive airway pressure (CPAP). Since obesity is associated with obstructive sleep apnea, other treatments for this patient would include weight loss. Use of stimulants and withdrawal from sedatives are associated with wakefulness rather than the daytime sleepiness seen here. Also, most sleep apnea patients are middle aged (age 40–60 years). Although depression and anxiety are associated with sleep problems, this man's snoring indicates that his sleep problem is more likely to have a physical cause.

11-D. Sawtooth waves are seen primarily in REM sleep.

12-B. Sleep spindles and K-complexes are seen primarily in stage 2 sleep.

13-A. Theta waves are seen primarily in stage 1 sleep.

14-B. In young adults, 45% of total sleep time is spent in stage 2 sleep. Five percent is spent in stage 1, 25% in REM and 25% in delta sleep.

15-C. Bedwetting occurs in stage 3-4 (delta) sleep.

16-C. This child is experiencing sleep terrors which occur in delta sleep and are characterized by screaming during the night and the inability to be awakened or to remember these experiences in the morning.

17-B. This child is experiencing nightmare disorder which occurs during REM sleep. In contrast to the child with sleep terror disorder, this child wakes up and can relate the nature of his frightening dreams.

18-A. The fact that patient is an adolescent, as well as the recurrent periods of hypersomnia and hyperphagia each lasting 1–3 weeks, indicate that this patient is suffering from Kleine-Levin syndrome.

11

Schizophrenia and Other Psychotic Disorders

*Typical **B**oard **Q**uestion*

A 26-year-old medical student is brought to the emergency department by her husband. The husband tells the doctor that his wife, who has been studying for final examinations, has shown odd behavior over the past two weeks. In particular, she told him that people are trying to poison her. The wife has no prior history of psychiatric disorder. What is the most appropriate diagnosis for this patient?

(A) Schizophrenia
(B) Schizoaffective disorder
(C) Schizophreniform disorder
(D) Brief psychotic disorder
(E) Delusional disorder
(F) Shared delusional disorder

(See "Answers and Explanations" at end of Chapter)

I. Schizophrenia

A. Overview

1. Schizophrenia is a **chronic** (lasting at least 6 months), **debilitating mental disorder** that is characterized by periods of loss of touch with reality (psychosis), persistent disturbances of thought, behavior, appearance and speech, abnormal affect, and social withdrawal.

2. Peak age of **onset** of schizophrenia is **15–25 years of age for men and 25–35 years of age for women.**

3. Schizophrenia occurs **equally in men and women** and equally in **all cultures and ethnic groups** studied.

4. The patient shows intact memory capacity and **is oriented to person, place,** and **time.**

B. Symptoms of schizophrenia can be classified as **positive** or **negative.**

1. **Positive symptoms** are things **additional to expected behavior** and include delusions, hallucinations, agitation, and talkativeness.

2. **Negative symptoms** are things **missing from expected behavior** and include lack of motivation, social withdrawal, flattened affect, cognitive disturbances, poor grooming, and poor speech content.

3. These classifications can be useful in predicting the effects of antipsychotic medication.

   a. **Positive symptoms** respond well to most **traditional antipsychotic agents.**

   b. **Negative symptoms** respond better to **atypical** than to traditional antipsychotics (see Chapter 16).

C. **Course.** Schizophrenia has **3 phases:** prodromal, psychotic, and residual.

1. **Prodromal** signs and symptoms occur prior to the first psychotic episode and include avoidance of social activities, physical complaints, and new interest in religion, the occult, or philosophy.

2. In the **psychotic phase,** the patient loses touch with reality. Disorders of perception, thought content, thought processes, and form of thought (Table 11-1) occur during an acute psychotic episode.

3. In the **residual phase** (time period between psychotic episodes), **the patient is in touch with reality** but does not behave normally. Residual

Table 11-1. Symptoms of Psychosis: Disorders of Perception, Thought Content, Thought Processes, and Form of Thought

Disorder of	Symptom	Definition	Example
Perception	Illusion	Misperception of real external stimuli	Interpreting the appearance of a coat in a dark closet as a man
	Hallucination	False sensory perception	Hearing voices when alone in a room
Thought content	Delusion	False belief not shared by others	The feeling of being followed by the FBI
	Idea of reference	False belief of being referred to by others	The feeling of being discussed by someone on television
Thought processes	Impaired abstraction ability	Problems discerning the essential qualities of objects or relationships	When asked what brought her to the emergency room, the patient says "an ambulance"
	Neologisms	Inventing new words	The patient refers to her doctor as the "medocrat"
Form of thought	Loose associations	Shift of ideas from one subject to another in an unrelated way	The patient begins to answer a question about her health and then shifts to a statement about baseball
	Tangentiality	Getting further away from the point as speaking continues	The patient begins to answer a question about her own health and ends up talking about her sister's abortion

signs and symptoms include social withdrawal, flat or inappropriate affect, and peculiar thinking.

D. Prognosis

1. Schizophrenia usually involves repeated psychotic episodes and a **chronic, downhill course** over years. The illness often stabilizes in midlife.

2. **Suicide is common** in patients with schizophrenia. More than 50% attempt suicide (often during post-psychotic depression or when having hallucinations "commanding" them to harm themselves), and 10% of those die in the attempt.

3. The **prognosis is better** and the **suicide risk is lower** if the patient is older at onset of illness, is married, has social relationships, is female, has a good employment history, has mood symptoms, has positive symptoms, and has few relapses.

E. Etiology. While the etiology of schizophrenia is not known, certain factors have been implicated in its development.

1. **Genetic factors**

   a. Schizophrenia **occurs in 1% of the population.** Persons with a **close genetic relationship** to a patient with schizophrenia are more likely than those with a more distant relationship to develop the disorder (Table 11-2).

   b. In some studies, markers on **chromosome 6, 8 and 13** have been associated with schizophrenia.

2. **Other factors**

   a. The **season of birth** is related to the incidence of schizophrenia. More people with schizophrenia are **born during cold weather months** (i.e., January through April in the northern hemisphere and July through September in the southern hemisphere). One possible explanation for this finding is **viral infection of the mother** during the second trimester of pregnancy, since infections occur seasonally.

   b. **No social or environmental factor causes schizophrenia.** However, because patients with schizophrenia tend to drift down the socioeconomic scale as a result of their social deficits (the **"downward drift" hypothesis**), they are often found in lower socioeconomic groups (e.g., homeless people).

F. Neural pathology

1. **Anatomy**

   a. **Abnormalities of the frontal lobes,** as evidenced by decreased use of glucose in the frontal lobes on positron emission tomography (PET) scans are seen in the brains of schizophrenics.

   b. **Lateral and third ventricle enlargement,** abnormal cerebral symmetry, and changes in brain density also may be present.

Table 11-2. The Genetics of Schizophrenia

Group	Approxiamte occurrence (%)
The general population	1%
Child who has one schizophrenic parent or sibling (or dizygotic twin)	12%
Child who has two schizophrenic parents	40%
Monozygotic twin of a schizophrenic person	50%

2. Neurotransmitter and other abnormalities

a. The dopamine hypothesis of schizophrenia states that schizophrenia results from **excessive dopaminergic activity** (e.g., excessive number of dopamine receptors, excessive concentration of dopamine, hypersensitivity of receptors to dopamine). As evidence for this hypothesis, stimulant drugs which increase dopamine availability (e.g., amphetamines and cocaine) can cause psychotic symptoms (see Chapter 9). Laboratory tests may show **elevated levels of homovanillic acid (HVA),** a metabolite of dopamine, in the body fluids of patients with schizophrenia (see Chapter 4).

b. Serotonin hyperactivity is implicated in schizophrenia because hallucinogens that increase serotonin levels cause psychotic symptoms and because some new, effective antipsychotics like clozapine (see Chapter 16) have anti-serotonergic-2 (5-HT_2) activity.

c. Eye movements are abnormal (e.g., poor smooth visual pursuit) in 50%–80% of schizophrenic patients and their relatives.

F. Subtypes. The **Diagnostic and Statistical Manual of Mental Disorders,** 4th edition **(DSM-IV),** lists five subtypes of schizophrenia (Table 11-3).

G. Differential Diagnosis

1. **Medical illnesses** that can cause psychotic symptoms and thus mimic schizophrenia (i.e., psychotic disorder caused by a general medical condition) include neurologic infection, neoplasm, trauma, disease (e.g., Huntington's disease, multiple sclerosis), temporal lobe epilepsy, and endocrine disorders (e.g., Cushing's syndrome, acute intermittent porphyria).

2. **Medications** that can cause psychotic symptoms include analgesics, antibiotics, anticholinergics, antihistamines, antineoplastics, cardiac glycosides (e.g., digitalis), and steroid hormones.

3. **Psychiatric illnesses** other than schizophrenia that may be associated with psychotic symptoms include:

   a. Other psychotic disorders (see below)

   b. The manic phase of bipolar disorder (see Chapter 12)

Table 11-3. DSM-IV Subtypes of Schizophrenia

Subtype	Characteristics
Disorganized	• Poor grooming and disheveled personal appearance, • Inappropriate emotional responses, disinhibition • Onset before 25 years of age
Catatonic	• Stupor or agitation, lack of coherent speech • Bizarre posturing (waxy flexibility) • Rare since the introduction of antipsychotic agents
Paranoid	• Delusions of persecution • Better functioning and older age at onset than other subtypes
Undifferentiated	• Characteristics of more than one subtype
Residual	• One previous schizophrenic episode • Subsequent residual symptoms but no psychotic symptoms

      c. Cognitive disorders (e.g., delirium, dementia, and amnestic disorder) (see Chapter 14).

      d. Substance-related disorders (see Chapter 10).

H. Treatment

    1. Pharmacologic treatments are the first line of treatment for schizophrenia and include traditional antipsychotics [dopamine-2 (D_2)-receptor antagonists] and atypical antipsychotic agents (see Chapter 16).

    2. Psychological treatments, including individual, family, and group psychotherapy (see Chapter 17), are useful to **provide long-term support** and to foster **compliance** with the drug regimen.

II. Other Psychotic Disorders

  A. Overview. Psychotic disorders are all characterized at some point during their course by a loss of touch with reality. However, the other psychotic disorders do **not include all of the criteria** required for the diagnosis of schizophrenia.

  B. Other psychotic disorders include (Table 11-4):

    1. Brief psychotic disorder

    2. Schizophreniform disorder

    3. Schizoaffective disorder

    4. Delusional disorder

    5. Shared psychotic disorder (folie à deux)

Table 11-4. Schizophrenia and Other Psychotic Disorders

Disorder	Characteristics	Prognosis
Schizophrenia	Psychotic and residual symptoms lasting >6 months	Lifelong social and occupational impairment
Brief psychotic disorder	Psychotic symptoms lasting >1 day, but <1 month; often precipitating psychosocial factors	50%–80% recover completely
Schizophreniform disorder	Psychotic and residual symptoms lasting 1–6 months	33% recover completely
Schizoaffective disorder	Symptoms of a mood disorder as well as psychotic symptoms	Lifelong social and occupational impairment (somewhat higher overall level of functioning than schizophrenia)
Delusional disorder	Fixed, persistent, nonbizarre delusional system [paranoid in the persecutory type and romantic (often with a famous person) in the erotomanic type]; few if any other thought disorders	50% recover completely; many have relatively normal social and occupational functioning
Shared delusional disorder (folie à deux)	Development of delusions in a person in a close relationship (e.g., spouse, child) with someone with delusional disorder (the inducer)	10%–40% recover completely when separated from the inducer

Review Test

Directions: Each of the numbered items or incomplete statements in this section is followed by answers or by completions of the statement. Select the **one** lettered answer or completion that is **best** in each case.

Questions 1–3

A 28-year-old man who lives in a group home says that his roommates are spying on him by listening to him through the television set. For this reason, he has changed roommates a number of times over the last 5 years. He dresses strangely, shows poor grooming, and seems preoccupied. He reports that has trouble paying attention to the doctor's questions because "I am listening to Abraham Lincoln talking to me in my head."

1. Neuropsychological evaluation of this patient is most likely to reveal

(A) memory impairment
(B) lack of orientation to person
(C) mental retardation
(D) frontal lobe dysfunction
(E) lack of orientation to place

2. Hearing the voice of Abraham Lincoln is an example of

(A) an illusion
(B) a neologism
(C) a hallucination
(D) a delusion
(E) an idea of reference

3. Analysis of neurotransmitter availability in the brain of this patient is most likely to reveal

(A) increased dopamine
(B) decreased dopamine
(C) increased acetylcholine
(D) decreased acetylcholine
(E) decreased serotonin

4. A 27-year-old schizophrenic patient shows extreme psychomotor agitation to the point of physical exhaustion. At times, he holds unusual uncomfortable-looking body positions. This patient is most likely to be suffering from which of the following subtypes of schizophrenia?

(A) Catatonic
(B) Disorganized
(C) Paranoid
(D) Residual
(E) Undifferentiated

Questions 5–6

A 36-year-old schizophrenic patient tells you that the government has been listening in on all of his phone conversations for the past year.

5. This symptom indicates that the patient is most likely to be suffering from which of the following types of schizophrenia?

(A) Catatonic
(B) Disorganized
(C) Paranoid
(D) Residual
(E) Undifferentiated

6. This belief is an example of a disorder of

(A) thought processes
(B) thought content
(C) form of thought
(D) perception
(E) affect

7. Which of the following symptoms of schizophrenia will respond best to traditional antipsychotic medication?

(A) Delusions
(B) Flattening of affect
(C) Poor speech content
(D) Lack of motivation
(E) Social withdrawal

8. Which of the following symptoms of schizophrenia will respond best to atypical antipsychotic medication?

(A) Hallucinations
(B) Delusions
(C) Agitation
(D) Talkativeness
(E) Social withdrawal

9. A 20-year-old woman tells you that sometimes she become frightened when her room is dark because her computer looks like a lion lurking in the corner. This is an example of

(A) an illusion
(B) a neologism
(C) a hallucination
(D) a delusion
(E) an idea of reference

10. A 53-year-old hospitalized schizophrenic patient tells you that a newscaster was talking about her when he said on television "A woman was found shoplifting today". This patient's statement is an example of

(A) an illusion
(B) a neologism
(C) a hallucination
(D) a flight of ideas
(E) an idea of reference

11. A 20-year-old man reports that he just found out that his mother (whom he believed had died when he was a child) has been in an institution for the past 15 years suffering from schizophrenia. He asks what the chances are that he will develop schizophrenia over the course of his life. The most correct answer is approximately

(A) 1%
(B) 5%
(C) 12%
(D) 50%
(E) 80%

12. A patient reports that his 19-year-old identical twin brother has just been diagnosed with schizophrenia and wants to know what the likelihood is that he will develop this disorder. The most correct answer is approximately

(A) 1%
(B) 5%
(C) 12%
(D) 50%
(E) 80%

13. The percentage of patients with schizophrenia who attempt suicide is approximately

(A) 1%
(B) 5%
(C) 12%
(D) 50%
(E) 80%

14. Which of the following is most closely associated with a good prognosis in schizophrenia?

(A) Younger age of onset
(B) Catatonic symptoms
(C) Negative symptoms
(D) Mood symptoms
(E) Many relapses

15. The most common type of hallucination seen in schizophrenia is

(A) visual
(B) gustatory
(C) auditory
(D) olfactory
(E) hypnogogic

16. A 45-year-old man with a history of severe depression and psychotic symptoms has held different jobs, but none of them for more than 6 months. He is successfully treated for his severe depressive symptoms, but he remains withdrawn and odd. What is the most appropriate diagnosis for this patient?

(A) Schizophrenia
(B) Schizoaffective disorder
(C) Schizophreniform disorder
(D) Brief psychotic disorder
(E) Delusional disorder
(F) Shared delusional disorder

17. A 68-year-old patient tells you that for the last 15 years his neighbor has been trying to get him evicted from his apartment by telling lies about him to the landlord. The patient is married and is retired from his job which he held for over 30 years. What is the most appropriate diagnosis for this patient?

(A) Schizophrenia
(B) Schizoaffective disorder
(C) Schizophreniform disorder
(D) Brief psychotic disorder
(E) Delusional disorder
(F) Shared delusional disorder

18. A 60-year-old woman whose husband believes (in the absence of any evidence) that their house is filled with radioactive dust, worries about her ability to clear the house of the dust when he is hospitalized. What is the most appropriate diagnosis for this woman?

(A) Schizophrenia
(B) Schizoaffective disorder
(C) Schizophreniform disorder
(D) Brief psychotic disorder
(E) Delusional disorder
(F) Shared delusional disorder

Answers and Explanations

TBQ-D. This patient is suffering from brief psychotic disorder. This disorder is characterized by psychotic symptoms lasting >1 day, but <1 month; she has had symptoms for the past 2 weeks. Also, the stress of final examinations is likely to be a precipitating psychosocial factor in this patient. Schizoaffective disorder is characterized by symptoms of a mood disorder as well as psychotic symptoms and lifelong social and occupational impairment. In schizophrenia, psychotic and residual symptoms last >6 months and there is lifelong social and occupational impairment. Schizophreniform disorder is characterized by psychotic and residual symptoms lasting 1–6 months. In delusional disorder, which often lasts for years, there is a fixed, nonbizarre delusional system; few if any other thought disorders; and relatively normal social and occupational functioning. In shared delusional disorder, a person develops the same delusion as a person with delusional disorder with whom they are in a close relationship.

1-D. This man who has dressed strangely, showed poor grooming, and had paranoid delusions and auditory hallucinations over a prolonged period is most likely to be suffering from schizophrenia. Neuropsychological evaluation of a schizophrenic patient is most likely to reveal frontal lobe dysfunction. Schizophrenics usually show intact memory, orientation to person, place and time, and normal intelligence.

2-C. Hearing the voice of Abraham Lincoln is an example of an auditory hallucination. An illusion is a misperception of real external stimuli, a delusion is a false belief not shared by others, an idea of reference is the false belief of being referred to by others and a neologism is an invented new word. All of these phenomena can be seen in psychotic patients.

3-A. Analysis of neurotransmitter availability in the brain of this schizophrenic patient is most likely to reveal increased dopamine or increased serotonin. Acetylcholine is not believed to be directly involved in the psychopathology of schizophrenia.

4-A. This patient who shows extreme psychomotor agitation and unusual uncomfortable-looking body positions is most likely to be suffering from catatonic schizophrenia. Disorganized schizophrenia is characterized by disinhibition, poor grooming and poor personal appearance, and inappropriate emotional responses. Paranoid schizophrenia is characterized by delusions of persecution; undifferentiated schizophrenia has the characteristics of more than one subtype. In residual schizophrenia, there is one previous schizophrenic episode and residual symptoms but no psychotic symptoms.

5-C. This patient is most likely to be suffering from paranoid schizophrenia which is characterized by delusions of persecution (also see Question 4).

6-B. This paranoid belief is a delusion, an example of a disorder of thought content. An idea of reference is also an example of a disorder of thought content. Illusions and hallucinations are disorders of perception and loose associations and tangentiality are disorders of form of thought. Problems with affect or mood are characteristic of the affective disorders (see Chapter 12).

7-A. Delusions are positive symptoms of schizophrenia. Positive symptoms respond best to traditional antipsychotic. Flattening of affect, poor speech content, lack of motivation, and social withdrawal are negative symptoms of schizophrenia and respond better to atypical antipsychotics.

8-E. Social withdrawal is a negative symptom of schizophrenia. Negative symptoms respond best to atypical antipsychotic medication. Hallucinations, delusions, agitation, and talkativeness are positive symptoms of schizophrenia.

9-A. An illusion is a misperception of a real external stimulus (e.g., a computer looking like a lion lurking in the corner in a darkened room). A hallucination is a false sensory perception and

104

a delusion is a false belief not shared by others. An idea of reference is the false belief of being referred to by others and a neologism is an invented new word.

10-E. An idea of reference is the false belief of being referred to by others (e.g., the President talking about the patient on television) (see also answers to Questions 1 and 9).

11-C. The chance that the son (or other first degree relative) of a schizophrenic will develop schizophrenia over the course of his life is approximately 12%.

12-D. The chance that the identical twin of a schizophrenic will develop schizophrenia over the course of his life is approximately 50%.

13-D. Approximately 50% of patients with schizophrenia attempt suicide at some point in their lives.

14-D. Mood symptoms are associated with a good prognosis in schizophrenia. A good prognosis is associated also with older age of onset, positive symptoms and few relapses. Catatonic symptoms are associated with a poor prognosis.

15-C. Auditory hallucinations are the most common type of hallucinations seen in schizophrenia.

16-B. This patient is suffering from schizoaffective disorder. This disorder is characterized by symptoms of a mood disorder as well as psychotic symptoms and lifelong social and occupational impairment (see also answer to TBQ).

17-E. This patient is suffering from delusional disorder, persecutory type. In this disorder there is a fixed, nonbizarre delusional system (paranoid in the persecutory type), few if any other thought disorders and relatively normal social and occupational functioning (e.g., this patient is married and held a job for over 30 years) (see also answer to TBQ).

18-F. This patient is suffering from shared delusional disorder. She has developed the same delusion that her husband has (i.e., that their house is filled with radioactive dust). If separated for a period of time from her husband (the inducer) her delusion will probably disappear (see also answer to TBQ).

12

Mood Disorders

*Typical **Board Question***

A 35-year-old physician tells his internist that he has lost interest in playing in the hospital string quartet, an activity he formerly enjoyed. He reports that over the past 3 months he commonly wakes up a few hours before his alarm goes off and cannot fall back to sleep, and has lost 12 pounds. He states "maybe everyone would be better off without me." He says that although he has lots of aches and pains and often feels tired, he feels somewhat better as the day progresses. This patient is most likely to be suffering from

(A) dysthymic disorder
(B) major depressive disorder
(C) bipolar disorder
(D) hypochondriasis
(E) cyclothymic disorder

(See "Answers and Explanations" at end of Chapter)

I. Overview

A. Definitions

1. The mood or affective disorders are characterized by a primary **disturbance** in **internal emotional state** causing subjective distress and problems in functioning.

2. **Given the patient's current social and occupational situation** he or she emotionally feels

—somewhat worse than would be expected (**dysthymia**)

—very much worse than would be expected (**depression**)

—somewhat better than would be expected (**hypomania**)

—very much better than would be expected (**mania**)

3. The **categories** of mood disorders are: major depressive disorder, bipolar disorder (I and II), dysthymic disorder, and cyclothymic disorder.

B. Epidemiology

1. There are **no differences** in the occurrence of mood disorders associated with ethnicity, education, marital status, or income.

2. The **lifetime prevalence** of mood disorders is
   a. Major depressive disorder: 5%–12% for men; 10%–20% for women
   b. Bipolar disorder: 1% overall; no sex difference
   c. Dysthymic disorder: 6% overall; up to 3 times more common in women
   d. Cyclothymic disorder: less than 1% overall; no sex difference

II. Classification of Mood Disorders

A. **Major depressive disorder**
   1. **Characteristics**
      a. Recurrent episodes of depression, each continuing **for at least 2 weeks.**
      b. **Symptoms** of depression are listed and described in **Table 12-1.**
   2. **Masked depression**
      a. As many as 50% of depressed patients seem unaware of or deny depression and thus are said to have **"masked depression."**
      b. Patients with masked depression often visit primary care doctors complaining of **vague physical symptoms.**
      c. These complaints may be **mistaken for hypochondriasis (see Chapter 14).**
      d. In contrast to patients with hypochondriasis, depressed patients show other symptoms of depression (i.e., severe weight loss, sleep problems) in addition to their physical complaints.
   3. **Seasonal affective disorder (SAD)**
      1. **SAD** is a subtype of major depressive disorder associated with the winter season and short days.
      2. Many SAD patients improve in response to **full-spectrum light exposure.**
   4. **Suicide risk**
      a. Patients with major depressive disorder are at increased **risk for suicide.**
      b. Certain demographic, psychosocial, and physical factors affect this risk (**Table 12-2**).
      c. The 5 top risk factors for suicide from highest to lowest risk are: 1) **serious prior suicide attempt,** 2) **age older than 45 years,** 3) alcohol dependence, 4) history of rage and violent behavior, and 5) male sex.

B. **Bipolar disorder**
   1. In bipolar disorder, there are episodes of **both mania and depression (bipolar I disorder)** or **both hypomania and depression (bipolar II disorder).**
   2. There is no simple manic disorder because depressive symptoms eventually occur. Therefore, **one episode of symptoms of mania (see Table 12-1) or hypomania** defines bipolar disorder.
   3. In some patients, (e.g., poor patients with low access to health care) a

Table 12-1. Symptoms of Depression and Mania

Type of Episode	Symptom	Likelihood of occurrence
Depression	• Depressed mood (has feelings of sadness, hopelessness, helplessness, low self-esteem, and excessive guilt)	++++ Hallmark
	• Reduced interest or pleasure in most activities (in severe form this is called anhedonia, the inability to respond to pleasurable stimuli)	++++
	• Reduced energy and motivation	++++
	• Anxiety (is apprehensive about imagined dangers)	++++
	• Sleep problems (wakes frequently at night and too early in the morning)	++++
	• Cognitive problems (has difficulty with memory and concentration)	+++
	• Psychomotor retardation (is slowed down) (seen particularly in the elderly) or agitation (is speeded up)	+++
	• Decreased appetite (has less interest in food and sex; in atypical depression, patients overeat)	+++
	• Diurnal variation in symptoms (feels worse in the morning and better in the evening)	++
	• Suicidal ideation (has thoughts of killing himself)	++
	• Suicide (takes his own life)	+
	• Psychotic symptoms (has delusions of destruction and fatal illness)	+
Mania	• Elevated mood (has strong feelings of happiness and physical well-being)	++++ Hallmark
	• Grandiosity and expansiveness (has feelings of self-importance)	++++
	• Irritability and impulsivity (is easily bothered and quick to anger)	++++
	• Disinhibition (shows uncharacteristic lack of modesty in dress or behavior)	++++
	• Assaultiveness (cannot control aggressive impulses; has problems with the law)	++++
	• Distractibility (cannot concentrate on relevant stimuli)	++++
	• Flight of ideas (thoughts move rapidly from one to the other)	++++
	• Pressured speech (seems compelled to speak quickly)	
	• Impaired judgment [provides unusual responses to hypothetical questions, (e.g., says she would buy a blood bank if she inherited money)]	++++
	• Delusions [has false beliefs which are often grandiose (e.g., of power and influence)]	+++

Approximate percentage of patients in which the sign or symptom is seen: +, less than 25%; ++, 50%; +++, 70%; ++++, more than 90%.

Table 12-2. Risk Factors for Suicide

Category	Factor	Increased Risk	Decreased Risk
History	Previous suicidal behavior	• Serious suicide attempt (about 30% of people who attempt suicide try again and 10% succeed) • Less than 3 months' time has passed since the previous attempt • Possibility of rescue was remote	• Suicidal gesture, but not a serious attempt, was made • More than 3 months' time has passed since the suicidal gesture • Rescue was very likely
	Family history	• Close family member (especially parent) committed suicide • Having divorced parents (especially for adolescents) • Being younger than 11 years old at the time of a parent's death	• No family history of suicide • Intact family • Parents alive through childhood
Current psychological, physical, and social factors	Psychiatric symptoms	• Severe depression • Psychotic symptoms • Hopelessness • Impulsiveness	• Mild depression • No psychotic symptoms • Some hopefulness • Thinks things out
	Depth of depression	• Initial stages of recovery from deep depression; recovering patients may have enough energy to commit suicide	• The depth of severe depression; patients rarely have the clarity of thought or energy needed to plan and commit suicide
	Substance use	• Alcohol and drug dependence • Current intoxication	• Little or no substance use
	Physical health	• Serious medical illness (cancer, AIDS). • Perception of serious illness (most patients have visited a physician in the 6 months prior to suicide)	• Good health • No recent visit to a physician
	Social relationships	• Divorced (particularly men) • Widowed • Single, never married • Lives alone	• Married • Strong social support systems • Has children • Lives with others
Demographic factors	Age	• Elderly (persons 65 years of age and older, especially elderly men) • Middle-aged (over 55 years of age in women and 45 years in men) • Adolescents (suicide is the third leading cause of death in those 15–24 years of age; rates increase after	• Children (up to age 15 years) • Young adults (age 25–40 years)

continued

Table 12-2. Risk Factors for Suicide (continued)

Category	Factor	Increased Risk	Decreased Risk
		neighborhood suicide of a teen or after television shows depicting teenage suicide)	
	Sex	• Male sex (men successfully commit suicide three times more often than women) • Professional women	• Female sex (although women attempt suicide three times more often than men)
	Occupation	• Physicians (especially women and psychiatrists) • Dentists • Police officers • Attorneys • Musicians • Unemployed	• Non-professionals • Employed
	Race	• Caucasian; 66% of successful suicides are Caucasian males	• Non-caucasian
	Religion	• Jewish • Protestant	• Catholic • Muslim
	Economic conditions	• Economic recession or depression	• Strong economy
Lethality	Plan and means	• A plan for suicide (e.g., decision to stockpile pills) • A means of committing suicide (e.g., access to a gun) • Sudden appearance of peacefulness in an agitated, depressed patient (he has reached an internal decision to kill himself and is now calm)	• No plan for suicide, • No means of suicide
	Method	• Shooting oneself • Crashing one's vehicle • Hanging oneself • Jumping from a high place	• Taking pills • Slashing one's wrists

mood disorder with psychotic symptoms can become severe enough to be **misdiagnosed as schizophrenia.**

    a. Psychotic symptoms such as **delusions** can occur in **depression** (depression with psychotic features) as well as in mania.

    b. In contrast to schizophrenia and schizoaffective disorder in which patients are chronically impaired, in mood disorders the patient's mood and functioning usually **return to normal** between episodes.

C. Dysthymic disorder and **cyclothymic disorder**

    1. Dysthymic disorder involves **dysthymia continuing over a 2-year period** with no discrete episodes of illness.

    2. Cyclothymic disorder involves periods of **hypomania and dysthymia occurring over a 2-year period** with no discrete episodes of illness.

3. In contrast to major depressive disorder and bipolar disorder respectively, dysthymic disorder and cyclothymic disorder are less severe, nonepisodic, chronic, and **never associated with psychosis.**

III. Etiology

A. The **biologic** etiology of mood disorders includes:
1. **Altered neurotransmitter activity** (see Chapter 4).
2. A **genetic component,** strongest in **bipolar disorder (Table 12-3).**
3. Physical **illness and related factors (Table 12-4).**
4. Abnormalities of the limbic-hypothalamic-pituitary-adrenal axis (see Chapter 5).

B. The **psychosocial** etiology of depression and dysthymia can include:
1. **Loss of a parent** in childhood;
2. **Loss of a spouse or child** in adulthood;
3. **Low self-esteem** and negative interpretation of life events;
4. **"Learned helplessness"** (i.e., because attempts to escape bad situations in the past have proven futile, the person now feels helpless; see Chapter 7).

C. Psychosocial factors are **not involved** in **the etiology of mania** or hypomania.

IV. Treatment

A. **Overview**
1. Depression is **successfully treated in most patients.**

Table 12-3. The Genetics of Bipolar Disorder

Group	Approximate Occurrence(%)
The general population	1%
Child who has one bipolar parent or sibling (or dizygotic twin)	20%
Child who has two bipolar parents	60%
Monozygotic twin of a person with bipolar disorder	75%

Table 12-4. Differential diagnosis of depression

Medical Conditions	Psychiatric and Pharmacologic conditions
• Cancer, particularly pancreatic and other gastrointestinal tumors • Viral illness [e.g., pneumonia, influenza, acquired immune deficiency syndrome (AIDS)] • Endocrinologic abnormalities, particularly hypothyroidism • Neurologic illness [e.g., Parkinson's disease, multiple sclerosis, stroke (particularly left frontal)] • Nutritional deficiency • Renal or cardiopulmonary disease	• Schizophrenia (particularly after an acute psychotic episode) • Anxiety disorders • Somatoform disorders • Eating disorders • Drug and alcohol abuse (particularly use of sedatives and withdrawal from stimulants) • Prescription drug use (e.g., reserpine, steroids, antihypertensives, antineoplastics)

2. Only about **25% of patients with depression seek and receive treatment.**

   a. Patients do not seek treatment in part because Americans often believe that mental illness indicates **personal failure or weakness.**

   b. As in other illnesses, **women are more likely than men to seek treatment.**

3. Untreated episodes of depression and mania are **usually self-limiting** and last approximately 6–12 months and 3 months, respectively.

4. The **most effective treatments** for the mood disorders are **pharmacologic.**

B. **Pharmacologic treatment** (see Chapter 16)

   1. Treatment for depression and dysthymia includes **antidepressant agents, (i.e., heterocyclics, selective serotonin reuptake inhibitors** (SSRIs) and **monoamine oxidase inhibitors** (MAOIs), and stimulants).

   2. Antimanics

      a. Lithium and anticonvulants such as carbamazepine [Tegretol] and valproic acid [Depakene] are used to treat mania.

      b. Antimanic agents in doses similar to those used to treat bipolar disorder are the primary treatment for **cyclothymic disorder.**

C. **Psychological treatment (see Chapter 17)**

   1. Psychological treatment for depression and dysthymia includes psychoanalytic, interpersonal, family, behavioral, and cognitive therapy.

   2. **Psychological treatment in conjunction with medication is more effective** than either type of treatment alone.

D. **Electroconvulsive therapy (ECT)** (and see Chapter 16). The primary indication for ECT is **major depressive disorder.** It is used when:

   1. The symptoms **do not respond to antidepressant medications.**

   2. Antidepressants are too dangerous or **have intolerable side effects.** Thus, ECT may be particularly useful for **elderly patients.**

   3. **Rapid resolution** of symptoms is necessary (i.e., the patient is acutely suicidal).

Review Test

Directions: Each of the numbered items or incomplete statements in this section is followed by answers or by completions of the statement. Select the **one** lettered answer or completion that is **best** in each case.

Questions 1–3

A 22-year-old male college student is taken to the emergency department by police because he tried to enter a state office building to "have a conference with the Governor" about conducting a fund drive to "finance my cure for cancer." When police prevent him from entering the building, he becomes irritable and hostile and resists attempts to restrain him.

1. This patient is most likely to be suffering from

(A) dysthymic disorder
(B) major depressive disorder
(C) bipolar disorder
(D) hypochondriasis
(E) cyclothymic disorder

2. The most effective long-term treatment for this patient is

(A) a heterocyclic antidepressant
(B) lithium
(C) electroconvulsive therapy
(D) psychotherapy
(E) a monoamine oxidase inhibitor

3. The chances that this patient's identical twin brother has or will develop the same disorder are about

(A) 1%
(B) 5%
(C) 25%
(D) 55%
(E) 75%

Questions 4 and 5

For the past 4 months, a 30-year-old woman has seemed full of energy and optimism for no obvious reason. For a few years before this, friends say she was often pessimistic and seemed tired and "washed out." There is no evidence of a thought disorder.

4. This patient is most likely to be suffering from

(A) dysthymic disorder
(B) major depressive disorder
(C) bipolar disorder
(D) hypochondriasis
(E) cyclothymic disorder

5. The most effective long term treatment for this patient is

(A) a heterocyclic antidepressant
(B) lithium
(C) electroconvulsive therapy
(D) psychotherapy
(E) a monoamine oxidase inhibitor

Questions 6 and 7

6. A severely depressed 52-year-old dentist is referred to you for a physical examination. Of the following signs and symptoms, which is most likely to be seen in this patient?

(A) Weight gain
(B) Flight of ideas
(C) Auditory hallucinations
(D) Feeling better in the morning than in the evening
(E) Poor grooming

7. Analysis of neurotransmitter availability in the brain of this patient is most likely to reveal

(A) increased dopamine
(B) decreased histamine
(C) increased acetylcholine
(D) decreased acetylcholine
(E) decreased serotonin

8. A 25-year-old male patient who is slow-moving and has a flat affect is put on fluoxetine [Prozac]. Within two weeks, the patient is showing greatly increased activity level, flight of ideas, and pressured speech. In this patient, the medication has

(A) precipitated a manic episode
(B) had a toxic effect
(C) had a delayed effect
(D) increased anxiety
(E) increased depression

9. The percentage of depressed patients who seek treatment for their symptoms is about

(A) 1%
(B) 5%
(C) 25%
(D) 55%
(E) 75%

10. A 28-year-old man comes in complaining of headaches and a variety of aches and pains which have been present for the past 6 months. He denies that he is sad or hopeless. After a 4-week trial of antidepressant medication, the patient's physical complaints have disappeared. This patient was probably

(A) suffering from hypochondriasis
(B) suffering from dysthymic disorder
(C) suffering from cyclothymic disorder
(D) suffering from masked depression
(E) faking his symptoms for attention

Questions 11–13

A 65-year-old Catholic male patient has been abusing alcohol for the past 15 years. His history reveals that his wife recently asked him for a separation.

11. Which of the following characteristics is this patient's greatest risk factor for suicide?

(A) Alcoholism
(B) Male sex
(C) Marital separation
(D) Religion
(E) Age

12. This man is at the lowest risk for suicide if he works as a

(A) messenger
(B) policeman
(C) physician
(D) lawyer
(E) dentist

13. If this patient tries to commit suicide, the method most likely to fail is

(A) shooting himself with a gun
(B) crashing his car
(C) slashing his wrists
(D) jumping from a high place
(E) hanging himself

Answers and Explanations

TBQ-B. This patient is most likely to be suffering from major depressive disorder. Evidence for this is that he has lost interest in his usual activities, wakes up too early in the morning, has vague physical symptoms, shows diurnal variation in symptoms (worse in the morning), has lost a significant amount of weight and is showing suicidal ideation (e.g., "maybe everyone would be better off without me"). Also, his symptoms have been present for a discrete, identified amount of time. Dysthymic disorder involves mild or moderate depression most of the time occurring over a 2-year period with no discrete episodes of illness. Bipolar disorder involves episodes of both mania and depression. Cyclothymic disorder involves episodes of hypomania and dysthymia occurring over a 2-year period with no discrete episodes of illness. In hypochondriasis, patients believe that normal body functions or minor illnesses are serious or life-threatening (see Chapter 13).

1-C, 2-B, 3-E. This patient is most likely to be suffering from bipolar I disorder. While this disorder involves episodes of both mania and depression, a single episode of mania defines the illness. The belief that one is important enough to demand a conference with the Governor and cure cancer are grandiose delusions. Schizophrenic delusions are commonly paranoid in nature. Irritability and hostility are also common in a manic episode (see also answer and explanation for **TBQ**). Of the listed treatments, the one most effective for bipolar disorder is lithium. Heterocyclic antidepressants, electroconvulsive therapy, monoamine oxidase inhibitors, and psychotherapy are used primarily to treat depression. Antidepressants and psychotherapy are used to treat dysthymia. The chance of the monozygotic twin of this bipolar patient developing the disorder is about 75%.

4-E, 5-B. This patient is probably suffering from cyclothymic disorder. This disorder involves periods of both hypomania (energy and optimism) and dysthymia (pessimism and feeling "washed out") occurring over a 2-year period with no discrete episodes of illness. Of the listed treatments, the one most effective for cyclothymic disorder, as for bipolar disorder, is lithium. Heterocyclic antidepressants, electroconvulsive therapy, monoamine oxidase inhibitors and psychotherapy are primarily used to treat depression. Antidepressants and psychotherapy are used to treat dysthymia.

6-E, 7-E. This severely depressed dentist is likely to show poor grooming. She is also more likely to show weight loss, and to feel better in the evening than in the morning. Auditory hallucinations are common in schizophrenia but uncommon in depression. Flight of ideas is characteristic of mania. Analysis of neurotransmitter availability in this patient is most likely to reveal decreased serotonin, commonly reflected in decreased plasma levels of its major metabolite 5-HIAA. Increased dopamine is seen in schizophrenia and decreased acetylcholine is seen in Alzheimer's disease.

8-A. In this depressed patient, the antidepressant fluoxetine has precipitated a manic episode (i.e., greatly increased activity level, flight of ideas, and pressured speech). This indicates that the patient has bipolar disorder rather than major depressive disorder. There is no evidence of increased depression, increased anxiety, or a delayed or toxic effect in this patient.

9-C. Only about 25% of depressed patients seek treatment although treatment (antidepressants, psychotherapy, electroconvulsive therapy) is effective in most depressed patients.

10-D. This patient's physical complaints (i.e., headaches and aches and pains) were relieved by antidepressant medication. This indicates that these symptoms were manifestations of masked (hidden) depression rather than hypochondriasis. There is no evidence in this patient for bipolar disorder, dysthymic disorder, cyclothymic disorder or factitious disorder (i.e., fabricating symptoms for attention) (see Chapter 13).

11-E, 12-A, 13-C. Although male sex, alcohol abuse and marital separation all are risk factors for suicide, the highest risk factor of those mentioned is age. Catholic religion is associated with a reduced risk of suicide. Nonprofessionals are at a lower suicide risk than professionals. Among professionals, those at the highest risk for suicide are policemen, physicians, lawyers, and dentists. The method of suicide most likely to fail is slashing the wrists. Shooting, crashing a car, jumping from a high place and hanging are more lethal methods of committing suicide.

13

Anxiety, Somatoform and Factitious Disorders, and Malingering

Typical Board Question

A 35-year-old woman who was raped 5 years ago has recurrent vivid memories of the incident accompanied by intense anxiety. These memories frequently intrude during her daily activities, and nightmares about the event often wake her. Her symptoms intensified when a coworker was raped 2 months ago. This patient's symptoms most closely suggest

(A) post-traumatic stress disorder
(B) panic disorder
(C) adjustment disorder
(D) acute stress disorder
(E) malingering

(See "Answers and Explanations" at end of Chapter)

I. Anxiety Disorders

A. Fear and anxiety

1. **Fear** is a normal reaction to a known, external source of danger.

2. In **anxiety,** the individual is frightened but the source of the danger is not known, not recognized, or **inadequate to account for the symptoms.**

3. The **physiologic manifestations** of anxiety are similar to those of fear.

They include

a. Shakiness and sweating

b. Palpitations (subjective experience of tachycardia)

c. Tingling in the extremities and numbness around the mouth

d. Dizziness and syncope (fainting)

e. Mydriasis (pupil dilation)

f. Gastrointestinal and urinary disturbances (e.g., diarrhea and urinary frequency.

B. Classification and occurrence of the anxiety disorders

1. The *DSM-IV classification* of anxiety disorders includes
   a. Panic disorder (with or without agoraphobia)
   b. Phobias (specific and social)
   c. Obsessive-compulsive disorder (OCD)
   d. Generalized anxiety disorder (GAD)
   e. Post-traumatic stress disorder (PTSD)
   f. Acute stress disorder (ASD)
2. Descriptions of these disorders can be found in **Table 13-1. Adjustment disorder** is included in this table because it often must be distinguished from post-traumatic stress disorder.
3. The anxiety disorders are the most commonly treated mental health problems.

C. The organic basis of anxiety

1. Neurotransmitters involved in the development of anxiety include Δ-aminobutyric acid (GABA) (decreased activity), serotonin (decreased activity), and norepinephrine (increased activity) (see also Chapter 4).
2. The **locus ceruleus** (site of noradrenergic neurons), **raphe nucleus** (site of serotonergic neurons), caudate nucleus (particularly in OCD) temporal cortex and frontal cortex are brain areas likely to be involved in anxiety disorders.
3. Organic causes of symptoms of anxiety include **excessive caffeine intake,** substance abuse, hyperthyroidism, vitamin B_{12} deficiency, hypo- or hyperglycemia, cardiac arrhythmia, anemia, pulmonary disease, and **pheochromocytoma** (an adrenal medullary tumor).

D. Treatment of the anxiety disorders

1. **Antianxiety agents** (and see Chapter 16) including benzodiazepines, buspirone, and β-blockers, are used to treat the symptoms of anxiety.
   a. Benzodiazepines (e.g., diazepam [Valium]), are fast-acting antianxiety agents.
      —Because they carry a high risk of dependence and addiction, they are usually **used for only a limited amount of time** to treat acute exacerbations of anxiety symptoms.
      —Because they work quickly, benzodiazepines, particularly **alprazolam [Xanax],** are used for emergency department treatment of **panic attacks.**
   b. **Buspirone [BuSpar]** is a relatively new antianxiety agent.
      —Because of its **low abuse potential,** buspirone is useful as **long term maintenance** therapy for patients with **GAD.**
      —Because it **takes up to 2 weeks to work,** buspirone has little immediate effect on anxiety symptoms.
   c. **β-blockers** such as propranolol are used to control **autonomic symptoms** (i.e., tachycardia) in anxiety disorders, particularly for anxiety about performing in public or taking an examination.

2. **Antidepressants**
   Antidepressants including monoamine oxidase inhibitors (MAOIs), tricyclics and especially **selective serotonin reuptake inhibitors (SSRIs)** like fluoxetine (Prozac) are the most effective long-term (maintenance) therapy for panic disorder and for OCD (see Chapter 16).

Table 13-1. DSM-IV Classification of the Anxiety Disorders and Adjustment Disorder

Panic disorder (with or without agoraphobia)
- Episodic (about twice weekly) periods of intense anxiety (panic attacks)
- Cardiac and respiratory symptoms and the conviction that one is about to die
- Sudden onset of symptoms, increasing in intensity over a period of approximately 10 minutes, and lasting about 30 minutes
- Attacks can be induced by administration of sodium lactate or CO_2 (see Chapter 5)
- Strong genetic component
- More common in young women in their twenties
- In panic disorder with agoraphobia, characteristics and symptoms of panic disorder (see above) are associated with fear of open places or situations in which the patient cannot escape or obtain help (agoraphobia)
- Panic disorder with agoraphobia it is associated with separation anxiety disorder in childhood (see Chapter 15)

Phobias (specific and social)
- In specific phobia, there is an irrational fear of certain things (e.g., elevators, snakes, or closed in areas)
- In social phobia, there is an exaggerated fear of social situations (e.g., public speaking, eating in public, using public restrooms)
- Because of the fear, the patient avoids the object or situation
- Avoidance leads to social and occupational problems
- Phobias are the most common mental health problem

Obsessive-compulsive disorder (OCD)
- Recurring intrusive feelings, thoughts, and images (obsessions) which cause anxiety
- Anxiety is relieved in part by performing repetitive actions (compulsions)
- A common obsession is avoidance of hand contamination
- A common compulsion includes the need to wash the hands after touching things
- Patients usually have insight (i.e., they realize that these thoughts and behaviors are irrational and want to eliminate them)
- Usually starts in early adulthood, but may begin in childhood
- Genetic factors are involved
- Increased in first-degree relatives of Tourette's disorder patients

Generalized anxiety disorder
- Persistent anxiety symptoms lasting 6 months or more
- Gastrointestinal symptoms are common
- Symptoms are not related to a specific person or situation (i.e., free-floating anxiety)
- Commonly starts during the third decade of life

Post-traumatic stress disorder (PTSD) and acute stress disorder (ASD)
- Symptoms occurring after a catastrophic (life-threatening or potentially fatal) event (e.g., war, earthquake, serious accident, rape, robbery) affecting the patient or the patient's close friend or relative
- Symptoms include anxiety, recurrent nightmares, intrusive memories of the event (flashbacks), increased startle response, hypervigilance, survivor's guilt, dissociation, and social withdrawal
- In PTSD, symptoms last for more than 1 month and can last for years
- In ASD, symptoms last only between 2 days and 4 weeks

Adjustment disorder
- Emotional symptoms (e.g., anxiety, depression, conduct problems) causing social, school, or work impairment occurring within 3 months and lasting less than 6 months after a serious (but usually not life-threatening) life event (e.g., divorce, bankruptcy, changing residence)

3. **Psychological treatment** (see also Chapter 17)

    a. Systematic desensitization with reciprocal inhibition and cognitive therapy are the most effective treatment for phobias and are useful adjuncts to pharmacotherapy in other anxiety disorders.

    b. Behavioral therapies like flooding and implosion are also useful.

    c. Support groups (e.g., victim survivor groups) are particularly useful for ASD and PTSD.

II. Somatoform Disorders

    A. Characteristics and classification

        1. Somatoform disorders are characterized by **physical symptoms without sufficient organic cause.**

        2. The patient thinks that the symptoms have an organic cause but they are believed to be **unconscious expressions of unacceptable feelings.**

        3. Most somatoform disorders are **more common in women,** although **hypochondriasis occurs equally** in men and women.

        4. The *DSM-IV* **categories** of somatoform disorders and their characteristics are listed in Table 13-2.

    B. Differential diagnosis

        1. The most important differential diagnosis of the somatoform disorders is **unidentified organic disease.**

        2. Factitious disorder, malingering (faking illness) and masked depression (see Chapter 12) also must be excluded.

    C. Treatment

        1. Treatment of somatoform disorders includes **individual and group psychotherapy.** Useful strategies for treatment include

Table 13-2. DSM-IV Classification of the Somatoform Disorders

Classification	Characteristics
Somatization disorder	• History of many physical complaints over years including at least 2 gastrointestinal symptoms (e.g., nausea), 4 pain symptoms, 1 sexual symptom (e.g., menstrual problems) and one pseudoneurotic symptom (e.g., paralysis) • Onset before 30 years of age
Hypochondriasis	• Exaggerated concern with health and illness lasting > 6 months • Concern persists despite medical evaluation and reassurance • More common in middle and old age • Goes to many different doctors seeking help ("doctor shopping")
Conversion disorder	• Sudden, dramatic loss of sensory or motor function (e.g., blindness, paralysis); often associated with a stressful event • More common in unsophisticated adolescents and young adults • Patients appear relatively unworried ("la belle indifference")
Body dysmorphic disorder	• Excessive focus on a minor or imagined physical defect • Onset usually in the late teens
Pain disorder	• Intense, prolonged pain not explained completely by physical disease • Onset usually in the 30s and 40s

   a. Forming a good physician-patient relationship (e.g., scheduling regular appointments, providing reassurance)

   b. Identifying and decreasing the social difficulties in the patient's life that may intensify the symptoms

  2. Antianxiety agents, hypnosis, and **behavioral relaxation therapy** may also be useful.

III. Factitious Disorder (Formerly Munchausen's Syndrome), Factitious Disorder by Proxy, and Malingering

  A. Characteristics

    1. While individuals with somatoform disorders truly believe that they are ill, patients with factitious disorders and malingering **feign mental** or **physical illness** or actually **induce physical illness** in themselves or others for psychological gain (factitious disorder) or tangible gain (malingering) (Table 13-3).

    2. Patients often have worked in the medical field (e.g., nurses, technicians) and know how to persuasively simulate an illness.

  B. Feigned symptoms most commonly include abdominal pain, fever (by heating the thermometer), blood in the urine (by adding blood from a needle stick), induction of tachycardia (by drug administration), skin lesions (by injuring easily reached areas), and seizures.

Table 13-3. Factitious Disorder, Factitious Disorder by Proxy, and Malingering

Disorder	Characteristics
Factitious disorder (formerly Munchausen syndrome)	• Conscious simulation of physical or psychiatric illness to gain attention from medical personnel • Undergoes unnecessary medical and surgical procedures • Has a "grid abdomen" (multiple crossed scars from repeated surgeries)
Factitious disorder by proxy	• Conscious simulation of illness in another person, typically in a child by a parent, to obtain attention from medical personnel • Is a form of child abuse (see also Chapter 18) because the child undergoes unnecessary medical and surgical procedures • Must be reported to child welfare authorities (state social service agency)
Malingering	• Conscious simulation or exaggeration of physical or psychiatric illness for financial (e.g., insurance settlement) or other obvious gain (e.g., avoiding incarceration) • Avoids treatment by medical personnel • Health complaints cease as soon as the desired gain is obtained

Review Test

Directions: Each of the numbered items or incomplete statements in this section is followed by answers or by completions of the statement. Select the **one** lettered answer or completion that is **best** in each case.

Questions 1–3

A 23-year-old female medical student comes to the emergency room with increased heart rate, sweating, and shortness of breath. She is convinced that she is having an asthma attack and that she will suffocate. The symptoms started suddenly during a car ride to school. She has no history of asthma and, other than an increased pulse rate, physical findings are normal.

1. Which of the following disorders best fits this clinical picture?

(A) Hypochondriasis
(B) Obsessive-compulsive disorder
(C) Panic disorder
(D) Generalized anxiety disorder
(E) Acute stress disorder

2. Of the following, the most effective immediate treatment for this patient is

(A) an antidepressant
(B) psychotherapy
(C) a benzodiazepine
(D) buspirone
(E) a β-blocker

3. Of the following, the most effective long-term treatment for this patient is

(A) an antidepressant
(B) psychotherapy
(C) a benzodiazepine
(D) buspirone
(E) a β-blocker

Questions 4–5

A 50-year-old man tells the doctor that he is tired all day because he gets out of bed at least 20 times a night to check the locks on the doors and to be sure the gas jets on the stove are turned off.

4. Which of the following disorders best fits this clinical picture?

(A) Hypochondriasis
(B) Obsessive–compulsive disorder
(C) Panic disorder
(D) Generalized anxiety disorder
(E) Acute stress disorder

5. Of the following, the most effective long-term treatment for this patient is

(A) an antidepressant
(B) psychotherapy
(C) a benzodiazepine
(D) buspirone
(E) a β-blocker

Questions 6–8

A 45-year-old woman says that she frequently feels "nervous" and often has an "upset stomach" which includes heartburn, indigestion and diarrhea. She has had this problem since she was 25 years of age and notes that other family members also are "tense and nervous."

6. Which of the following disorders best fits this clinical picture?

(A) Hypochondriasis
(B) Obsessive-compulsive disorder
(C) Panic disorder
(D) Generalized anxiety disorder
(E) Acute stress disorder

7. Which of the following additional signs or symptoms is this patient most likely to show?

(A) Flight of ideas
(B) Hallucinations
(C) Tingling in the extremities
(D) Ideas of reference
(E) Neologisms

8. The most effective long-term treatment for this patient is

(A) An antidepressant
(B) psychotherapy
(C) a Benzodiazepines
(D) buspirone
(E) a β-blocker

9. A 39-year-old woman claims that she injured her hand at work. She asserts that the pain caused by her injury prevents her from working. She has no further hand problems after she receives a $30,000 workmen's compensation settlement. This clinical presentation is an example of

(A) factitious disorder
(B) conversion disorder
(C) factitious disorder by proxy
(D) somatization disorder
(E) malingering

10. Which of the following events is most likely to result in post-traumatic stress disorder (PTSD)?

(A) Divorce
(B) Bankruptcy
(C) Illness
(D) Changing residence
(E) Robbery at knifepoint

Questions 11–12

A 39-year-old woman takes her 6-year-old son to a physician's office. She says that the child often experiences episodes of breathing problems and abdominal pain. The child's medical record shows many office visits and four abdominal surgical procedures that resulted in cross-hatched abdominal scarring although no abnormalities were ever found. When the doctor confronts the mother with the suspicion that she is fabricating the illness in the child, the mother angrily grabs the child and leaves the office immediately.

11. This clinical presentation is an example of

(A) factitious disorder
(B) conversion disorder
(C) factitious disorder by proxy
(D) somatization disorder
(E) malingering

12. In this situation, what is the first thing the physician should do?

(A) Take the child aside and ask him how he really feels
(B) Call a pediatric pulmonologist to determine the cause of the dyspnea
(C) Call a pediatric gastroenterologist to determine the cause of the abdominal pain
(D) Notify the appropriate state social service agency to report the physician's suspicions
(E) Wait until the child's next visit before taking any action

13. A 45-year-old woman has a 20-year history of vague physical complaints including nausea, painful menses, and loss of feeling in her legs. Physical examination and laboratory workup are unremarkable. She says that she has always had physical problems but that her doctors never seem to identify their cause. Which disorder best fits this clinical picture?

(A) Post-traumatic stress disorder
(B) Hypochondriasis
(C) Obsessive-compulsive disorder
(D) Panic disorder
(E) Somatization disorder
(F) Generalized anxiety disorder
(G) Body dysmorphic disorder
(H) Conversion disorder
(I) Specific phobia
(J) Social phobia
(K) Adjustment disorder
(L) Masked depression

14. Three months after moving, a teenager who was formerly outgoing and a good student seems sad, loses interest in friends, and begins to do poor work in school. Which disorder best fits this clinical picture?

(A) Post-traumatic stress disorder
(B) Hypochondriasis
(C) Obsessive-compulsive disorder
(D) Panic disorder
(E) Somatization disorder
(F) Generalized anxiety disorder
(G) Body dysmorphic disorder
(H) Conversion disorder
(I) Specific phobia
(J) Social phobia
(K) Adjustment disorder
(L) Masked depression

15. A 28-year-old woman experiences a sudden loss of vision, but appears unconcerned. She reports that just before the onset of her blindness, she saw her 2-year-old child run out the front door of their home. Physical examination fails to reveal evidence of a physiologic problem. Which disorder best fits this clinical picture?

(A) Post-traumatic stress disorder
(B) Hypochondriasis
(C) Obsessive-compulsive disorder
(D) Panic disorder
(E) Somatization disorder
(F) Generalized anxiety disorder
(G) Body dysmorphic disorder
(H) Conversion disorder
(I) Specific phobia
(J) Social phobia
(K) Adjustment disorder
(L) Masked depression

16. A 41-year-old man says that he has been "sickly" for most of his life. He has seen many doctors but is angry with most of them because they ultimately referred him for psychological help. He now fears that he has stomach cancer because his stomach makes noises after he eats. Physical examination is unremarkable. Which disorder best fits this clinical picture?

(A) Post-traumatic stress disorder
(B) Hypochondriasis
(C) Obsessive-compulsive disorder
(D) Panic disorder
(E) Somatization disorder
(F) Generalized anxiety disorder
(G) Body dysmorphic disorder
(H) Conversion disorder
(I) Specific phobia
(J) Social phobia
(K) Adjustment disorder
(L) Masked depression

17. A 41-year-old man says that he has been "sickly" for the past 3 months. He fears that he has stomach cancer. The patient is unshaven and appears thin and "slowed down." Physical examination including a gastrointestinal workup is unremarkable except that the patient has lost 15 pounds since his last visit 1 year ago. Which disorder best fits this clinical picture?

(A) Post-traumatic stress disorder
(B) Hypochondriasis
(C) Obsessive-compulsive disorder
(D) Panic disorder
(E) Somatization disorder
(F) Generalized anxiety disorder
(G) Body dysmorphic disorder
(H) Conversion disorder
(I) Specific phobia
(J) Social phobia
(K) Adjustment disorder
(L) Masked depression

18. A 28-year-old woman seeks facial reconstructive surgery for her "sagging" eyelids. She rarely goes out in the daytime because she believes that this characteristic makes her look "like a grandmother." On physical examination, her eyelids appear completely normal. Which disorder best fits this clinical picture?

(A) Post-traumatic stress disorder
(B) Hypochondriasis
(C) Obsessive-compulsive disorder
(D) Panic disorder
(E) Somatization disorder
(F) Generalized anxiety disorder
(G) Body dysmorphic disorder
(H) Conversion disorder
(I) Specific phobia
(J) Social phobia
(K) Adjustment disorder
(L) Masked depression

19. A 29-year-old man is upset because he must take a client to dinner in a restaurant. Although he knows the client well, he is so afraid of making a mess while eating that he says he is not hungry and sips from a glass of water instead of ordering a meal. Which disorder best fits this clinical picture?

(A) Post-traumatic stress disorder
(B) Hypochondriasis
(C) Obsessive-compulsive disorder
(D) Panic disorder
(E) Somatization disorder
(F) Generalized anxiety disorder
(G) Body dysmorphic disorder
(H) Conversion disorder
(I) Specific phobia
(J) Social phobia
(K) Adjustment disorder
(L) Masked depression

Answers and Explanations

TBQ-A. This patient is most likely to be suffering from post-traumatic stress disorder (PTSD) characterized by symptoms of anxiety and intrusive memories and nightmares of this life-threatening rape. This disorder can last for many years in chronic form and may have been intensified in this patient by reexperiencing her own rape through the rape of her coworker.

1-C, 2-C, 3-A. This patient is most likely to be suffering from panic disorder. Panic disorder is characterized by panic attacks which include increased heart rate, dizziness, sweating, shortness of breath, and fainting, and the conviction that one is about to die. Attacks commonly occur twice weekly and last about 30 minutes and are most common in young women. While the most effective immediate treatment for this patient is a benzodiazepine because it works quickly, the most effective long-term (maintenance) treatment for this patient is an antidepressant, particularly a selective serotonine-reuptake inhibitor (SSRI) like paroxetine [Paxil].

4-B, 5-A. This patient is most likely to be suffering from obsessive–compulsive disorder (OCD). Rechecking the locks on the doors and the gas jets are typical compulsions of OCD. As for the patient with panic disorder (above), the most effective long-term treatment for this OCD patient is an antidepressant, particularly a selective serotonin reuptake inhibitor (SSRI).

6-D, 7-C, 8-D. This patient is most likely to be suffering from generalized anxiety disorder (GAD). This disorder includes chronic symptoms of anxiety (heartburn, indigestion, and diarrhea) over a prolonged period with no distinct attacks. Genetic factors are seen in the observation that other family members have similar problems with anxiety. Additional signs or symptoms of anxiety that this patient is likely to show include tingling in the extremities. Flight of ideas, hallucinations, ideas of reference, and neologisms are psychotic symptoms which are not seen in the anxiety disorders or the somatoform disorders. The most effective long-term treatment for this patient is buspirone because, unlike benzodiazepines it does not cause dependence or withdrawal symptoms with long-term use. Antidepressants, psychotherapy, and β-blockers can be used as adjuncts to treat GAD but are not the most effective long-term treatments.

9-E. This presentation is an example of malingering, feigning illness for obvious gain (the $30,000 workmen's compensation settlement). Evidence for this is that the woman has no further hand problems after she receives the money. In conversion disorder, somatization disorder, factious disorder, and factitious disorder by proxy there is no obvious gain related to the symptoms.

10-E. Robbery at knifepoint, a life-threatening event, is most likely to result in post-traumatic stress disorder (PTSD). While life events like divorce, bankruptcy, illness, and changing residence are stressful, they are not life-threatening. Psychological symptoms occurring after events like these are more likely to be evidence of adjustment disorder, not PTSD or acute stress disorder (ASD).

11-C, 12-D. This presentation is an example of factitious disorder by proxy. The mother has faked the child's illness (episodes of breathing problems and abdominal pain) for attention from medical personnel. This faking has resulted in four abdominal surgical procedures in which no abnormalities were found, and the child now has a "grid abdomen." Since she knows she is lying, the mother will become angry and flee when confronted with the truth. The first thing the physician must do is to notify the state social service agency since factitious disorder by proxy is a form of child abuse. Waiting until the child's next visit before acting could result in the child's further injury or even death. Calling in specialists may be done in the future but the physician must first report his suspicions to the state. It is not appropriate to take the child aside and ask him how he really feels. He probably has no knowledge of his mother's behavior.

13-E. This woman with a 20-year history of unexplained vague and chronic physical complaints is probably suffering from somatization disorder. This can be distinguished from hypochondriasis which is an exaggeration of normal physical sensations and minor ailments.

14-K. This teenager who was formerly outgoing and a good student and now seems sad, loses interest in friends, and begins to do poor work in school is probably suffering from adjustment disorder (with depressed mood). It is likely that he is having problems adjusting to his new school. In contrast to adjustment disorder, masked depression has no obvious environmental cause and the symptoms are often more severe (i.e., significant weight loss).

15-H. This woman who experiences a sudden loss of vision triggered by seeing her child run outside, is likely to be suffering from conversion disorder. This disorder also may be characterized by an apparent lack of concern about the symptoms (i.e., la belle indifference).

16-B. This man who says that he has been "sickly" for most of his life and fears that he has stomach cancer is probably suffering from hypochondriasis, exaggerated concern over normal physical sensations (e.g., stomach noises) and minor ailments. There are no physical findings or evidence of depression in this patient.

17-L. This man who says that has been "sickly" for the past 3 months and fears that he has stomach cancer is probably suffering from masked depression. In contrast to the hypochondriacal man in the previous question, evidence for depression in this patient includes the fact that, in addition to the somatic complaints, he shows symptoms of depression [e.g., he is ungroomed, appears "slowed down" (psychomotor retardation), and has lost a significant amount of weight].

18-G. This woman is probably suffering from body dysmorphic disorder, which is characterized by overconcern about a physical feature ("sagging" eyelids) despite normal appearance.

19-J. This man is probably suffering from social phobia. He is afraid of humiliating himself in a public situation (i.e., eating dinner in front of others in a restaurant).

14

Other Psychiatric Disorders

Typical Board Question

A 28-year-old stockbroker who is married and has 2 children usually dresses conservatively. She receives a letter containing a recent photograph of herself in a skimpy black leather outfit. She does not remember the man who signed the letter or posing for the photograph. This woman is most likely to be suffering from

(A) dissociative amnesia
(B) dissociative fugue
(C) dissociative identity disorder
(D) depersonalization disorder
(E) derealization

(See "Answers and Explanations" at end of Chapter)

I. Cognitive Disorders

A. Characteristics

1. Cognitive disorders (formerly called "organic mental syndromes") involve problems in **memory,** orientation, **level of consciousness,** and other cognitive functions.

   a. These difficulties are due to abnormalities in neural chemistry, structure, or physiology **originating in the brain** or **secondary to systemic illness.**

   b. Patients with cognitive disorders may show **psychiatric symptoms secondary to the cognitive problems** (e.g., depression, anxiety, paranoia, hallucinations, and delusions).

2. The major cognitive disorders are **delirium, dementia,** and **amnestic disorder.** Characteristics of these disorders can be found in Table 14-1.

B. Dementia of the Alzheimer's Type (Alzheimer's disease)

1. Diagnosis

   a. Alzheimer's is the **most common type** of dementia and is diagnosed when other obvious causes for the symptoms have been eliminated.

Table 14-1. Characteristics and Etiology of the Cognitive Disorders

Characteristic	Delirium	Dementia	Amnestic disorder
Hallmark	Impaired consciousness	Loss of memory and intellectual abilities	Loss of memory with few other cognitive problems
Etiology	• CNS disease (e.g., Huntington's or Parkinson's disease) • CNS trauma • CNS infection (e.g. meningitis) • Systemic disease (e.g., hepatic, cardiovascular) • High fever • Substance abuse • Substance withdrawal	• Alzheimer's disease (about 55% of all dementias) • Vascular disease (about 10% of all dementias) • CNS disease (e.g., Huntington's or Parkinson's disease) • CNS trauma • CNS infection (e.g., HIV or Creutzfeldt-Jakob)	• Thiamine deficiency due to long-term alcohol abuse leading to destruc of mediotemporal lobe structures (e.g., mammillary bodies) • Temporal lobe trauma, vascular disease or infection (e.g., herpes simplex encephalitis)
Occurrence	• More common in children and the elderly • Most common etiology of psychiatric symptoms in medical and surgical hospital units	• More common in the elderly • Seen in about 20% of individuals over 65 years of age (5% in severe form, 15% in mild form)	• Patients commonly have a history of alcohol abuse
Associated physical findings	• Acute medical illness • Autonomic dysfunction • Abnormal EEG (fast wave activity or generalized slowing)	• No medical illness • Little autonomic dysfunction • Normal EEG	
Associated psychological findings	• Impaired consciousness • Illusions or hallucinations (often visual and disorganized) • Anxiety with psychomotor agitation • "Sundowning" (symptoms are worse at night)	• Normal consciousness • No psychotic symptoms in early stages • Depression • Little diurnal variability • Confabulation (untruths told to hide memory loss) in amnestic disorder	
Course	• Develops quickly • Fluctuating course with lucid intervals	• Develops slowly • Progressive course	
Treatment and Prognosis	• Removal of the underlying medical problem will allow the symptoms to resolve	• No effective treatment • Pharmacotherapy and supportive therapy to treat associated psychiatric symptoms • Rarely reversible	

CNS= central nervous system; *EEG*=electroencephalogram

b. Patients show a **gradual loss of memory and intellectual abilities,** inability to control impulses, and lack of judgment. Depression and anxiety are often seen.

c. Later in the illness, symptoms include confusion and psychosis that progress to coma and **death (usually within 8–10 years of diagnosis).**

d. Because all are associated with aging and memory problems, it is important for patient management and prognosis to make the distinction between **Alzheimer's** and both **pseudodementia** (depression that mimics dementia) and **normal aging** (Table 14-2).

2. **Genetic associations** in dementia of the Alzheimer's type include

   a. Abnormalities of **chromosome 21** (Down patients ultimately develop Alzheimer's)

   b. Abnormalities of **chromosomes 1 and 14** (implicated particularly in **early onset Alzheimer's** (i.e., occurring before 65 years of age)

   c. Possession of at **least one copy of the apolipoprotein E4 (apoE4)** gene on chromosome 19

   d. Gender—there is a higher occurrence of Alzheimer's in **women**

3. **Neurophysiological factors**

   a. Decreased activity of acetylcholine (ACh) and reduced brain levels of **choline acetyltransferase** (i.e., the enzyme needed to synthesize ACh) are seen in Alzheimer's (see Chapter 4).

   b. Abnormal processing of amyloid precursor protein.

4. **Gross anatomical changes** occur in Alzheimer's.

   a. **Brain ventricles** become **enlarged.**

   b. Diffuse atrophy and flattened sulci appear.

5. **Microscopic anatomical changes** occur in Alzheimer's.

   a. **Senile (amyloid) plaques** and **neurofibrillary tangles** are seen (seen also in Down syndrome and, to a lesser extent, in normal aging).

   b. Loss of cholinergic neurons occurs in the basal forebrain.

   c. Neuronal loss and degeneration are seen in the hippocampus and cortex.

6. Alzheimer's has a **progressive, irreversible, downhill** course. The most effective initial interventions involve **providing a structured environment** including visual orienting cues. Such cues include labels over the doors of rooms identifying their function; daily posting of the day of the week, date, and year; daily written activity schedules, and practical safety measures (e.g., disconnecting the stove).

7. **Pharmacologic** interventions include:

   a. **Acetylcholinesterase inhibitors** [e.g., tacrine (Cognex) and donepezil (Aricept)] to temporarily **slow progression** of the disease. These agents cannot restore function already lost.

   b. **Psychotropic agents** are used to treat associated symptoms of anxiety, depression, or psychosis.

Table 14-2. Memory Problems in the Elderly: Comparison of Dementia of the Alzheimer's Type, Pseudodementia, and Normal Aging

Condition	Etiology	Clinical Example	Major Manifestations	Medical Interventions
Dementia of the Alzheimer's Type	Brain dysfunction	A 65-year-old former banker cannot remember to turn off the gas jets on the stove nor can he name the object in his hand (a comb)	• Severe memory loss • Other cognitive problems • Decrease in IQ • Disruption of normal life	• Structured environment • Acetylcholine-sterase inhibitors (e.g., tacrine) • Ultimately, nursing home placement
Pseudodementia (depression that mimics dementia)	Depression of mood	A 65-year-old dentist cannot remember to pay her bills. She also appears to be physically "slowed down" (psychomotor retardation) and sad	• Moderate memory loss • Other cognitive problems • No decrease in IQ • Disruption of normal life	• Antide-pressants • Electro-convulsive therapy (ECT) • Psychotherapy
Normal aging	Minor changes in the normal aging brain	A 65-year-old woman forgets new phone numbers and names but functions well living on her own	• Minor forget-fulness • Reduction in the ability to learn new things quickly • No decrease in IQ • No disruption of normal life	• No medical intervention • Practical and emotional support from the physician

II. Personality Disorders (PDs)

A. Characteristics

1. Individuals with PDs show **chronic, lifelong, rigid, unsuitable patterns of relating to others** that cause social and occupational problems (i.e., few friends, job loss).

2. Persons with PDs generally are not aware that they are the cause of their own problems (**do not have "insight"**), do not have frank psychotic symptoms, and **do not seek psychiatric help.**

B. Classification

1. Personality disorders are categorized by the ***DSM-IV*** into clusters **A** (paranoid, schizoid, schizotypal), **B** (histrionic, narcissistic, borderline, and antisocial), and **C** (avoidant, obsessive–compulsive, dependent, and passive aggressive)

2. Each cluster has its own hallmark characteristics and genetic or familial associations, (i.e., relatives of people with PDs have a higher likelihood of having certain disorders) (Table 14-3).

Table 14-3. DSM-IV Classification and Characteristics of the Personality Disorders

Personality Disorder	Characteristics
CLUSTER A	
Hallmark:	Avoids social relationships, is "peculiar" but not psychotic
Genetic or familial association:	Psychotic illnesses
Paranoid	• Distrustful, suspicious, litigious • Attributes responsibility for own problems to others
Schizoid	• Long-standing pattern of voluntary social withdrawal
Schizotypal	• Peculiar appearance • Magical thinking (i.e., believing that one's thoughts can affect the course of events) • Odd thought patterns and behavior
CLUSTER B	
Hallmark:	Dramatic, emotional, inconsistent
Genetic or familial association:	Mood disorders and substance abuse
Histrionic	• Theatrical, extroverted, emotional, sexually provocative, "life of the party" • In men, "Don Juan" dress and behavior • Cannot maintain intimate relationships
Narcissistic	• Pompous, with a sense of special entitlement • Lacks empathy for others
Antisocial	• Refuses to conform to social norms and shows no concern for others • Associated with conduct disorder in childhood and criminal behavior in adulthood ("psychopaths" or "sociopaths")
Borderline	• Erratic, impulsive, unstable behavior and mood • Feeling bored, alone and "empty" • Suicide attempts for relatively trivial reasons • Self-mutilation (cutting or burning oneself) • Mini-psychotic episodes (i.e., brief periods of loss of contact with reality)
CLUSTER C	
Hallmark:	Fearful, anxious
Genetic or familial association:	Anxiety disorders
Avoidant	• Sensitive to rejection, socially withdrawn • Feelings of inferiority
Obsessive–compulsive	• Perfectionistic, orderly, inflexible • Indecisive
Dependent	• Allows other people to make decisions and assume responsibility for them • Poor self-confidence
Passive-aggressive	• Procrastinates and is inefficient • Shows outward compliance, but feels inward defiance • Is no longer an official DSM-IV diagnosis

C. Treatment

1. For those who seek help, individual and group psychotherapy may be useful.

2. Pharmacotherapy can also be used to treat symptoms such as depression and anxiety that may be associated with the PDs.

III. Dissociative Disorders

A. Characteristics

1. The dissociative disorders are characterized by abrupt but temporary **loss of memory (amnesia) or identity** or by feelings of detachment due to psychological factors.

2. Dissociative disorders are commonly related to **disturbing emotional experiences** in the patient's **recent or remote past.**

3. Besides dissociative disorders, causes of amnesia may include physiological factors such as head injury, substance abuse, sequelae of general anesthesia, and dementia.

B. Classification and treatment

1. The *DSM-IV* categories of dissociative disorders are listed in Table 14-4.

2. Treatment of the dissociative disorders includes **hypnosis and amobarbital sodium interviews** (see Chapter 5) and long-term **psychoanalytically oriented psychotherapy** (see Chapter 16) to recover "lost" (repressed) memories of disturbing emotional experiences.

Table 14-4. *DSM-IV* Classification and Characteristics of Dissociative Disorders

Classification	Characteristics
Dissociative amnesia	• Failure to remember important information about oneself • Amnesia usually resolves in minutes or days but may last years
Dissociative fugue	• Amnesia combined with sudden wandering from home and taking on a different identity • The person is not consciously aware that he has done this
Dissociative identity disorder (formerly multiple personality disorder)	• At least two distinct personalities ("alters") in an individual • More common in women (particularly those sexually abused in childhood) • In a forensic (e.g., jail) setting, malingering and alcohol abuse must be considered and excluded
Depersonalization disorder	• Recurrent, persistent feelings of detachment from one's own body, the social situation, or the environment (derealization)

Table 14-5. Physical and Psychological Characteristics and Treatment of Anorexia Nervosa and Bulimia Nervosa

Disorder	Physical characteristics	Psychological characteristics	Treatment (in order of highest to lowest utility)
Anorexia nervosa	• Extreme weight loss (15% or more of normal body weight) • Amenorrhea (3 or more consecutive missed menstrual periods) • Metabolic acidosis • Hypercholesterolemia • Mild anemia and leukopenia • Lanugo (downy body hair on the trunk) • Melanosis coli (blackened area of the colon if there is laxative abuse)	• Refusal to eat despite normal appetite because of an overwhelming fear of being obese • Abnormal behavior dealing with food (e.g., simulating eating) • Lack of interest in sex • Was a "perfect child" (e.g., good student) • Interfamily conflicts (e.g., patient's problem draws attention away from parental marital problem or an attempt to gain control to separate from the mother) • Excessive exercising	• Hospitalization directed at reinstating nutritional condition (starvation can result in death) • Family therapy (aimed particularly at the mother-daughter relationship) • Psychoactive drugs such as amitriptyline [Elavil] and cyproheptadine [Periactin]
Bulimia nervosa	• Relatively normal body weight • Esophageal varices caused by repeated vomiting • Tooth enamel erosion due to gastric acid in the mouth • Swelling or infection of the parotid glands • Callouses on the dorsal surface of the hand from the teeth because the hand is used to induce gagging • Electrolyte disturbances • Menstrual irregularities	• Binge eating (in secret) of high-calorie foods, followed by vomiting or other purging behavior to avoid weight gain (binge eating and purging also occurs in 50% of patients with anorexia nervosa) • Poor self-image • Distress over the binge eating • Depression • Excessive exercising	• Cognitive and behavioral therapies • Average to high doses of antidepressants • Psychotherapy

IV. Obesity and Eating Disorders

A. Obesity

1. Overview

    a. Obesity is defined as being **more than 20% over ideal weight** based on common height and weight charts.

    b. At least **25% of adults** in the United States are obese.

    c. **Genetic factors are most important** in obesity; adult weight is closer to that of biologic rather than of adoptive parents.

    d. Obesity is more common in lower socioeconomic groups and is associated with **increased risk** for cardiorespiratory problems, hypertension, diabetes mellitus, and orthopedic problems.

2. Treatment

    a. Most weight loss achieved using commercial dieting and weight loss programs is **regained within a 5-year-period.**

    b. Gastric stapling and other **surgical techniques** are initially effective but are of **little value** in maintaining long-term weight loss.

    c. A combination of **sensible dieting and exercise** is the most effective to way to maintain long term weight loss.

B. Eating disorders: anorexia nervosa and bulimia nervosa

1. In anorexia nervosa and bulimia nervosa, the patient shows abnormal behavior associated with food despite **normal appetite.**

2. Eating disorders are **more common in women** and in **higher socioeconomic groups** and are much more common in the **United States** than in other developed countries.

3. Physical and psychological characteristics and treatment of anorexia nervosa and bulimia can be found in Table 14-5.

Review Test

Directions: Each of the numbered items or incomplete statements in this section is followed by answers or by completions of the statement. Select the **one** lettered answer or completion that is **best** in each case.

Questions 1–2

A 75-year-old man is brought to the emergency department after being burned in a house fire. This is the patient's third emergency visit in 2 months. His other visits occurred after he inhaled natural gas when he left the stove on without a flame and because he fell down the stairs after wandering out of the house in the middle of the night. There is no evidence of physical illness and no history of substance abuse. His wife is distressed and begs the doctor to let her husband come home.

1. This patient is most likely to be suffering from

(A) delirium
(B) pseudodementia
(C) dementia of the Alzheimer's type
(D) dissociative fugue
(E) amnestic disorder

2. Of the following, the most effective initial intervention for this patient is

(A) antipsychotic medication
(B) provision of a structured environment
(C) antidepressant medication
(D) tacrine
(E) reassurance

3. A doctor conducts a yearly physical on a normal 85-year-old patient. Which of the following mental characteristics is the doctor most likely to see in this patient?

(A) Impaired consciousness
(B) Abnormal level of arousal
(C) Minor forgetfulness
(D) Psychosis
(E) Depression

4. The new pharmacological treatments for Alzheimer's disease (donepezil and tacrine) are effective because they act to

(A) increase dopamine availability
(B) decrease dopamine availability
(C) increase acetylcholine availability
(D) decrease acetylcholine availability
(E) decrease serotonin availability

5. A 43-year-old woman says that she feels as if she is "outside of herself" and is watching her life as though it were a play. She knows that this perception is only a feeling and that she is really living her life. This woman is most likely to be suffering from

(A) dissociative amnesia
(B) dissociative fugue
(C) dissociative identity disorder
(D) depersonalization disorder
(E) derealization

Questions 6–7

A 78-year-old retired female physician reports that she has been confused and forgetful over the past 10 months. She also has difficulty sleeping, her appetite is poor, and she has lost 12 pounds. Questioning reveals that her 18-year-old dog died 10 months ago.

6. This woman is most likely to be suffering from

(A) delirium
(B) pseudodementia
(C) dementia of the Alzheimer's type
(D) dissociative fugue
(E) amnestic disorder

7. Of the following, the most effective intervention for this patient is

(A) antipsychotic medication
(B) provision of a structured environment
(C) antidepressant medication
(D) tacrine
(E) reassurance

8. A 38-year-old man asks his doctor to refer him to a physician who attended a top-rated medical school. He says that he knows the doctor will not be offended because he understands that he is "better" than her other patients. Which of the following disorders best fits this picture?

(A) Borderline personality disorder
(B) Histrionic personality disorder
(C) Obsessive-compulsive personality disorder
(D) Avoidant personality disorder
(E) Antisocial personality disorder
(F) Dependent personality disorder
(G) Dissociative identity disorder
(H) Adjustment disorder
(I) Paranoid personality disorder
(J) Passive-aggressive personality disorder
(K) Narcissistic personality disorder
(L) Schizotypal personality disorder
(M) Schizoid personality disorder

9. A 20-year-old female college student tells the doctor that because she was afraid to be alone, she tried to commit suicide after a man with whom she had had two dates did not call her again. After the interview, she tells him that all of the other doctors she has seen were terrible and that he is the only doctor who has ever understood her problems. Which of the following disorders best fits this picture?

(A) Borderline personality disorder
(B) Histrionic personality disorder
(C) Obsessive-compulsive personality disorder
(D) Avoidant personality disorder
(E) Antisocial personality disorder
(F) Dependent personality disorder
(G) Dissociative identity disorder
(H) Adjustment disorder
(I) Paranoid personality disorder
(J) Passive-aggressive personality disorder
(K) Narcissistic personality disorder
(L) Schizotypal personality disorder
(M) Schizoid personality disorder

10. A 28-year-old woman comes to the doctor's office bringing gifts for the receptionist and the nurses. When she hears that one of the nurses has taken another job, she begins to sob loudly. When the doctor sees her, she reports that she is so hot that she must have "a fever of at least 106°." Which of the following disorders best fits this picture?

(A) Borderline personality disorder
(B) Histrionic personality disorder
(C) Obsessive-compulsive personality disorder
(D) Avoidant personality disorder
(E) Antisocial personality disorder
(F) Dependent personality disorder
(G) Dissociative identity disorder
(H) Adjustment disorder
(I) Paranoid personality disorder
(J) Passive-aggressive personality disorder
(K) Narcissistic personality disorder
(L) Schizotypal personality disorder
(M) Schizoid personality disorder

11. Two weeks after a 50-year-old, overweight, hypertensive woman agreed to start an exercise program, she gained 4 pounds. She reports that she has not exercised yet because "the gym was so crowded that I couldn't get in." Which of the following disorders best fits this picture?

(A) Borderline personality disorder
(B) Histrionic personality disorder
(C) Obsessive-compulsive personality disorder
(D) Avoidant personality disorder
(E) Antisocial personality disorder
(F) Dependent personality disorder
(G) Dissociative identity disorder
(H) Adjustment disorder
(I) Paranoid personality disorder
(J) Passive-aggressive personality disorder
(K) Narcissistic personality disorder
(L) Schizotypal personality disorder
(M) Schizoid personality disorder

12. The parents of a 26-year-old woman say that they are concerned about her because she has no friends and spends most of her time hiking in the woods and working on her computer. The doctor examines her and finds that she is content with her solitary life and has no evidence of a formal thought disorder. Which of the following disorders best fits this picture?

(A) Borderline personality disorder
(B) Histrionic personality disorder
(C) Obsessive-compulsive personality disorder
(D) Avoidant personality disorder
(E) Antisocial personality disorder
(F) Dependent personality disorder
(G) Dissociative identity disorder
(H) Adjustment disorder
(I) Paranoid personality disorder
(J) Passive-aggressive personality disorder
(K) Narcissistic personality disorder
(L) Schizotypal personality disorder
(M) Schizoid personality disorder

13. A 18-year-old gymnast who is currently 5 feet, 5 inches tall and weighs 100 pounds tells the doctor that she needs to lose another 15 pounds to pursue a career in the sport. Her mood appears good. Findings on physical examination are normal except for excessive growth of downy body hair. She reports that she has not menstruated in more than 1 year. Which of the following is most likely to characterize this teenager?

(A) Lack of appetite
(B) Low socioeconomic group
(C) High sexual interest
(D) Conflict with her mother
(E) Poor school performance

Answers and Explanations

TBQ-C. This stockbroker is most likely to be suffering from dissociative identity disorder (formerly multiple personality disorder). She does not remember the man who signed the letter or posing for the photograph because these events occurred when she was in another personality. Dissociative amnesia involves a failure to remember important information about oneself and dissociative fugue is amnesia combined with sudden wandering from home and taking on a different identity. Depersonalization disorder is a persistent feeling of detachment from one's own body, the social situation or the environment (derealization). None of these disorders involves multiple personalities.

1-C, 2-B. This patient is most likely to be suffering from dementia of the Alzheimer's type. He is having accidents because he is forgetful (e.g., forgetting to turn off the gas jet) and wanders out of the house because he does not know which is the closet or bathroom door and which is the outside door. There is no evidence of a medical cause for his symptoms as there would be in delirium. There is no evidence of depression as in pseudodementia or of a history of alcohol abuse as in amnestic disorder. The most effective initial intervention for this patient is provision of a structured environment [e.g., giving the patient visual cues for orientation (labeling doors for function)] and taking practical measures (e.g., removing the gas stove). Medications and reassurance may be useful for associated symptoms but that will not change the patient's forgetful and potentially dangerous behavior.

3-C. This normal 85-year-old patient is likely to show minor forgetfulness, such as forgetting new names and phone numbers. Impaired consciousness, psychosis, and abnormal level of arousal are seen in delirium which is associated with a variety of physical illnesses. While seen more commonly in the elderly than in younger people, depression is an illness (see Chapter 12) not a natural consequence of normal aging.

4-C. Low levels of acetylcholine (ACh) are associated with the symptoms of dementia of the Alzheimer's type. The new pharmacological treatments for Alzheimer's, donepezil and tacrine, are acetylcholinesterase inhibitors (i.e., they block the breakdown of ACh, increasing its availability). These agents can thus be effective in slowing down the progression of the illness, but not in restoring function already lost.

5-D. This woman, who feels as if she is "outside of herself" watching her life as though it were a play is suffering from depersonalization disorder, a persistent feeling of detachment from one's own body or the social situation. In contrast to some of the other dissociative disorders (see answer to TBQ), and psychotic disorders (see Chapter 11) this woman knows that this perception is only a feeling and that she is really living her life.

6-B, 7-C. This woman is most likely to be suffering from pseudodementia—depression which mimics dementia. In the elderly, depression is often associated with cognitive problems as well as sleep and eating problems. Strong evidence for depression is provided by the fact that this patient's symptoms began with the loss of an important relationship (i.e., the death of her dog). Delirium and dementia are caused by physiological abnormalities. Dissociative fugue involves wandering away from home and amnestic disorder is associated with a history of alcoholism. The most effective intervention for this depressed patient is antidepressant medication. When the medication relieves the depressive symptoms, her memory will improve. Antipsychotic medication, provision of a structured environment, tacrine, and simple reassurance are not appropriate for this patient.

8-K. This 38-year-old man who asks to be referred to a physician who attended a top-rated medical school because he is "better" than your other patients is demonstrating narcissistic personality disorder.

9-A. This 20-year-old college student who made a suicide attempt after a relatively trivial relationship broke up and who uses splitting as a defense mechanism (e.g., all of the other doctors she has seen were terrible and he is the best) is demonstrating borderline personality disorder.

10-B. This 28-year-old woman who brings gifts for the receptionist and the nurses because she needs to have everyone like her is demonstrating histrionic personality disorder. Patients with this personality disorder tend to exaggerate their physical symptoms for dramatic effect (e.g., "a fever of at least 106°").

11-J. This 50-year-old woman who agreed to start an exercise program and then makes weak excuses for her failure to follow the program is demonstrating passive-aggressive personality disorder. She really never intended to follow the doctor's exercise program (was inwardly defiant) but agreed to do it (was outwardly compliant).

12-M. This 26-year-old woman who shows no evidence of a thought disorder, has no friends, and spends most of her time at solitary pursuits is demonstrating schizoid personality disorder. In contrast to those with avoidant personality disorder, schizoid patients are content with their solitary lifestyle.

13-D. This teenager is already underweight yet wants to lost more weight, and she has developed lanugo (growth of downy body hair) and amenorrhea (absence of menses). These symptoms show that she is suffering from anorexia nervosa. Because gymnasts must be small and slim, gymnastics is the sport most closely associated with the development of anorexia nervosa. Anorexia is also characterized by family conflicts particularly with the mother, normal appetite, high socioeconomic group, low sexual interest, good school performance and excessive exercising.

15

Psychiatric Disorders in Children

*Typical **B**oard **Q**uestion*

A 4-year-old child who has never spoken voluntarily shows no interest in or connection to his parents, other adults, or other children. His hearing is normal. His mother tells the doctor that he persistently turns on the taps to watch the water running and that he screams and struggles fiercely when she tries to dress him. Which of the following disorders best fits this clinical picture?

(A) Autistic disorder
(B) Rett's disorder
(C) Attention deficit hyperactivity disorder (ADHD)
(D) Tourette's disorder
(E) Selective mutism

(See "Answers and Explanations" at end of Chapter)

I. Pervasive Developmental Disorders of Childhood

A. Overview

1. Pervasive developmental disorders are characterized by the **failure to acquire** (e.g., autistic disorder, Asperger disorder) or the **early loss** (e.g., Rett's disorder, childhood disintegrative disorder) of **social skills and language** resulting in lifelong **problems** in **social and occupational functioning.**

2. These disorders are **not reversible.** Treatment involves **behavioral therapy** to increase social and communicative skills, decrease behavior problems (e.g., self-injury) and improve self-care skills as well as supportive therapy and counseling to parents.

3. The prototype of these disorders is **autistic disorder.**

B. Autistic disorder

1. **Characteristics** of autistic disorder include

   a. Severe **problems with communication** (despite normal hearing)

    b. Significant **problems forming social relationships** (including those with caregivers)

    c. **Repetitive behavior** (e.g., spinning, self-injury)

    d. Subnormal intelligence in most children

    e. **Unusual abilities** in some children (e.g., exceptional memory or calculation skills). These children are referred to as "savants."

  2. Occurrence

    a. Autistic disorder occurs in about 5 children per 10,000.

    b. It begins **before 3 years of age.**

    c. The disorder is much **more common in boys.**

  3. The etiology of autistic disorder includes

    a. **Cerebral dysfunction** (no psychological causes have been identified)

    b. A history of **perinatal complications**

    c. A **genetic component** (e.g., the concordance rate for autism in monozygotic twins is 35% and is lower in dizygotic twins)

C. Other pervasive developmental disorders

  1. Asperger disorder involves

    a. Significant problems forming social relationships

    b. Repetitive behavior

    c. In contrast to autistic disorder, in Asperger disorder there is **normal cognitive development** and little or no developmental language delay.

  2. Rett's disorder involves

    a. **Diminished social, verbal,** and **cognitive development** after up to 4 years of normal functioning

    b. Occurs **only in girls**

    c. Stereotyped, hand-wringing movements

    d. Mental retardation

  3. Childhood disintegrative disorder involves

    a. **Diminished social, verbal, cognitive,** and **motor development** after at least 2 years of normal functioning

    b. Mental retardation

II. Attention-Deficit Hyperactivity Disorder (ADHD) and Disruptive Behavior Disorders of Childhood

A. Overview

  1. ADHD and the **disruptive behavior disorders (i.e., conduct disorder and oppositional defiant disorder)** are characterized by **inappropriate behavior** that causes problems in social relationships and school performance.

  2. There is **no frank mental retardation.**

3. These disorders are **not uncommon** and are **seen more often in boys.**

4. **Differential diagnosis** includes **mood disorders and anxiety disorders.**

5. **Characteristics** of these disorders can be found in Table 15-1.

B. Etiology

1. **Genetic factors** are involved. Relatives of children with conduct disorder and ADHD have an increased incidence of these disorders and of **antisocial personality disorder and substance abuse.**

2. Although evidence of serious structural problems in the brain is not present, children with conduct disorder and ADHD may have **minor brain dysfunction.**

3. Substance abuse, serious marital discord, mood disorders and **child abuse** are seen in some parents of children with these disorders.

C. Treatment

1. Pharmacologic treatment for **ADHD** consists of use **of central nervous system stimulants** including methylphenidate [Ritalin], dextroamphetamine sulfate [Dexedrine], and pemoline [Cylert].

   a. For ADHD, CNS stimulants apparently help to **reduce activity level and increase attention span** and the ability to concentrate; antidepressants also may be useful.

   b. Since stimulant drugs **decrease appetite** (see Chapter 9), they may inhibit growth and lead to **failure to gain weight;** both growth and weight usually return to normal once the child stops taking the medication.

2. **Family therapy** is the most effective treatment for conduct disorder and oppositional defiant disorder (see Chapter 17).

Table 15-1. Characteristics of Attention-Deficit Hyperactivity Disorder and the Disruptive Behavior Disorders

Attention-Deficit Hyperactivity Disorder (ADHD)	Conduct Disorder	Oppositional Defiant Disorder
• Hyperactivity, limited attention span, • Propensity for accidents • Impulsiveness • Emotional lability • Irritability • History of excessive crying, high sensitivity to stimuli, and irregular sleep patterns in infancy • Hyperactivity is the first symptom to disappear as the child gets older • Most children show remission in adolescence	• Behavior that violates social norms (e.g., torturing animals, stealing, truancy, setting fires) • Criminal behavior, antisocial personality disorder, substance abuse, and mood disorder in adulthood	• Behavior that, while defiant, negative, and noncompliant, does not grossly violate social norms (e.g., anger, argumentativeness, resentment toward authority figures) • Remits by adulthood in 25% of children • May progress to conduct disorder

III. Other Disorders of Childhood

A. Tourette's disorder

1. Tourette's disorder is characterized by **involuntary movements and vocalizations (tics),** often including the involuntary use of profanity. While these behaviors can be controlled briefly, they must ultimately be expressed.

2. The disorder, which is **lifelong and chronic,** begins before age 18, usually between the ages of 7 and 8.

3. While the manifestations are behavioral, the **etiology** of Tourette's is neurological. **It is believed to involve dysfunctional regulation of dopamine in the caudate nucleus.**

4. The disorder is three times **more common in males** and has a **strong genetic component.**

5. There is a **genetic relationship** between Tourette's and both **ADHD** and **obsessive-compulsive disorder** (see Chapter 13).

6. **Haloperidol** and some other antipsychotic agents are the most effective treatment for Tourette disorder.

B. Separation anxiety disorder

1. Often incorrectly called "school phobia," because the child refuses to go to school, this disorder is characterized by an **overwhelming fear of loss of a major attachment figure,** particularly the mother.

2. The child often complains of **physical symptoms,** (e.g., stomach pain or headache) to avoid going to school and leaving the mother.

3. Individuals with a history of separation anxiety disorder in childhood are at **greater risk for anxiety disorders in adulthood,** particularly agoraphobia.

C. Selective mutism

1. Children (more commonly girls) with this rare disorder **speak in some social situations** (e.g., at home) **but not in others** (e.g., at school); the child may whisper or communicate with hand gestures.

2. Selective mutism must be distinguished from normal shyness.

Review Test

Directions: Each of the numbered items or incomplete statements in this section is followed by answers or by completions of the statement. Select the **one** lettered answer or completion that is **best** in each case.

Questions 1–2

Since the age of 8, a 13-year-old boy has shown a number of repetitive motor movements. He recently has begun to have outbursts in which he curses and shrieks. When asked if he can control the vocalizations and movements he says "For a short time only; it is like holding your breath—eventually you have to let it out."

1. This child is most likely to be suffering from

(A) autistic disorder
(B) Rett's disorder
(C) attention-deficit hyperactivity disorder (ADHD)
(D) Tourette's disorder
(E) selective mutism

2. The most effective treatment to reduce the unwanted vocalizations and movements is

(A) antipsychotic medication
(B) provision of a structured environment
(C) antidepressant medication
(D) tacrine
(E) reassurance

3. A 9-year-old boy with normal intelligence has a history of fighting with other children and catching and torturing birds, squirrels, and rabbits. When asked why he engages in this behavior, he says "it's just fun." The best description of this child's behavior is

(A) normal
(B) attention-deficit hyperactivity disorder (ADHD)
(C) autistic disorder
(D) oppositional defiant disorder
(E) conduct disorder

Questions 4–6

A 9-year-old boy with normal intelligence frequently gets into trouble at school because he interrupts the teacher, disturbs the other students and cannot seem to sit still in class. However, the child works well and productively when alone with his tutor.

4. The best description of this child's behavior is

(A) normal
(B) attention-deficit hyperactivity disorder (ADHD)
(C) autistic disorder
(D) oppositional defiant disorder
(E) conduct disorder

5. Which of the following is most closely involved in the etiology of this child's problem?

(A) Neurological dysfunction
(B) Improper diet
(C) Food allergy
(D) Excessive punishment
(E) Excessive leniency

6. The most effective treatment for this child is

(A) lithium
(B) a stimulant
(C) an antidepressant
(D) a sedative
(E) psychotherapy

7. A 3-year-old boy with normal intelligence cannot seem to sit still for more than 15 minutes at a time in nursery school. He squirms in his seat and often gets out of his seat to walk around. The best description for this child's behavior is

(A) normal
(B) attention-deficit hyperactivity disorder (ADHD)
(C) autistic disorder
(D) oppositional defiant disorder
(E) conduct disorder

Answers and Explanations

TBQ-A. This child who has never spoken voluntarily and who shows no interest in or connection to his parents, other adults, or other children despite normal hearing is suffering from autistic disorder, a pervasive developmental disorder of childhood. He turns on the tap to watch the water running because, as with many autistic children, repetitive motion calms him. Any change in his environment, such as being dressed, leads to intense discomfort, struggling, and screaming. Selective mutism, speaking in some social situations but not in others, is associated with otherwise normal development. Attention-deficit hyperactivity disorder (ADHD) involves normal development of speech and social interaction but difficulty paying attention or sitting still. Rett's disorder occurs after a period of normal function and only occurs in girls. Tourette's disorder involves unwanted vocalizations and motor tics but otherwise normal motor and social development.

1-D, 2-A. This child is most likely to be suffering from Tourette's disorder, a chronic neurological condition with behavioral manifestations. The unwanted vocalizations and motor tics can be controlled only briefly and then they must be expressed (see also answer to TBQ above). The most effective treatment for this child is antipsychotic medication such as haloperidol. There is no evidence that provision of a structured environment, antidepressant medication, or an acetylcholinesterase inhibitor (i.e., tacrine) are helpful for control of motor or vocal tics. Reassurance can help patients with many disorders but is not the most effective treatment for the symptoms of Tourette's disorder.

3-E. This child is demonstrating conduct disorder. Children with this disorder have no concern for others or for animals (i.e., this child finds torturing animals "fun"). Children with conduct disorder generally have normal intelligence. They often set fires and are truant. Children with attention-deficit hyperactivity disorder (ADHD) have trouble controlling their behavior but do not intentionally cause harm. Children with oppositional defiant disorder have problems dealing with authority figures but not with other children or animals. See TBQ for a discussion of autistic disorder.

4-B, 5-A, 6-B. This 9-year-old boy who gets into trouble at school because he disturbs the teacher and the other students and cannot seem to sit still is suffering from attention-deficit hyperactivity disorder (ADHD) (see also answer to Question 3). Children with ADHD can often learn well when there are few distractions (i.e., alone with a tutor). ADHD is believed to result from neurological dysfunction. Although anecdotal evidence has been put forward, scientific studies have not revealed an association between ADHD and either improper diet (e.g., excessive sugar intake) or food allergy (e.g., to artificial colors or flavors). The disorder also is not a result of parenting style (e.g., excessive punishment or leniency). However, in part because of their difficult behavior, children with ADHD are more likely to be physically abused by parents. The most effective treatment for children with ADHD is use of central nervous system stimulants including methylphenidate [Ritalin], dextroamphetamine sulfate [Dexedrine], and pemoline [Cylert]. Lithium is used to treat bipolar disorder, antidepressants are used primarily to treat depression, and sedatives are used primarily to treat anxiety. While psychotherapy may help, it is not the most effective treatment since the disorder is caused by neurological dysfunction.

7-A. The best description for this child's behavior is normal. A normal 3-year-old child cannot be expected to sit still for more than 15 minutes at a time (see also answer to Question 3). Normal school age children should be able to sit still and pay attention for longer periods of time.

16

Biologic Therapies: Psychopharmacology and Electroconvulsive Therapy

Typical Board Question

A 26-year-old man comes to the emergency department with elevated blood pressure, sweating, headache, and vomiting. His companion tells you that the patient became ill at a party where he ate pizza and drank punch. The drug that this patient is most likely to be taking is

(A) fluoxetine
(B) lithium
(C) nortriptyline
(D) phenelzine
(E) haloperidol

(See "Answers and Explanations" at end of Chapter)

I. Overview

    A. Neurotransmitter abnormalities are involved in the etiology of many psychiatric illnesses (e.g., psychotic disorders, mood disorders, anxiety disorders) (see Chapter 4).

    B. Normalization of such levels by **pharmacologic agents** can ameliorate many of the symptoms of these disorders.

    C. Psychopharmacologic agents also may be useful in the **treatment of symptoms of certain medical conditions** (e.g., gastrointestinal problems, pain, seizures).

II. Antipsychotic Agents

    A. Overview

        1. Antipsychotic agents (formerly called neuroleptics or major tranquilizers) are used in the treatment of **schizophrenia** as well as in the treatment of psychotic symptoms associated with other **psychiatric and physical disorders.**

2. **Antipsychotics are also used medically to treat** nausea, hiccups, intense anxiety and agitation, and Tourette's disorder.

3. Although antipsychotics commonly are taken daily by mouth, noncompliant patients can be treated with long-acting **"depot"** forms such as **haloperidol decanoate** administered intramuscularly every 4 weeks.

4. Antipsychotic agents can be classified as **"traditional"** or **"atypical"** depending on their mode of action and side effect profile.

B. **"Traditional"** antipsychotic agents

1. Traditional antipsychotic agents act primarily by **blocking central D_2** receptors.

2. Although negative symptoms of schizophrenia, such as withdrawal, **may** improve with continued treatment, traditional antipsychotic agents **are most effective against positive symptoms** such as hallucinations and delusions (see Chapter 11).

3. Traditional antipsychotics are classified according to their potency.
   a. **Low-potency** agents, (e.g., chlorpromazine [Thorazine], and thioridazine [Mellaril]) are associated primarily with **non-neurologic** adverse effects (Table 16-1).
   b. **High-potency** agents, (e.g. haloperidol [Haldol], trifluoperazine [Stelazine], pimozide [Orap] and perphenazine [Trilafon]) are associated primarily with **neurologic** adverse effects (see Table 16-1).

C. **"Atypical"** antipsychotic agents, (e.g., clozapine [Clozaril], risperidone [Risperdal], olanzapine [Zyprexa], and quetiapine [Seroquel])

1. Atypical agents are used to treat psychosis in patients who cannot use traditional antipsychotics because of **treatment resistance (inadequate clinical response to other agents) or adverse effects.**

2. In contrast to traditional antipsychotic agents, a **major mechanism of action** of atypical antipsychotics appears to be on **serotonergic systems.** They also affect dopaminergic systems, primarily as D_4-receptor antagonists.

3. **Advantages** of atypical agents over traditional agents
   a. Atypical agents may be **more effective** when used to treat the **negative,** chronic, and refractory **symptoms** of schizophrenia (see Chapter 11).
   b. They are **less likely to cause extrapyramidal symptoms, tardive dyskinesia,** and **neuroleptic malignant syndrome.**

4. **Disadvantages** of atypical agents
   a. Atypical agents may increase the likelihood of hematologic problems, such as **agranulocytosis** (with clozapine as the most problematic agent).
   b. They may also increase the likelihood of **seizures** and anticholinergic side effects.

Table 16-1. Adverse Effects of Antipsychotic Agents

System	Adverse Effects
Non-neurological adverse effects. More common with traditional, low-potency agents	
Circulatory	• Orthostatic (postural) hypotension • Electrocardiogram abnormalities • Thioridazine is most cardiotoxic in overdose
Endocrine	• Increase in prolactin level results in gynecomastia (breast enlargement), galactorrhea, erectile dysfunction, amenorrhea, and decreased libido
Hematologic	• Leukopenia; agranulocytosis (decreased number of certain white blood cells, particularly polymorphonuclear leukocytes) • Usually occur in the first 3 months of treatment
Hepatic	• Jaundice; elevated liver enzyme levels • Usually occur in the first month of treatment • More common with chlorpromazine
Dermatologic	• Skin eruptions, photosensitivity, and blue-gray skin discoloration • More common with chlorpromazine
Ophthalmologic	• Irreversible retinal pigmentation with thioridazine • Deposits in lens and cornea with chlorpromazine
Anticholinergic	• Peripheral effects: Dry mouth, constipation, urinary retention, and blurred vision • Central effects: Agitation and disorientation
Antihistaminergic	• Weight gain and sedation • Chlorpromazine is most sedating
Neurological adverse effects: More common with traditional high-potency agents	
Extrapyramidal	• Pseudoparkinsonism (muscle rigidity, shuffling gait, resting tremor, mask-like facial expression) • Akathisia (subjective feeling of motor restlessness) • Acute dystonia (prolonged muscular spasms; more common in men under age 40) • Treat with anticholinergic (e.g., benztropine) or antihistaminergic (e.g., diphenhydramine) agent
Other	• Tardive dyskinesia (abnormal writhing movements of the tongue, face, and body; more common in women and after at least 6 months of treatment); to treat, substitute low potency or atypical antipsychotic agent • Neuroleptic malignant syndrome (high fever, sweating, increased pulse and blood pressure, muscular rigidity; more common in men and early in treatment; mortality rate about 20%); to treat, stop agent and provide medical support • Decreased seizure threshold

III. Antidepressant Agents

A. Overview

1. **Heterocyclic antidepressants** (tricyclic and tetracyclic), **selective serotonin reuptake inhibitors (SSRIs), monoamine oxidase inhibitors (MAOIs),** and **atypical antidepressants** are used to treat depression. These agents also have other clinical uses (Table 16-2).

2. While heterocyclics were once the mainstay of treatment, because of their more **positive side effect profile, SSRIs** (e.g., fluoxetine [Prozac]) are now used as **first-line agents.**

3. All antidepressants **take about 3–6 weeks to work** and **all have equal efficacy.**

Table 16-2. Antidepressant Agents (grouped alphabetically by category)

Agent [brand name]	Effects	Clinical Uses in Addition to Depression
Heterocyclic Agents (HCAs)		
Amytriptyline [Elavil]	• Sedating • Anticholinergic	• Depression with insomnia • Chronic pain
Clomipramine [Anafranil]	• Most serotonin-specific of the HCAs	• Obsessive-compulsive disorder (OCD)
Desipramine [Norpramin, Pertofrane]	• Least sedating of the HCAs • Least anticholinergic of the HCAs • Stimulates appetite	• Depression in the elderly • Enuresis • Eating disorders
Doxepin [Adapin, Sinequan]	• Sedating, antihista-minergic • Anticholinergic	• Generalized anxiety disorder • Peptic ulcer disease
Imipramine [Tofranil]	• Likely to cause orthostatic hypotension	• Panic disorder with agoraphobia • Enuresis • Eating disorders
Maprotiline [Ludiomil]	• Low cardiotoxicity • May cause seizures	• Anxiety with depressive features
Nortriptyline [Aventyl, Pamelor]	• Least likely of the HCAs to cause orthostatic hypotension	• First choice for depression in the elderly • Patients with cardiac diseases
Selective Serotonin Reuptake Inhibitors (SSRIs)		
Fluoxetine [Prozac]	• May cause agitation and insomnia initially • Sexual dysfunction • May uniquely cause weight loss	• OCD • Premature ejaculation • Panic disorder • Premenstrual syndrome • Social phobia (paroxative)
Paroxetine [Paxil]	• Most serotonin-specific and sedative of the SSRIs • Sexual dysfunction	
Sertraline [Zoloft]	• Most likely of the SSRIs to cause gastrointestinal disturbances (e.g., diarrhea) • Sexual dysfunction	
Fluvoxamine [Luvox]	• Currently indicated only for OCD	
Monoamine Oxidase Inhibitors (MAOIs)		
Isocarboxazid [Marplan] Phenelzine [Nardil] Tranylcypromine [Parnate]	• Hyperadrenergic crisis precipitated by ingestion of pressor amines in tyramine-containing foods or sympatho-mimetic drugs	• Atypical depression • Pain disorders • Eating disorders • Panic disorder • Social phobia (phenelzine)

continued

Table 16-2. Antidepressant Agents (*continued*)

Agent [brand name]	Effects	Clinical Uses in Addition to Depression
Other Antidepressants		
Amoxapine [Asendin]	• Antidopaminergic effects (e.g., parkinsonian symptoms, galactorrhea, sexual dysfunction) • Most dangerous in overdose	• Depression with psychotic features
Bupropion [Wellbutrin, Zyban]	• Insomnia • Seizures • Sweating • Fewer adverse sexual effects	• Refractory depression (inadequate clinical response to other antidepressants) • Smoking cessation • Seasonal affective disorder (SAD) • Adult attention-deficit hyperactivity disorder
Mirtazapine [Remeron]	• Targets specific serotonin receptors and causes fewer adverse effects	• Refractory depression • Lack of appetite
Nefazodone [Serzone]	• Related to trazodone, but causes less sedation and priapism	• Refractory depression • Depression with anxiety • Insomnia
Trazodone [Desyrel]	• Sedation • Priapism • Safe in overdose	• Insomnia
Venlafaxine [Effexor]	• Serotonergic • Noradrenergic • Low cytochrome P450 effects	• Refractory depression • Generalized anxiety disorder

4. Antidepressant agents **do not elevate mood in nondepressed people** and **have no abuse potential.**

5. **Stimulants,** such as **methylphenidate** or **dextroamphetamine,** may also be useful in treating depression. They work quickly, and thus may help to improve mood in terminally ill or elderly patients. They are also useful in patients with depression refractory to other treatments and in those at risk for the development of adverse effects of other agents for depression. Disadvantages include their addiction potential.

B. **Heterocyclic Agents**

1. **Heterocyclic antidepressants block reuptake of norepinephrine and serotonin** at the synapse, increasing the availability of these neurotransmitters and improving mood. (see Chapter 4)

    a. These agents also block muscarinic acetylcholine receptors, resulting in **anticholinergic effects,** (e.g., dry mouth, blurred vision, urine retention, constipation)

    b. Histamine receptors are also blocked by heterocyclic agents, resulting in antihistiminergic effects (e.g., **weight gain and sedation**).

2. Other adverse effects include precipitation of manic episodes in potentially bipolar patients, cardiovascular effects such as orthostatic hypotension, neurologic effects such as tremor, weight gain, and sexual dysfunction.

3. **Heterocyclics are dangerous in overdose.**

C. SSRIs

1. **SSRIs selectively block the reuptake of serotonin,** increasing its availability in the synapse and improving mood. (see Chapter 4)

2. SSRIs have little effect on dopamine, norepinephrine, acetylcholine, or histamine systems.

3. Because of this selectivity, **SSRIs cause fewer side effects** and are **safer in overdose** than heterocyclics or MAOIs.

D. MAOIs

1. MAOIs inhibit the breakdown of neurotransmitters by monoamine oxidase (MAO) in the brain in an irreversible reaction, thereby **increasing norepinephrine and serotonin availability** in the synapse and improving mood.

2. These agents may be particularly useful in the treatment of **atypical depression** (see Chapter 12) and treatment resistence to other agents.

3. A major drawback of use of MAOIs is **a potentially fatal reaction** when they are taken **in conjunction with certain foods.** This reaction occurs because

   a. **MAO metabolizes tyramine, a pressor,** in the gastrointestinal tract.

   b. If MAO is inhibited, ingestion of **tyramine-rich foods** (e.g., aged cheese, beer, wine, broad beans, beef or chicken liver, and smoked or pickled meats or fish) or **sympathomimetic drugs** (e.g., ephedrine, methylphenidate [Ritalin], phenylephrine [Neo-Synephrine], pseudoephedrine [Sudafed]) can increase tyramine levels.

   c. Increase in tyramine can cause elevated blood pressure, sweating, headache, and vomiting (i.e., a **hypertensive crisis**), which in turn can lead to **stroke and death.**

4. MAOIs and SSRIs used together can cause a potentially life-threatening drug-drug interaction, **the serotonin syndrome,** marked by autonomic instability, hyperthermia, convulsions, coma, and death.

5. Other adverse effects of MAOIs are similar to those of the heterocyclics, including danger in overdose.

IV. Mood Stabilizers: Agents Used to Treat Mania

A. **Lithium** (carbonate and citrate)

1. Lithium is a mood stabilizer which is used **to prevent** both the manic and depressive phases of bipolar disorder.

2. It may be used also to **increase the effectiveness of antidepressant agents** in depressive illness and to **control aggressive behavior.** (see Chapter 20)

3. **Adverse effects** of chronic use of lithium include

   a. congenital abnormalities (particularly of the cardiovascular system)

   b. hypothyroidism

   c. tremor

    d. renal dysfunction

    e. cardiac conduction problems

    f. gastric distress

    g. mild cognitive impairment

  4. Lithium **takes 2–3 weeks to work.** Haloperidol is therefore the initial treatment for psychotic symptoms in an acute manic episode.

  5. Because of **potential toxicity,** blood levels of lithium must be maintained at 0.8–1.3 mEqL.

B. Anticonvulsants: Carbamazepine [Tegretol] and Valproic Acid [Depakene, Depakote]

  1. Anticonvulsants are also used to treat mania, particularly **rapid cycling bipolar disorder** (i.e., more than 4 episodes annually) and **mixed episodes** (mania and depression occurring at the same time).

  2. Carbamazepine may be associated with severe adverse effects such as **aplastic anemia and agranulocytosis.**

  3. Valproic acid may be particularly useful for treating bipolar symptoms resulting from cognitive disorders (see Chapter 14) and for prophylaxis of migraine headaches.

  4. Adverse effects of valproic acid include gastrointestinal and liver problems, congenital neural tube defects, and alopecia (hair loss).

V. Antianxiety Agents. These agents are also known as anxiolytics or minor tranquilizers.

A. Benzodiazepines

  1. These agents have a short, intermediate, or long onset and duration of action and may be used to treat disorders other than anxiety disorders (Table 16-3).

  2. Their characteristics of action are related to their clinical indications and their potential for abuse; for example, short-acting agents are good hypnotics (sleep inducers) but have a higher potential for abuse than longer acting agents.

  3. Benzodiazepines commonly cause **sedation** but have few other adverse effects.

  4. Tolerance and dependence may occur with chronic use of these agents.

  5. Flumazenil [Mazicon, Romazicon] is a benzodiazepine receptor antagonist which can reverse the effects of benzodiazepines in cases of overdose or when used for a surgical procedure.

B. Nonbenzodiazepines

  1. Buspirone [BuSpar], an azaspirodecanedione, is not related to the benzodiazepines.

    a. In contrast to benzodiazepines, buspirone is **nonsedating,** and is **not associated with dependence, abuse,** or **withdrawal** problems.

    b. It is used primarily to treat conditions causing chronic anxiety in

Table 16-3. Antianxiety Agents (grouped alphabetically by duration of action and category)

Agent [brand name]	Duration of Action	Clinical Uses in Addition to Anxiety
Benzodiazepines		
Chlorazepate [Tranxene]	Short	Management of partial seizures
Lorazepam [Ativan]	Short	Psychotic agitation, alcohol withdrawal (particularly for hallucinations), status epilepticus (persistent seizures)
Oxazepam [Serax]	Short	Alcohol withdrawal
Triazolam [Halcion]	Short	Insomnia
Alprazolam [Xanax]	Intermediate	Depression; panic disorder; social phobia
Temazepam [Restoril]	Intermediate	Insomnia
Chlordiazepoxide [Librium]	Long	First choice for alcohol withdrawal (particularly for agitation and delirium)
Clonazepam [Klonopin]	Long	Seizures, mania, social phobia, panic disorder, aggression, adjuncts with mood stabilizers
Diazepam [Valium]	Long	Muscle relaxation, analgesia, anticonvulsant, alcohol withdrawal (particularly for seizures)
Flurazepam [Dalmane]	Long	Insomnia
Nonbenzodiazepines		
Zolpidem (Ambien)	Short	Insomnia
Buspirone (BuSpar)	Very long	Anxiety in the elderly, generalized anxiety disorder

      which benzodiazepine dependence can become a problem (e.g., **generalized anxiety disorder** (see Chapter 13).

    c. Buspirone **takes up to 2 weeks to work** and may not be acceptable to patients who are accustomed to taking the fast acting benzodiazepines for their symptoms.

  2. Zolpidem tartrate (Ambien) is a short acting agent unrelated to the benzodiazepines and used primarily to treat insomnia.

  3. Carbamates (e.g., meprobamate [Miltown]) are used only rarely because they have a greater potential for abuse and a lower therapeutic index than benzodiazepines.

VI. Electroconvulsive Therapy (ECT)

  A. Uses of ECT

    1. ECT provides **rapid, effective, safe** treatment for some psychiatric disturbances.

      a. It is most commonly used to treat **major depressive disorder** that **is refractory to antidepressants.**

      b. ECT may be indicated also for serious **depressive symptoms from any cause,** particularly when rapid symptom resolution is imperative because of **suicide risk** (see Chapter 12).

      c. ECT is particularly useful for treating **depression in the elderly** because it may be safer than long-term use of antidepressant agents.

  2. ECT may alter neurotransmitter function in a manner similar to that of treatment with antidepressant drugs.

B. Administration

  1. ECT involves inducing a **generalized seizure** lasting 25–60 seconds by **passing an electric current across the brain.**

  2. Prior to seizure induction, the patient is **premedicated** (e.g., with atropine) followed by general anesthesia and a muscle relaxant to prevent injury during the seizure.

  3. ECT can be **unilateral** (two electrodes placed on the nondominant hemisphere) or **bilateral** (one electrode placed on each temple). With unilateral ECT, there are fewer side effects but less efficacy than with bilateral ECT.

  4. Improvement in mood typically **begins after a few ECT treatments.** A maximum response to ECT is usually seen after 5–10 treatments given over a 2–3 week period.

B. Problems associated with ECT

  1. The **major adverse effect** of ECT is **retrograde amnesia** (i.e., forgetting past events). In most patients, this memory impairment resolves within 6 months after treatment concludes.

  2. **Increased intracranial pressure is the major contraindication** for ECT.

  3. The mortality rate associated with ECT is comparable to that associated with the induction of general anesthesia.

Review Test

Directions: Each of the numbered items or incomplete statements in this section is followed by answers or by completions of the statement. Select the **one** lettered answer or completion that is **best** in each case.

1. A 25-year-old male schizophrenic patient reports that he has difficulty staying awake during the daytime and waking up in the morning. The antipsychotic agent that this patient is most likely to be taking is

(A) haloperidol
(B) chlorpromazine
(C) perphenazine
(D) clozapine
(E) trifluoperazine

2. A 30-year-old male schizophrenic patient is taking an antipsychotic agent which is helping him to be more outgoing and sociable. However, the patient is experiencing seizures and a blood test reveals agranulocytosis. The antipsychotic agent that this patient is most likely to be taking is:

(A) haloperidol
(B) chlorpromazine
(C) perphenazine
(D) clozapine
(E) trifluoperazine

Questions 3–4

A 54-year-old chronic schizophrenic patient has begun to show involuntary chewing and lip-smacking movements.

3. These signs indicate that the patient is experiencing a side effect of antipsychotic medication known as

(A) tardive dyskinesia
(B) neuroleptic malignant syndrome
(C) pseudoparkinsonism
(D) dystonia
(E) akathisia

4. The side effect described in Question 3 is best treated initially

(A) by changing to a low potency antipsychotic agent
(B) with an antianxiety agent
(C) with an antidepressant agent
(D) with an anticonvulsant
(E) by stopping the antipsychotic agent

Questions 5–6

5. A 25-year-old patient who has taken haloperidol for the past 2 months is brought to the hospital with a temperature of 104°F, blood pressure of 190/110, and muscular rigidity. These signs indicate that the patient has an antipsychotic medication side effect known as

(A) tardive dyskinesia
(B) neuroleptic malignant syndrome
(C) pseudoparkinsonism
(D) dystonia
(E) akathisia

6. The side effect described in Questions 5 is best treated initially

(A) by changing to a low potency antipsychotic agent
(B) with an antianxiety agent
(C) with an antidepressant agent
(D) with an anticonvulsant
(E) by stopping the antipsychotic agent

7. A 65-year-old patient taking haloperidol [Haldol] develops a resting tremor, mask-like facial expression, and difficulty initiating movement. After reducing the haloperidol, the next step the doctor should take to relieve these symptoms is to give the patient

(A) a high potency antipsychotic agent
(B) an anticholinergic agent
(C) an antianxiety agent
(D) an antidepressant agent
(E) an antimanic agent

8. A 30-year old woman tells you that she must drive over the route she takes home from work each day at least three times to be sure that she did not hit an animal in the road. Of the following, the most appropriate pharmacological treatment for this patient is:

(A) a high potency antipsychotic agent
(B) an anticholinergic agent
(C) an antianxiety agent
(D) an antidepressant agent
(E) an antimanic agent

9. A 45-year-old woman presents with the symptoms of a major depressive episode. The patient has never previously taken an antidepressant. Her physician decides to give her fluoxetine (Prozac). The most likely reason for this choice is that when compared to a heterocyclic antidepressant, fluoxetine

(A) is more effective
(B) works faster
(C) has fewer side effects
(D) is less likely to be abused
(E) is longer lasting

10. The best choice of antianxiety agent for a 40-year-old woman with generalized anxiety disorder and a history of benzodiazepine abuse is

(A) triazolam
(B) flurazepam
(C) clonazepam
(D) buspirone
(E) chlordiazepoxide

11. A 40-year-old businessman who has been a physician's patient for the past 5 years asks her for a medication to help him sleep on an overnight flight to Australia. The best antianxiety agent for this use is

(A) triazolam
(B) flurazepam
(C) clonazepam
(D) buspirone
(E) chlordiazepoxide

12. A 57-year-old male patient with a history of alcoholism has decided to stop drinking. The antianxiety agent most commonly used to treat anxiety and agitation associated with the initial stages of alcohol withdrawal is

(A) triazolam
(B) flurazepam
(C) clonazepam
(D) buspirone
(E) chlordiazepoxide

13. Which of the following psychotropic agents is most likely to be abused?

(A) Diazepam [Valium]
(B) Haloperidol [Haldol]
(C) Fluoxetine [Prozac]
(D) Buspirone [BuSpar]
(E) Lithium

14. An elderly, severely depressed, suicidal patient has not responded to any antidepressant medication. The physician's most appropriate next step is to recommend

(A) diazepam
(B) electroconvulsive therapy (ECT)
(C) psychotherapy
(D) buspirone (BuSpar)
(E) lithium

Questions 15–16

A 30-year-old patient is brought to the emergency department after being found running down the street naked. He is speaking very quickly and tells you that he has just given his clothing and all of his money to a homeless man. He states that God spoke to him and told him to do this. His history reveals that he is a practicing attorney who is married with 3 children.

15. The most effective immediate treatment for this patient is

(A) lithium
(B) fluoxetine
(C) amitriptyline
(D) diazepam
(E) haloperidol

16. The most effective long term treatment for this patient is

(A) lithium
(B) fluoxetine
(C) amitriptyline
(D) diazepam
(E) haloperidol

17. What is the most appropriate agent for a doctor to recommend for a 34-year-old overweight, depressed patient who needs to take an antidepressant but is afraid of gaining weight?

(A) Isocarboxazid
(B) Tranylcypromine
(C) Trazodone
(D) Doxepin
(E) Amoxapine
(F) Fluoxetine
(G) Desipramine
(H) Nortriptyline
(I) Amitriptyline
(J) Imipramine

18. What is the antidepressant agent most likely to cause persistent erections (priapism) in a 40-year-old male patient?

(A) Isocarboxazid
(B) Tranylcypromine
(C) Trazodone
(D) Doxepin
(E) Amoxapine
(F) Fluoxetine
(G) Desipramine
(H) Nortriptyline
(I) Amitriptyline
(J) Imipramine

19. Which of the following antidepressant agents is most likely to cause gynecomastia in a 45-year-old male patient?

(A) Isocarboxazid
(B) Tranylcypromine
(C) Trazodone
(D) Doxepin
(E) Amoxapine
(F) Fluoxetine
(G) Desipramine
(H) Nortriptyline
(I) Amitriptyline
(J) Imipramine

20. What is the most appropriate heterocyclic antidepressant agent for an 82-year-old woman?

(A) Isocarboxazid
(B) Tranylcypromine
(C) Trazodone
(D) Doxepin
(E) Amoxapine
(F) Fluoxetine
(G) Desipramine
(H) Nortriptyline
(I) Amitriptyline
(J) Imipramine

Answers and Explanations

TBQ-D. This patient who became ill at a pizza party is most likely to be taking phenelzine, a monoamine oxidase inhibitor (MAOI). These agents can cause a hypertensive crisis if certain foods (e.g., aged cheese, smoked meats, beer and wine) are ingested. A patient who eats in an unfamiliar place (e.g., a party) may unwittingly ingest forbidden foods. This patient unwittingly ate pizza that probably contained aged Parmesan cheese and drank punch that probably contained wine. This resulted in a hypertensive crisis (e.g., elevated blood pressure, sweating, headache, and vomiting). Fluoxetine, lithium, nortriptyline, and haloperidol do not interact negatively with food.

1-B. The antipsychotic agent that this somnolent patient is most likely to be taking is chlorpromazine. Chlorpromazine is more sedating than haloperidol, perphenazine, clozapine, or trifluoperazine.

2-D. The antipsychotic agent that this patient is most likely to be taking is clozapine. Clozapine, an atypical agent, is more effective against negative symptoms (e.g., withdrawal), but also is more likely to cause seizures and agranulocytosis than traditional agents like haloperidol, chlorpromazine, perphenazine or trifluoperazine.

3-A, 4-A. These involuntary chewing and lip smacking movements indicate that the patient has developed tardive dyskinesia, a side effect of treatment with antipsychotic medication. Other side effects particulary of high potency antipsychotic agents include neuroleptic malignant syndrome (high fever, sweating, increased pulse and blood pressure and muscular rigidity), pseudoparkinsonism (muscle rigidity, shuffling gait, resting tremor, and mask-like facial expression), akathisia (a subjective feeling of motor restlessness) and dystonia (prolonged muscular spasms). Tardive dyskinesia usually occurs after at least 6 months of starting a high potency antipsychotic and is best treated by changing to a low potency or atypical agent; stopping the antipsychotic medication will exacerbate the symptoms.

5-B. High body temperature and blood pressure and muscular rigidity indicate that the patient has an antipsychotic medication side effect known as neuroleptic malignant syndrome (and see answer to Question 3).

6-E. Neuroleptic malignant syndrome is seen with a high potency antipsychotic treatment and is best relieved by stopping the antipsychotic medication and providing medical support. After recovering from this life-threatening condition, the patient can be put on a low potency agent.

7-B. This patient is suffering from pseudoparkinsonism due to haloperidol treatment. After reducing the haloperidol, the next step the doctor should take is to give the patient an anticholinergic agent. Any antipsychotic (particularly high potency agents like haloperidol) can cause these symptoms. Benzodiazepines, antidepressants and antimanic agents are not the next step in treatment for this patient.

8-D. The most effective pharmacological treatment for this patient who is suffering from obsessive compulsive disorder is an antidepressant, particularly a selective serotonin reuptake inhibitor (see Chapter 13). Antipsychotics, antimanics, and antianxiety agents are less appropriate than an antidepressant for this patient.

9-C. The doctor probably decides to give this patient fluoxetine [Prozac] because, when compared to a heterocyclic antidepressant, fluoxetine has fewer side effects. Heterocyclics and selective serotonin reuptake inhibitors (SSRIs) like fluoxetine have equal efficacy, equivalent speed of action, and equivalent length of action. Neither SSRIs, nor heterocyclics are likely to be abused.

10-D. The best choice of antianxiety agent for a 40-year-old patient with generalized anxiety disorder and a history of benzodiazepine abuse is buspirone, a non-benzodiazepine with a very low abuse potential. All the other choices are benzodiazepines and thus all have more abuse potential.

11-A. Triazolam [Halcion], a short-acting, hypnotic benzodiazepine, is the best choice to aid sleep on an overnight flight.

12-E. Because it is long acting and has a relatively low abuse potential for a benzodiazepine, chlordiazepoxide is the antianxiety agent most commonly used to treat the anxiety and agitation associated with the initial stages of alcohol withdrawal.

13-A. Of the listed agents, benzodiazepines like diazepam are most likely to be abused. Antipsychotics such as haloperidol, antidepressants like fluoxetine, antimanics like lithium and nonbenzodiazepines like buspirone (see answer to Question 10) have little or no abuse potential.

14-B. The most appropriate next step is to recommend a course of electroconvulsive therapy (ECT) for this elderly, severely depressed patient. ECT is a safe, fast, effective treatment for major depression. Diazepam, lithium, buspirone, and psychotherapy are much less likely to be effective for this patient.

15-E, 16-A. This patient's good employment and relationship history suggest that his psychotic symptoms are an acute manifestation of a manic episode. While the most effective immediate treatment for this patient is haloperidol to control his hallucinations and delusions, lithium, which takes 2–3 weeks to work, would be more effective for long-term maintenance. Fluoxetine, amitriptyline, and diazepam are not appropriate primary treatments for this bipolar patient.

17-F. In contrast to most antidepressant agents which are associated with weight gain, fluoxetine (Prozac) is associated with weight loss. Thus it is the most appropriate antidepressant agent for a patient who is afraid of gaining weight.

18-C. Trazadone is the agent most likely to cause priapism in a male patient.

19-E. Amoxapine has antidopaminergic action and thus is the agent most likely to cause gynecomastia as well as parkinsonian symptoms in a male patient.

20-H. Because it has few cardiovascular effects and is unlikely to cause orthostatic hypotension, nortriptyline is the most appropriate heterocyclic agent for this elderly patient. Fluoxetine, while also appropriate, is an SSRI not a heteroyclic.

17

Psychological Therapies

Typical Board Question

A 35-year-old man who is afraid of heights is instructed to stand in the observation tower of the Empire State Building and look down until he is no longer afraid. This method of treatment is best described as

(A) implosion
(B) systematic desensitization
(C) cognitive therapy
(D) flooding
(E) token economy

I. Psychoanalysis and Related Therapies

A. Overview

1. Psychoanalysis and related therapies (e.g., psychoanalytically-oriented psychotherapy, brief dynamic psychotherapy) are **psychotherapeutic treatments** based on Freud's concepts of the **unconscious mind and defense mechanisms** (see Chapter 6).

2. The central strategy of these therapies is to **uncover experiences** that are **repressed in the unconscious mind** and integrate them into the person's conscious mind and personality.

B. Techniques that are used to recover repressed experiences include

1. **Free association**

   a. In psychoanalysis, the person **lies on a couch** in a reclined position facing away from the therapist and says whatever comes to mind.

   b. In therapies related to psychoanalysis, the person sits in a chair and talks while facing the therapist.

2. **Interpretation of dreams** is used to examine unconscious conflicts and impulses.

3. **Analysis of transference reactions** (i.e., the person's unconscious responses to the therapist) is used to examine important past relationships (see Chapter 6).

C. People who are appropriate for using psychoanalysis and related therapies should have the following characteristics:

1. Are younger than 40 years of age

2. Are intelligent and not psychotic

3. Have good relationships with others (e.g., no evidence of antisocial or borderline personality disorder)

4. Have a stable life situation (e.g., not be in the midst of divorce)

5. Have the time and money to spend on treatment

D. In **psychoanalysis,** people receive treatment **4–5 times weekly for 3–4 years;** related therapies are briefer and more direct (e.g., brief dynamic psychotherapy is limited to 12–40 weekly sessions).

II. Behavioral and Cognitive Therapies

A. Behavioral and cognitive therapies are based on **learning theory** (i.e., relieving the person's symptoms by unlearning maladaptive behavior patterns) (see Chapter 7).

B. In contrast to psychoanalysis and related therapies, the person's history and **unconscious conflicts are irrelevant** and thus are not examined in behavioral and cognitive therapies.

C. Characteristics of specific behavioral and cognitive therapies (e.g., systematic desensitization, aversive conditioning, flooding and implosion, token economy, and biofeedback) can be found in **Table 17-1.**

III. Other Therapies

Other therapies include group, family, marital, supportive, and interpersonal therapy. Specific uses of these therapies can be found in **Table 17-2.**

A. **Group therapy**

1. **Groups with therapists**

a. Groups of about 8 people usually meet weekly for 1–2 hours.

b. Members of the group provide the opportunity to express feelings as well as **feedback, support,** and **friendship** to each other.

c. **The therapist has little input.** He or she facilitates and observes the members interpersonal interactions.

2. **Leaderless groups**

a. In a leaderless group, **no one person is in authority.**

b. Members of the group provide each other with **support and practical help** for a shared problem (e.g., alcoholism, loss of a loved one, a specific illness).

c. Twelve-step groups like **Narcotics Anonymous** (NA) and **Overeaters Anonymous** (OA) are based on the Alcoholics Anonymous (AA) leaderless group model.

Table 17-1. Behavioral and Cognitive Therapies: Uses and Strategies

Most Common Use	Strategy
Systematic desensitization	
Treatment of phobias (irrational fears; see Chapter 13)	• In the past, through the process of classical conditioning (see Chapter 7), the person associated an innocuous object with a fear-provoking stimulus, until the innocuous object became frightening. • In the present, increasing doses of the fear provoking stimulus are paired with a relaxing stimulus to induce a relaxation response. • Because one cannot simultaneously be fearful and relaxed (reciprocal inhibition), the person shows less anxiety when exposed to the fear-provoking stimulus in the future.
Aversive conditioning	
Treatment of paraphilias or addictions (e.g., pedophilia, smoking)	• Classical conditioning is used to pair a maladaptive but pleasurable stimulus with an aversive or painful stimulus (e. g., a shock) so that the two become associated. • The person ultimately stops engaging in the maladaptive behavior, because it automatically provokes an unpleasant response.
Flooding and implosion	
Treatment of phobias	• The person is exposed to an actual (flooding) or imagined (implosion) overwhelming dose of the feared stimulus. • Through the process of habituation the person becomes accustomed to the stimulus and is no longer afraid.
Token economy	
To increase positive behavior in a person who is severely disorganized (e.g., psychotic), autistic, or mentally retarded	• Through the process of operant conditioning (see Chapter 7), desirable behavior (e. g., shaving, hair combing) is differentially reinforced by a reward or positive reinforcement (e. g., the token). • The person increases the desirable behavior to gain the reward.
Biofeedback	
To treat hypertension, Raynaud's disease, migraine and tension headaches, chronic pain, fecal incontinence, and temporomandibular joint pain	• Through the process of operant conditioning, the person is given ongoing physiologic information (e. g., blood pressure measurement) which acts as reinforcement (e.g., when blood pressure drops). • The person uses this information along with relaxation techniques to control visceral changes (e.g., heart rate, blood pressure, smooth muscle tone).
Cognitive therapy	
To treat mild to moderate depression, somatoform disorders, eating disorders	• Weekly, for as long as 25 weeks, the person is helped to identify distorted, negative thoughts about himself. • The person replaces these negative thoughts with positive, self-assuring thoughts and symptoms improve.

Table 17-2. Uses of Group, Family, Marital, Interpersonal, and Supportive Therapies

Type of therapy	Targeted population
Group therapy	• People with a common problem (e.g., rape victims) • People with personality disorders or other interpersonal problems • People who have trouble interacting with therapists as authority figures in individual therapy
Family therapy	• Children with behavioral problems • Families in conflict • People with eating disorders • People who abuse substances
Marital therapy	• Couples with communication problems • Couples with psychosexual problems • Couples with differences in values
Supportive therapy	• People who are experiencing a life crisis • Chronically mentally ill people dealing with ordinary life situations
Interpersonal therapy	• People with emotional difficulties due to problems with interpersonal skills

B. Family therapy

1. **Family systems theory**

   a. Family therapy is based on the family systems idea that psychopathology in one family member (i.e., the identified patient) reflects **dysfunction of the entire family system.**

   b. Because all members of the family cause behavioral changes in other members, **the family (not the identified patient) is really the patient.**

   c. **Strategies** of family therapy include identifying dyads (i.e., subsystems between two family members), triangles (i.e., dysfunctional alliances between two family members against a third member), and boundaries (i.e., barriers between subsystems) which may be too rigid or too permeable.

2. **Specific techniques** are used in family therapy.

   a. **"Mutual accommodation"** is encouraged. This is a process in which family members work toward meeting each other's needs.

   b. **Normalizing boundaries** between subsystems and reducing the likelihood of triangles is encouraged.

   c. **Redefining "blame"** (i.e., encouraging family members to reconsider their own responsibility for problems) is another important technique.

C. Supportive and interpersonal therapy

1. **Supportive therapy** is aimed not at insight into problems, but rather at **helping people feel protected** and supported during life crises (e.g., serious illness of a loved one). For **chronically mentally ill people,** supportive therapy may be used over many years along with medication.

2. Based on the idea that psychiatric problems like anxiety and depression are based on **difficulties in dealing with others,** interpersonal therapy aims to develop interpersonal skills in 12–16 weekly sessions.

Review Test

Directions: Each of the numbered items or incomplete statements in this section is followed by answers or by completions of the statement. Select the **one** lettered answer or completion that is **best** in each case.

1. A 30-year-old man who is afraid to ride in an elevator is put into a relaxed state and then is shown a film of people entering elevators in a high rise building. This method of treatment is best described as

(A) implosion
(B) systematic desensitization
(C) cognitive therapy
(D) flooding
(E) token economy

2. A 28-year-old woman joins ten other women who have been abused by their husbands. The women meet weekly and are led by a psychotherapist who is trained in domestic violence issues. This type of therapy is best described as

(A) group therapy
(B) leaderless group therapy
(C) brief dynamic psychotherapy
(D) family therapy
(E) supportive therapy

3. A 9-year-old boy who is angry and resentful toward adults (oppositional defiant disorder; see Chapter 15) meets with a therapist for 2 hours each week along with his parents and his sister. This type of therapy is best described as

(A) group therapy
(B) leaderless group therapy
(C) brief dynamic psychotherapy
(D) family therapy
(E) supportive therapy

4. Ten arthritis patients meet once per week to talk with each other and to inform each other of new devices and services to help disabled people with everyday tasks. This type of therapy is best described as

(A) group therapy
(B) leaderless group therapy
(C) brief dynamic psychotherapy
(D) family therapy
(E) supportive therapy

5. A 50-year-old male hypertensive patient is given ongoing blood pressure readings as he uses mental relaxation techniques to try to lower his blood pressure. This method of blood pressure reduction is based primarily on

(A) reciprocal inhibition
(B) classical conditioning
(C) aversive conditioning
(D) operant conditioning
(E) stimulus generalization

6. Each time she combs her hair and brushes her teeth, an autistic woman receives a coupon which can be exchanged for dessert in the cafeteria. Her grooming then improves. Which of the following treatment techniques does this example illustrate?

(A) Implosion
(B) Biofeedback
(C) Aversive conditioning
(D) Token economy
(E) Flooding
(F) Systematic desensitization
(G) Cognitive therapy

7. A man who is afraid to drive is told to imagine driving a car from the northernmost border to the southernmost border of the state of New Jersey. Which of the following treatment techniques does this example illustrate?

(A) Implosion
(B) Biofeedback
(C) Aversive conditioning
(D) Token economy
(E) Flooding
(F) Systematic desensitization
(G) Cognitive therapy

8. A 30-year-old depressed man is told to replace each self-deprecating thought with a mental image of victory and praise. Which of the following treatment techniques does this example illustrate?

(A) Implosion
(B) Biofeedback
(C) Aversive conditioning
(D) Token economy
(E) Flooding
(F) Systematic desensitization
(G) Cognitive therapy

9. A 42-year-old man with sexual interest in children (pedophilia) is given an electric shock each time he is shown a videotape of children. Later, he feels tense around children, and avoids them. Which of the following treatment techniques does this example illustrate?

(A) Implosion
(B) Biofeedback
(C) Aversive conditioning
(D) Token economy
(E) Flooding
(F) Systematic desensitization
(G) Cognitive therapy

Answers and Explanations

TBQ-D. This method of treatment is best described as flooding, a treatment technique for phobias in which a person is exposed to an overwhelming dose of the feared stimulus or situation—in this case, heights. In implosion, a person is exposed to an imagined, rather than actual, overwhelming dose of a feared stimulus or situation. In systematic desensitization, increasing doses of the frightening stimulus are paired with a relaxing stimulus to provoke a relaxation response in situations involving the frightening stimulus. In cognitive therapy, a person is helped to identify distorted, negative thoughts and to replace them with positive, self-assuring thoughts. In token economy a person's desired behavior is reinforced by a reward or positive reinforcement; the person then increases the desired behavior in order to get the reward.

1-B. This method of treatment is best described as systematic desensitization. The film of people entering elevators in a high rise building is a low level exposure to the feared stimulus. Later on in treatment, the person will be encouraged to look into a real elevator and finally to ride in one. (See also the answer to the TBQ).

2-A. This type of therapy is best described as group therapy, a treatment technique in which people with a common problem (e.g., victims of abuse), get together with a psychotherapist. In leaderless groups there is no therapist or other person in authority; members of the group provide each other with support and practical help for a shared problem. Brief dynamic psychotherapy is a form of psychoanalytically oriented therapy in which a person works with a therapist to gain insight into the cause of his problems. In supportive therapy a therapist helps a person feel protected and supported during life crises.

3-D. This type of therapy in which a child with a behavior problem and his family meet with a therapist is best described as family therapy. Family therapy is based on the idea that psychopathology in one family member (i.e., the child) reflects dysfunction of the entire family system (see also answer to Question 2).

4-B. This type of therapy in which patients with a particular illness (e.g., arthritis) meet for communication and practical help is best described as leaderless group therapy (and see answer to question 2 above).

5-D. The technique described here (i.e., biofeedback) is based primarily on operant conditioning (see Chapter 7 for a discussion of classical conditioning, stimulus generalization, and operant conditioning). Reciprocal inhibition is the mechanism which prevents one from feeling two opposing emotions at the same time (e.g., relaxation and fear, and is associated with systematic desensitization). In aversive conditioning, classical conditioning is used to pair a maladaptive but pleasurable stimulus with an aversive or painful stimulus so that the two become associated and the person stops engaging in the maladaptive behavior.

6-D. The treatment technique described here is token economy. The desirable behavior (e.g., grooming) is reinforced by a reward (e. g., dessert) and the person increases her behavior to gain the reward.

7-A. The treatment technique described here is implosion, a treatment technique related to flooding (see answer to TBQ above) in which the person is instructed to imagine extensive exposure to a feared stimulus (driving a car—or New Jersey, depending on your outlook) until he is no longer afraid.

8-G. The treatment technique described here is cognitive therapy, a short-term behavioral treatment technique in which the person is instructed to replace each negative thought with a positive mental image.

9-C. The treatment technique described here is aversive conditioning in which a maladaptive but pleasurable stimulus (for this man, sexual interest in children) is paired with painful stimulus (e.g., a shock) so that the two become associated. The person associates sexual interest in children with pain and stops this maladaptive behavior.

18

The Family, Culture, and Illness

Typical Board Question

The daughter of a 65-year-old Vietnamese woman brings her mother in for treatment of a serious medical condition. The older woman, who lives in the same house with her daughter, is alert and oriented. The necessary treatment regimen is quite complex and the older woman does not speak English. To best convey the needed information to this patient, the physician should

(A) write the instructions down in English to be translated later
(B) explain the instructions to the daughter and have her monitor her mother's treatment
(C) call in a translator to explain the instructions to the mother
(D) ask the daughter to translate the instructions to the mother
(E) refer the patient to a doctor who speaks Vietnamese

(See "Answers and Explanations" at end of Chapter)

I. Overview of the Family

A. Definition

1. A group of people related by **blood, adoption,** or **marriage** is a family.

2. The interpersonal relationships in families play a significant role in the health of family members.

B. Nuclear and extended families

1. The **traditional nuclear family** includes a mother, a father, and dependent children (i.e., under age 18) living together in one household.

2. The **extended family** includes family members such as grandparents, aunts, uncles, and cousins who live outside of the household.

II. Demographics and Current Trends

A. Marriage and children

1. In the United States, the average **age of first marriage** is **24.5** years for **women** and **26.7** years for **men.**

2. More than **75%** of people **30–54 years of age** are married.

3. A good marriage is an important predictor of health. Married people are

167

mentally and **physically healthier** and have **higher self-esteem** than nonmarried people.

4. Approximately **40% of children** live in families with **two working parents;** only **23% of children live in the "traditional family"** in which the father works outside of the home and the mother remains at home.

5. Raising children is expensive. The total cost of raising a child to age 17 in the United States is currently about **$90,000–$180,000.** An education at a private college can add more than $80,000 to these figures.

6. About 25% of married couples are childless; half of these are childless by choice.

B. **Divorce and single-parent families**

1. **Close to half of all marriages in the United States end in divorce.**

   a. Factors associated with divorce include short courtship, lack of family support, premarital pregnancy, marriage during teenage years, divorce in the family, differences in religion or socioeconomic background, and serious illness or death of a child.

   b. Divorced **men are more likely to remarry** than are divorced women.

   c. **Physicians have a higher divorce rate** than people in other occupations. Much of this difference may be due to the lifestyle and stresses associated with a career in medicine.

2. **Single-parent families**

   a. Single-parent families often have **lower incomes** and **less social support** and, therefore, face increased chances of physical and mental illness.

   b. While many unmarried mothers belong to low socioeconomic groups, the fastest growing population of single mothers is **educated professional women.**

   c. Among single parent families, **87% are headed by women** and 13% are headed by men. This ratio and the percentage of children living in single parent families vary by ethnic group (Table 18-1).

3. **Children in single-parent families**

   a. **Children in single-parent families** are at **increased risk** for failure in school, depression, drug abuse, suicide, criminal activity, and divorce.

   b. Even if the non-custodial parent does not provide financial support, **children who continue to have regular contact with that parent** have fewer of these problems than those who have no contact.

Table 18-1. Distribution by Ethnic Group of Members of Single Parent Families in the United States

Ethnic group	Approximate percentage of single parent families headed by women	Approximate percentage of children (under 18 years of age) living in single parent families
African American	95%	62%
Hispanic American	88%	33%
White American	83%	21%
All Americans	**87%**	**28%**

    4. Child custody
- **a.** After divorce, the types of **child custody** that may be granted by the courts include joint, split, and sole custody; **fathers are increasingly being granted** joint or sole custody.
- **b.** **In sole custody,** the child lives with one parent while the other has visitation rights. Until quite recently, sole custody was the most common type of custody arrangement after divorce.
- **c.** In **joint residential custody,** which has recently become more popular, the child spends some time living with each parent.
- **d.** In **split custody,** each parent has custody of at least one child.

III. Culture in the United States

A. Characteristics

1. In 1998, there were **269 million people** in the United States. The population is made up of many **minority subcultures** as well as a **large, white middle class,** which is the major cultural influence (see Table 18-1).
2. Although many subcultures have formed the American culture, the culture seems to have certain characteristics of its own.
   - **a.** **Financial and personal independence** are valued at all ages and especially in the elderly. **Most elderly Americans** spend their last years **living on their own;** only about 20% live with family members and about 5% live in nursing homes.
   - **b.** Emphasis is placed on **personal hygiene** and cleanliness.
   - **c.** The **nuclear family** with few children is valued.

B. Culture and illness

1. While ethnic groups are **not homogeneous,** (i.e., their members have different backgrounds and different reasons for emigrating), groups often have **characteristic ways of dealing with illness.**
2. Although the major psychiatric disorders such as schizophrenia and depression are seen to about the same extent in all cultures, **the sorts of behavior considered abnormal may differ considerably by culture.**
3. While differences in presentation of symptoms may be due to the individual characteristics of a patient, they may also be due to the **characteristics of the particular ethnic group.**
4. A patient's belief system has much to do with compliance and response to treatment. The physician must have **respect for and work in the context of such beliefs** in order to help patients. For example:
   - **a.** In certain ethnic groups, it is believed that illness can be cured by **eating certain foods.** Therefore, if not contraindicated medically, the doctor should attempt **to make available the food** the ill patient believes can help him.
   - **b.** The idea that an **outside influence** (i.e., a hex or a curse imposed by the anger of an acquaintance or relative) **can cause illness** is seen in some ethnic groups. The doctor should not dismiss the pa-

tient's belief, but rather should ask the patient who can help to **remove the curse** and involve that person in the treatment plan.

C. Culture shock

1. Culture shock is a **strong emotional response** (which may involve **psychiatric symptoms**) related to geographic relocation and the need to adapt to unfamiliar social and cultural surroundings. Culture shock is reduced when groups of immigrants of a particular culture live in the same geographic area.

2. **Young immigrant men** appear to be at **higher risk for culture shock** including psychiatric symptoms, such as paranoia and depression, than other sex and age groups. This is in part because:
   a. Young men **lose the most status** on leaving their culture of origin.
   b. Unlike others in the group who can stay at home among familiar people, young men often **must get out into the new culture** and earn a living.

IV. Minority Subcultures

A. African Americans

1. There are approximately **32 million** African Americans (about 12% of the total population).

2. The **average income** of African American families is only about **half that of white families.** This lower socioeconomic status is associated with decreased access to health care services leading to **increased health risks.**

3. When compared to white Americans, **African Americans** have:
   a. A **shorter life expectancy** (see Table 3-1)
   b. **Higher rates** of **hypertension,** heart disease, stroke, obesity, asthma, tuberculosis, diabetes, prostate cancer, and AIDS. (African American men and women are 15 times and 5 times more likely to have AIDS than white men and women respectively).
   c. **Higher death rates** from heart disease and from all forms of cancer.

4. **Religion** and **strong extended family networks** play a major role in social and personal support among many African Americans. This may in part explain why the overall **suicide rate is lower** among African Americans than among white Americans.

   —While the overall suicide rate is lower, suicide in African-American teenagers, once rare, has more than doubled in the last 20 years. It is now the third leading cause of death in this group with homicide the leading cause and accidents second. In white teenagers, accidents are the leading cause of death, with homocide second and suicide third.

B. Hispanic Americans

1. Overview
   a. As a group, Hispanic Americans (those of Spanish-speaking background) place great value on the nuclear family and on **nuclear families with many children.**

   b. **Respect for the elderly is important.** Younger people are expected to care for elderly family members, to **protect elderly relatives from negative medical diagnoses,** and, often, to make medical decisions concerning the care of elderly relatives.

   c. Hispanic Americans may **seek health care from folk healers** (i.e., chamanes, curanderos, espiritistas). Treatment provided by these healers includes **herbal or botanical medicines,** magical remedies, or specific changes in diet. **Religious beliefs** also play an important role in these treatments.

   d. Hispanic-American women are less likely to get mammograms than white or African-American women.

2. There are over **15 million Mexican Americans** living in the United States, especially in the Southwest, making them the largest group of Hispanic Americans. Among some Mexican Americans, **"hot" and "cold" influences** are believed to relate to illness.

3. The second largest group of Hispanic Americans in the United States are **Puerto Rican Americans (2 million people).** Most live in the Northeastern states.

4. There are about **5 million** Hispanic Americans from places other than Mexico and Puerto Rico (e.g., Cuba, Central America, South America) in the United States.

C. Asian Americans

1. The largest groups of Asian Americans are **Chinese** (1.5 million), **Filipino** (1.4 million), and **Japanese** (1.0 million) Americans.

2. Other Asian American groups include **Korean** (0.8 million), **Asian Indian** (0.6 million), and **Vietnamese** (0.5 million) Americans.

3. Although **many groups are assimilated,** ethnic differences may still result in different responses to illness among different Asian-American groups.

4. Characteristics of these cultures include the following:
   a. As in Hispanic-American cultures, adult Asian-American children **show strong respect for** and **are expected to care for their elderly parents,** protect elderly relatives from negative medical diagnoses, and make medical decisions about elderly relatives' care.

   b. Patients may express emotional pain as physical illness.

   c. In some Asian American groups, the **abdominal-thoracic area** rather than the brain is thought to be the **spiritual core** of the person; thus, the concept of brain death and resulting organ transplant are generally not well accepted.

   d. Many Asian Americans **metabolize alcohol differently** from white Americans. When alcohol is consumed, they accumulate more acetaldehyde and show a characteristic flushing reaction.

   e. **Folk remedies are used** to heal illness (e.g., in coining, a coin is rubbed on the affected area; the resulting bruises are believed to aid the patient). Injuries occurring as a result of use of such remedies may be mistaken by medical personnel for abuse.

    f. Asian Americans are at higher risk for stomach and liver cancer than other Americans.

D. Native Americans: American Indians and Eskimos

    1. There are about **2 million Native Americans** in the United States.

    2. Native Americans have their own program of medical care under the direction of the **Indian Health Service** of the federal government.

    3. The distinction between mental and physical illness may be blurred; engaging in forbidden behavior and witchcraft are thought to result in illness.

    4. In general, Native Americans have low incomes and **high rates of alcoholism** and **suicide**.

V. Other Subcultures

—Studies of Americans of **European descent** indicate that members of different European groups may respond differently to illness. For example, **Anglo-Americans** (those originating in English-speaking European countries, mostly from Ireland) numbering about 47 million, are less emotional, more stoic, and less vocal about pain and illness than members of groups of Mediterranean origin (e.g., Jewish and Italian). Therefore, Anglo-Americans may become very ill before seeking treatment.

Review Test

Directions: Each of the numbered items or incomplete statements in this section is followed by answers or by completions of the statement. Select the **one** lettered answer or completion that is **best** in each case.

1. A 26-year-old woman and a 29-year-old man get married after a 2-year engagement. They are both Episcopalian and are both from middle class families. Both sets of their parents are divorced. Which of the following factors puts this couple at highest risk for divorce?

(A) Their ages
(B) The length of their engagement
(C) Their parents' marital histories
(D) Their socioeconomic backgrounds
(E) Their religious backgrounds

2. The principal of an elementary school is trying to estimate how many of the school's students live in a "traditional" family situation. If the school's population is representative of the United States population, her best guess is approximately

(A) 5%
(B) 10%
(C) 25%
(D) 45%
(E) 65%

3. Similarly, the principal's best guess about how many children in the school live in single parent families is approximately

(A) 5%
(B) 10%
(C) 25%
(D) 45%
(E) 65%

4. A large extended family emigrates to the United States. The person in the family who is at highest risk for psychiatric symptoms after the move is the

(A) 84-year-old great-grandfather
(B) 28-year-old uncle
(C) 36-year-old aunt
(D) 10-year-old sister
(E) 55-year-old grandmother

5. A 12-year-old child is told to write a report about his "nuclear family." To do this task correctly, the report must contain information on his

(A) 84-year-old great-grandfather
(B) 28-year-old uncle
(C) 36-year-old aunt
(D) 10-year-old sister
(E) 55-year-old grandmother

6. The percentage of Americans who are Native Americans is approximately

(A) 1%
(B) 10%
(C) 15%
(D) 20%
(E) 30%

7. Which of these patients is most likely to spend the last years of her life in a nursing home if she becomes incapacitated?

(A) An 80-year-old Anglo-American woman
(B) An 80-year-old Puerto Rican American woman
(C) An 80-year-old Japanese American woman
(D) An 80-year-old Mexican American woman
(E) An 80-year-old Vietnamese American woman

8. A physician has two 56-year-old male patients. One of them is African American and one is white. Statistically, the African American patient has a lower likelihood of

(A) stroke
(B) asthma
(C) hypertension
(D) suicide
(E) prostate cancer

9. Which of the following living situations is most common in the United States?

(A) A 34-year-old medical resident living with his parents
(B) A 46-year-old divorced man living with his 10-year-old son
(C) A 65-year-old man living with his daughter and her husband
(D) A 46-year-old single man living alone
(E) A 46-year-old man living with his wife and children

Answers and Explanations

TBQ-C. When the treatment regimen is complex and the patient does not speak English, the physician's best choice is to call in a translator so that he can explain the instructions directly to his patient (in this case, the elderly woman). Communicating as directly as possible with the patient is particularly important in cultures where adult children may protect an elderly relative from a negative medical diagnosis (e.g., Asian and Hispanic cultures). Thus, in translating the information, or monitoring the treatment, the daughter may not relay to the elderly patient the complete picture. Writing the instructions down in English to be translated later is not appropriate because it is uncertain how and when the translation will be done. Since the doctor can call in a translator, there is no reason to refer the patient to another doctor. Patients expect to receive care when they visit a physician, and referrals are usually made only for medical reasons.

1-C. Of the listed factors, their parents' histories of divorce is a risk factor for divorce for this couple. Teenage, short courtship, and differences in socioeconomic and religious backgrounds also put couples at risk for divorce.

2-C. Approximately 23% of American children live in a "traditional" family situation (the mother stays home and the father works).

3-C. Approximately 28% of American children live in single-parent families.

4-B. Young immigrant men, such as the 28-year-old uncle, are at higher risk for psychiatric symptoms when entering a new culture than any other gender or age group. This is because they lose the most status on leaving their old culture and because, unlike other groups which can stay at home among their families, young men often must get out into the new culture and make a living.

5-D. The "nuclear family" consists of parents and dependent children (e.g., the boy's sister) living in one household. The great-grandfather, uncle, aunt, and grandmother are part of the "extended family."

6-A. The percentage of Native Americans is approximately 1% of all Americans.

7-A. Asian and Hispanic Americans are more likely to be cared for by their adult children when they become incapacitated than are Anglo-American patients.

8-D. Statistically, a middle-aged African-American patient has a lower likelihood of suicide than a white patient of the same age. However, when compared to white patients, African American patients have a higher likelihood of stroke, asthma, hypertension, and prostate cancer.

9-E. Of the listed choices, a 46-year-old man living with his wife and children is the most common living situation in the United States. While the divorce rate is high, most people in their 40's are married, not single or divorced. It is relatively uncommon to see a self-supporting adult like the 34-year-old medical resident living with his parents. It is also relatively uncommon to see a 65-year-old man living with his children.

19

Sexuality

*Typical **B**oard **Q**uestion*

A 45-year-old physician states that he has been living with another man in a stable, sexual, love relationship for the past 10 years. This physician is most likely to have a history in adolescence of

(A) seduction by an older man
(B) mental illness
(C) sexual fantasies about men
(D) choosing to spend time alone
(E) wanting sex change surgery

(See "Answers and Explanations" at end of Chapter)

I. Sexual Development

A. Prenatal physical sexual development

1. Differentiation of the **gonads** is dependent on the presence or absence of the **Y chromosome,** which contains the testis-determining factor gene.

2. The androgenic secretions of the **testes** direct the differentiation of **male** internal and external genitalia.

   a. **In the absence of androgens** during prenatal life, internal and external **genitalia are female.**

   b. In **androgen insensitivity syndrome** (testicular feminization), despite an **XY genotype** and testes which secrete androgen, a genetic defect prevents the body cells from responding to androgen resulting in a female phenotype.

   c. In the presence of excessive adrenal androgen secretion prenatally **(adrenogenital syndrome),** female genitalia may be masculinized.

B. Prenatal psychological sexual development

1. Differential exposure to gonadal hormones during prenatal life also results in **gender differences in certain brain areas** (e.g., the hypothalamus, anterior commissure, corpus callosum, and thalamus).

2. **Gender identity, gender role,** and **sexual orientation** (Table 19-1) also may be affected by prenatal exposure to gonadal hormones.

   a. Individuals with **androgen insensitivity syndrome** commonly have

Table 19-1. Gender Identity, Gender Role, and Sexual Orientation

Term	Definition	Presumed Etiology	Comments
Gender identity	Sense of self as being male or female	• Sex of assignment and rearing • Differential exposure to prenatal sex hormones	• Developed by age 3 years (see Chapter 1) • May or may not agree with physiological sex or gender role (i.e., gender identity disorder)
Gender role	Expression of one's gender identity in society	• Societal pressure to conform to sexual stereotypes	• May or may not agree with gender identity or physiological sex
Sexual orientation	Persistent and unchanging preference for people of the same sex (homosexual) or the opposite sex (heterosexual) for love and sexual expression	• Societal expectations • Exposure to prenatal sex hormones	• Preference for people of either sex (bisexuality) is much less common than homosexuality or heterosexuality; most people have a sexual preference • Homosexuality is considered a normal variant of sexual expression

  a female gender identity and gender role and have sexual interest in men.

  b. Individuals with **adrenogenital syndrome** commonly have a female gender identity and gender role; about 1/3 have a **lesbian** sexual orientation.

  c. Individuals with **gender identity disorder** (transsexuality) have a pervasive psychological feeling of being born into the body of the wrong sex despite a body form normal for their physiological sex. It is associated with altered prenatal brain exposure to sex hormones. In adulthood, these individuals commonly take sex hormones and seek sex-change surgery.

II. The Biology of Sexuality in Adults

—In adults, alterations in circulating levels of gonadal hormones (estrogen, progesterone, and testosterone) can affect sexual interest and expression.

  A. Hormones and behavior in women

  1. Because estrogen is only minimally involved in libido, **menopause (i.e., cessation of ovarian estrogen production)** and **aging do not reduce sex drive** if a woman's general health is good (see also Chapter 3).

  2. **Testosterone is secreted by the adrenal glands** (as well as the

ovaries and testes) throughout adult life and is believed to **play an important role in sex drive** in both men and women.

3. **Progesterone,** which is contained in many oral contraceptives, may inhibit sexual interest and behavior in women.

B. Hormones and behavior in men

1. Testosterone levels in men generally **are higher than necessary** to maintain normal sexual functioning.

2. Psychological and physical **stress may decrease testosterone** levels.

3. Medical treatment with **estrogens, progesterone,** or **antiandrogens** (e.g., to treat prostate cancer) blocks androgen receptors resulting in **decreased sexual interest and behavior.**

C. Homosexuality (see Table 19-1)

1. **Etiology**

   a. The etiology of homosexuality is believed to be related to **alterations in levels of prenatal sex hormones** (i.e., increased androgens in females and decreased androgens in males) resulting in anatomic changes in some hypothalamic nuclei; sex hormone levels in adulthood are indistinguishable from those of heterosexual people of the same biological sex.

   b. Evidence for involvement of **genetic factors** includes markers on the X chromosome and higher concordance rate in monozygotic than in dizygotic twins.

   c. **Social factors, such as early sexual experiences, are not associated with the etiology** of homosexuality.

   d. Because homosexuality is not a dysfunction, **no treatment is needed.** If needed, psychological intervention is aimed mainly at helping people who are uncomfortable become comfortable with their sexual orientation.

2. **Occurrence**

   a. Homosexuality is present in 3%–10% of men and 1%–5% of women.

   b. There are **no significant ethnic differences** in the occurrence of homosexuality.

   c. Most gay or lesbian people have experienced heterosexual sex, and many have had children.

D. The Sexual Response Cycle

1. Masters and Johnson devised a **four-stage model** for sexual response in both men and women.

2. Stages of the sexual response cycle include **excitement, plateau, orgasm,** and **resolution** (Table 19-2).

3. Sexual dysfunctions involve difficulty with one or more aspects of the sexual response cycle.

Table 19-2. Characteristics of the Stages of the Sexual Response Cycle in Men and Women

Men	Women	Both Men and Women
Excitement Stage		
• Penile erection	• Clitoral erection • Labial swelling • Vaginal lubrication • Tenting effect (rising of the uterus in the pelvic cavity)	• Increased pulse, blood pressure, and respiration • Nipple erection
Plateau Stage		
• Increased size and upward movement of the testes • Secretion of a few drops of sperm-containing fluid	• Contraction of the outer one-third of the vagina, forming the orgasmic platform (enlargement of the upper one-third of the vagina)	• Further increase in pulse, blood pressure, and respiration • Flushing of the chest and face
Orgasm Stage		
• Forcible expulsion of seminal fluid	• Contractions of the uterus and vagina	• Contractions of the anal sphincter • Further increase in pulse, blood pressure, and respiration
Resolution Stage		
• Refractory, or resting, period (length varies by age and physical condition) when restimulation is not possible	• Little or no refractory period	• Muscle relaxation • Return of the sexual and cardiovascular systems to the prestimulated state over 10–15 minutes

III. Sexual Dysfunction

A. Characteristics

1. Sexual dysfunction can result from biological, psychological, or interpersonal causes or a combination of causes.

   a. **Biological causes** include an unidentified general medical condition (e.g., **diabetes** can cause erectile dysfunction; **pelvic adhesions** can cause dyspareunia), **side effects of medication** [e.g., selective serotonin reuptake inhibitors (SSRIs) can cause delayed orgasm], **substance abuse** (e.g., alcohol use can cause erectile dysfunction) and **hormonal** or **neurotransmitter alterations.**

   b. **Psychological causes** include current relationship problems, stress, depression, and anxiety (e.g., guilt, performance pressure). In men with **erectile disorder,** the presence of **morning erections,** erections during masturbation, or erections during rapid eye movement (REM) sleep suggests a psychological rather than a physical cause.

2. Dysfunctions may have always been present **(primary sexual dys-**

function), or they may occur after an interval when function has been normal **(secondary sexual dysfunction).**

    B. **DSM-IV classifications** of sexual dysfunctions

        1. The sexual desire disorders are **hypoactive sexual desire** disorder and **sexual aversion** disorder (disorders of the excitement phase).

        2. The sexual arousal disorders are **female sexual arousal disorder** and **male erectile disorder** (disorders of the excitement and plateau phases).

        3. The orgasmic disorders are **male orgasmic disorder, female orgasmic disorder,** and **premature ejaculation** (disorders of the orgasm phase).

        4. The sexual pain disorders are **dyspareunia** and **vaginismus** (not due to a general medical condition).

        5. **Table 19-3** shows characteristics of the sexual dysfunctions.

Table 19-3. Characteristics of the DSM-IV Sexual Dysfunctions

Disorder	Characteristics
Hypoactive sexual desire disorder	• Decreased interest in sexual activity
Sexual aversion disorder	• Aversion to and avoidance of sexual activity
Female sexual arousal disorder	• Inability to maintain vaginal lubrication until the sex act is completed, despite adequate physical stimulation (reported in as many as 20% of women)
Male erectile disorder (commonly called "impotence")	• Lifelong or primary (rare): Has never had an erection sufficient for penetration • Acquired or secondary (the most common of all male sexual disorders): Is currently unable to maintain erections despite normal erections in the past • Situational (common): Has difficulty maintaining erections in some situations, but not in others
Orgasmic disorder (male and female)	• Lifelong: Has never had an orgasm • Acquired: Is currently unable to achieve orgasm despite adequate genital stimulation and normal orgasms in the past • Female orgasmic disorder is reported more often than male organic disorder
Premature ejaculation	• Ejaculation occurs before the man would like it to • Plateau phase of the sexual response cycle is short or absent • Anxiety usually accompanies the problem • Is the second most common of all male sexual disorders
Vaginismus	• Painful spasms occur in the outer one-third of the vagina, which make intercourse or pelvic examination difficult
Dyspareunia	• Persistent pain occurs in association with sexual intercourse • Occurs much more commonly in women; can occur in men

C. Treatment

1. There is a growing tendency for **physicians to treat the sexual problems of patients** rather than to refer these patients to sex therapists.

2. **Behavioral treatment techniques**

   a. In **sensate-focus exercises** (used to treat sexual desire, arousal, and orgasmic disorders), the individual's awareness of touch, sight, smell, and sound stimuli are increased during sexual activity, and psychological pressure to achieve an erection or orgasm is decreased.

   b. In the **squeeze technique,** which is used **to treat premature ejaculation,** the man is taught to identify the sensation that occurs just before the emission of semen. At this moment, the man asks his partner to exert pressure on the coronal ridge of the glans on both sides of the penis until the erection subsides, thereby delaying ejaculation.

   c. **Relaxation techniques, hypnosis,** and **systematic desensitization** are used to reduce anxiety associated with sexual performance.

   d. **Masturbation** may be recommended (particularly for patients with **orgasmic disorders**) to help the patient learn what stimuli are most effective.

3. **Medical and surgical treatment**

   a. Because they delay orgasm, **SSRIs** (e.g., fluoxetine) are used to treat **premature ejaculation.**

   b. **Systemic administration of opioid antagonists** (e.g., naltrexone), vasodilators (e.g., yohimbine), or **sildenafil citrate** (i.e., Viagra), a new agent for erectile disorder. Viagra works by blocking an enzyme [phosphodiester (PDE) 5] which destroys cyclic guanosine monophosphate (cGMP), a vasodilator which is secreted in the penis with sexual stimulation. Thus, degradation of cGMP is slowed and the erection persists. These agents are used to treat **erectile dysfunction.**

   c. **Intracorporeal injection of vasodilators** (e.g., papaverine, phentolamine) or implantation of **prosthetic devices** also are used to treat **erectile dysfunction.**

IV. Paraphilias

A. **Definition.** Paraphilias are the preferential use of fantasies and behaviors involving **unusual objects** of sexual desire or engagement in **unusual sexual activity (Table 19-4).** To be in this category of sexual disorder, a paraphilia must be used over a period of at least 6 months, and cause impairment in occupational or social functioning.

B. **Occurrence and treatment**

1. Pedophilia, voyeurism, and exhibitionism are the most frequently seen types of paraphilias.

2. Paraphilias occur **almost exclusively in men.**

3. **Pharmacologic treatment** includes **antiandrogens** and **female sex hormones** for paraphilias that are characterized by hypersexuality.

Table 19-4. Sexual Paraphilias

Paraphilia	Obtaining sexual pleasure by
Exhibitionism	Revealing one's genitals to strangers so that they will be shocked
Fetishism	Using inanimate objects (e.g., women's shoes, rubber sheets)
Transvestic fetishism	Wearing women's clothing, particularly underclothing (exclusive to heterosexual men)
Frotteurism	Rubbing the penis against a clothed woman who is nonconsenting and not aware
Necrophilia	Engaging in sexual activity with dead bodies
Pedophilia	Engaging in fantasies or actual behaviors with children (under 14 years of age) of the opposite or same sex; is the most common paraphilia (the pedophile must be at least 16 years of age and 5 years older than the victim)
Sexual sadism or masochism	Giving (sadism) or receiving (masochism) physical pain or humiliation
Telephone scatologia	Making telephone calls to unsuspecting women and engaging them in conversations of a sexual nature
Voyeurism	Secretly watching other people (often by using binoculars) undressing or engaging in sexual activity

V. Illness, Injury, and Sexuality

A. Heart disease and myocardial infarction (MI)

1. Men who have a history of MI often have **erectile dysfunction.** Both men and women who have a history of MI may have **decreased libido** due to side effects of cardiac medications and to **fear that sexual activity will cause another heart attack.**

2. Generally, if exercise that raises the heart rate to **110–130 beats per minute** (i.e., exertion equal to climbing two flights of stairs) can be tolerated without severe shortness of breath or chest pain, sexual activity can be resumed after a heart attack.

3. **Sexual positions** that produce the least exertion in the patient (e.g., the **partner in the superior position**) are the safest after MI.

B. Diabetes

1. One quarter to one half of all diabetic men (more commonly older patients) have **erectile dysfunction. Orgasm and ejaculation are less likely to be affected.**

2. The major causes of erectile dysfunction in men with diabetes are **vascular changes** and **diabetic neuropathy** caused by damage to blood vessels and nerve tissue as a result of hyperglycemia.

   a. Erectile problems generally occur several years after diabetes is diagnosed but **may be the first symptom** of the disease.

   b. **Poor metabolic control** of diabetes is related to increased incidence of sexual problems.

    c. Although physiologic causes are most important, **psychological factors** may also influence erectile problems associated with diabetes.

    d. Sildenafil citrate (Viagra) is reported to be effective in diabetes-related erectile disorders.

    e. Although penile implants may be used to treat erectile dysfunction, diabetic men often have greater difficulties in wound-healing and **greater susceptibility to infection.**

C. Spinal cord injury

    1. Spinal cord injuries in **men** cause **erectile** and **orgasmic dysfunction, retrograde ejaculation** (into the bladder), reduced testosterone levels, and decreased fertility.

    2. Spinal cord injuries in **women** cause problems with **vaginal lubrication, pelvic vasocongestion,** and **orgasm.** Fertility is not usually adversely affected.

VI. Aging and Sexuality

A. Physical changes

—Alterations in sexual functioning normally occur with the aging process.

    1. In men, these changes include **slower erection, diminished intensity of ejaculation, longer refractory period,** and **need for more direct stimulation.**

    2. In **women,** these changes include **vaginal thinning, shortening of vaginal length,** and **vaginal dryness.** These changes can be reversed with estrogen replacement therapy.

B. Sexual interest and activity

    1. In spite of physical changes, societal attitudes, and loss of the sexual partner due to illness or death, **sexual interest usually does not change significantly with increasing age.**

    2. Continued sexual activity is associated with good health. Prolonged abstinence from sex leads to faster physical atrophy of the genital organs in old age **("use it or lose it").**

VII. Drugs and Sexuality

A. Prescription drugs affect libido, erection, orgasm, ejaculation, and other sexual functions, often as a result of their effects on neurotransmitter systems (Table 19-5).

B. Prescription drugs that lead to decreased sexual function **include:**

    1. Antihypertensives, particularly α-adrenergic agonists (e.g., methyldopa) and β-adrenergic blockers (e.g., propranolol); the fewest sexual problems are found with use of angiotensin-converting enzyme (ACE) inhibitors (e.g., captopril).

    2. Antidepressants, particularly SSRIs like fluoxetine since serotonin may depress sexuality.

    3. Antipsychotics, particularly D_2 receptor blockers

Table 19-5. The Effects of Some Prescription Drugs on Sexuality

Effect	Drug Type (Representative Agent)	Associated neuro-transmitter (↑ increased or ↓ decreased availability)
Reduced libido	Antidepressant (fluoxetine) Antihypertensive (propranolol) Antihypertensive (methyldopa)	↑ Serotonin ↓ Norepinephrine β ↑ Central norepinephrine α
Increased libido	Antiparkinsonian (L-dopa)	↑ Dopamine
Erectile dysfunction	Antihypertensive (propranolol) Antihypertensive (methyldopa) Antidepressant (fluoxetine) Antipsychotic (thioridazine)	↓ Norepinephrine β ↑ Central norepinephrine α ↑ Serotonin ↓ Dopamine
Vaginal dryness	Antihistamine (diphenhydramine) Anticholinergic (atropine)	↓ Histamine ↓ Acetylcholine
Inhibited orgasm (in men and women)	Antidepressant (fluoxetine)	↑ Serotonin
Priapism	Antidepressant (trazodone)	↑ Serotonin
Inhibited ejaculation	Antidepressant (fluoxetine) Antipsychotic (thioridazine)	↑ Serotonin ↓ Dopamine

      a. Dopamine may enhance sexuality; its blockade may decrease sexual functioning.

      b. Prolactin levels increase as a result of dopamine blockade; this may in turn **depress sexuality.**

  C. Drugs of abuse

    1. Alcohol and marijuana increase sexuality in the short term by decreasing psychological inhibitions.

      a. With long-term use, **alcohol may cause liver dysfunction,** resulting in increased estrogen availability and sexual dysfunction in men.

      b. Chronic use of **marijuana may reduce testosterone levels** in men and **pituitary gonadotropin** levels in women.

    2. Amphetamines and cocaine increase sexuality by stimulating dopaminergic systems. Cocaine use is associated also with **priapism** (persistent erection).

    3. Heroin and methadone (to a lesser extent) are associated with suppressed libido, retarded ejaculation, and failure to ejaculate.

    4. Amyl nitrite is a vasodilator that is used as an aphrodisiac to enhance the sensation of orgasm; however, cardiovascular accidents may result from its use.

VIII. The Human Immunodeficiency Virus (HIV) and Sexuality

  A. Occurrence of HIV

    1. Over 33 million people in the world are infected with HIV.

      a. 95% of HIV-infected people live in Africa, Asia and Eastern Europe.

Table 19-6. Route of Contact and Chance of Contracting the Human Immunodeficiency Virus (HIV)

Infection route	Approximate chance of contracting HIV
Sexual activity with an HIV-infected person	
Anal intercourse	1 in 10
Vaginal intercourse with an infected man	1 in 200
Vaginal intercourse with an infected woman	1 in 700
Direct contact with blood of an HIV-infected person	
Transfusion	1 in 1.05 (95 in 100)
Needle sharing	1 in 150
Needle stick	1 in 200
HIV-positive mother to fetus	
Mother to fetus (mother not taking AZT)	1 in 4
Mother to fetus (mother taking AZT)	<1 in 10

AZT= zidovudine; *HIV*=human immunodeficiency virus

> b. Less than **1 million infected people live in North America.**
>
> c. Less than **2 million** infected people live in Latin America and the Caribbean and about 0.5 million live in Western Europe.
>
> 2. There is a **sex difference** in the HIV viral load and the symptoms of **acquired immune deficiency syndrome** (AIDS); a woman with the same HIV viral load as a man is **likely to develop full-blown AIDS sooner than the man.**

B. Transmission of HIV

> 1. Because of the likelihood of tissue tearing leading to contact with the blood supply, **anal intercourse** is the sexual behavior that is **riskiest for transmitting HIV (Table 19-6).**
>
> 2. Patients who are HIV-positive **must protect their sexual partners from infection.** If they fail to do so (i.e., do not use a condom) and the physician has knowledge of such failure, the physician can inform the threatened partner (see also Chapter 22).

Review Test

Directions: Each of the numbered items or incomplete statements in this section is followed by answers or by completions of the statement. Select the **one** lettered answer or completion that is **best** in each case.

1. A 29-year-old woman says that she has always felt as if she was "a man in the body of a woman." Physical and pelvic examinations are normal. She is sexually attracted to heterosexual women and wants to wear men's clothes, take male hormones, and undergo a mastectomy and surgical sex reversal so that she can live as a man. The final diagnosis for this patient is most likely to be

(A) adrenogenital syndrome
(B) androgen insensitivity syndrome
(C) gender identity disorder
(D) transvestic fetishism
(E) normal

2. A 17-year-old woman comes to the doctor because she has never menstruated and because she has discovered labial masses. Initial examination reveals a tall, thin female with normal external genitalia and breast development. A pelvic examination is not performed. There are no Barr bodies in the buccal smear. The final diagnosis for this patient is most likely to be

(A) adrenogenital syndrome
(B) androgen insensitivity syndrome
(C) gender identity disorder
(D) transvestic fetishism
(E) normal

3. A 35-year-old man must wear women's high heels and lingerie to become aroused whenever he has sexual intercourse with a woman. The final diagnosis for this patient is most likely to be

(A) adrenogenital syndrome
(B) androgen insensitivity syndrome
(C) gender identity disorder
(D) transvestic fetishism
(E) normal

4. The best estimate of the occurrence of homosexuality in men is

(A) 0.5%–1%
(B) 3%–10%
(C) 12%–14%
(D) 15%–17%
(E) 20%–22%

5. A 50-year-old man shows breast enlargement after years of abusing a substance. The substance he is most likely to have abused is

(A) alcohol
(B) marijuana
(C) heroin
(D) amphetamine
(E) amyl nitrite

Questions 6–7

A 34-year-old man has been taking fluoxetine for treatment of depression for the past 4 months. His mood is now normal but he reports that he is having sexual problems.

6. Which of the following sexual dysfunctions is this man most likely to report?

(A) Primary erectile disorder
(B) Secondary erectile disorder
(C) Premature ejaculation
(D) Orgasmic disorder
(E) Dyspareunia

7. The neurotransmitter alteration most likely to be associated with this man's sexual problem is

(A) increased dopamine
(B) decreased dopamine
(C) increased serotonin
(D) decreased serotonin
(E) decreased norepinephrine

8. A 30-year-old male patient who is HIV-positive asks the doctor what type of sexual behavior poses the most risk for transmitting HIV to his partner. The doctor's best response is

(A) anal intercourse
(B) fellatio
(C) cunnilingus
(D) vaginal intercourse
(E) kissing

9. A husband and wife in their mid-30s state that they are having sexual problems. During the interview the doctor discovers that, while their sex life had been good, the last time they tried to have intercourse (4 weeks previously), the husband could not maintain an erection. Which of the following agents is most likely to have caused this sexual problem?

(A) Cocaine
(B) Propranolol
(C) Levodopa
(D) Amyl nitrate
(E) Dextroamphetamine

10. A 65-year-old married couple complain to the doctor that their sex life is not what it used to be. Which of the following problems are they most likely to report?

(A) Premature ejaculation
(B) Vaginal dryness
(C) Shorter refractory period
(D) Decreased sexual interest
(E) Vaginismus

11. A 32-year-old man complains that he has no problem with erection, but that he usually has an orgasm and ejaculates before he achieves vaginal penetration. This man's complaint

(A) is uncommon
(B) is associated with depression
(C) is associated with an absent excitement phase
(D) can be effectively treated with intensive psychotherapy
(E) can be effectively treated with the squeeze technique

12. A 62-year-old patient complains of erectile dysfunction. Which of the following illnesses is most likely to be associated with this problem?

(A) Dementia of the Alzheimer's type
(B) Untreated hypertension
(C) Untreated diabetes
(D) Myocardial infarction
(E) Untreated schizophrenia

13. A 25-year-old man masturbates by rubbing against women in crowded buses. This man is exhibiting which of the following paraphilias?

(A) Fetishism
(B) Exhibitionism
(C) Frotteurism
(D) Voyeurism
(E) Sexual masochism

14. The tenting effect begins in which stage of the sexual response cycle?

(A) Excitement
(B) Plateau
(C) Orgasm
(D) Resolution

15. Which stage of the sexual response cycle shows the greatest difference between men and women?

(A) Excitement
(B) Plateau
(C) Orgasm
(D) Resolution

16. Uterine contractions mainly occur in which stage of the sexual response cycle?

(A) Excitement
(B) Plateau
(C) Orgasm
(D) Resolution

17. The sex flush commonly first occurs in which stage of the sexual response cycle?

(A) Excitement
(B) Plateau
(C) Orgasm
(D) Resolution

Answers and Explanations

TBQ-C. Like other men with a homosexual sexual orientation, this physician is likely to have a history of sexual fantasies about men (heterosexual men commonly have a history of sexual fantasies about women). Homosexuality is a normal variant of sexual expression and is biologically based. There is no evidence that it is associated with a history in adolescence of seduction by an older man, mental illness, or a preference for being alone. While people with gender identity disorder (feeling of being born into the wrong body) may seek sex change surgery, in homosexuality there is no desire to change biological sex.

1-C. The final diagnosis for this patient who has always felt as if she was "a man in the body of a woman" in the presence of a normal female body is most likely to be gender identity disorder. Females with adrenogenital syndrome have masculinized genitalia and transvestic fetishists are always male. People with androgen insensitivity syndrome are genetic males with female bodies (with which they are content), and sexual interest in men. See also the explanations to Questions 2 and 3.

2-B. The final diagnosis for this patient who has a female phenotype despite a male genotype (i.e., no Barr bodies in the buccal smear) is most likely to be androgen insensitivity syndrome. In this genetic defect, body cells do not respond to the androgen being produced by the testes resulting in failure of physical masculinization. The masses noted by the patient are testes which have descended into the labia. People with androgen insensitivity syndrome are heterosexual with respect to phenotypic sex (i.e., women with sexual interest in men). See also the explanations to Questions 1 and 3.

3-D. The final diagnosis for this patient who must wear women's clothes to become sexually aroused is most likely to be transvestic fetishism. See also the explanations to Questions 1 and 2.

4-B. The best estimate of the occurrence of homosexuality in men is 3%–10%.

5-A. The substance that this 50-year-old man with breast enlargement is most likely to have abused is alcohol. Long term use of alcohol damages the liver resulting in accumulation of estrogens and feminization of the body. Marijuana, heroin, amphetamine, and amyl nitrite are much less likely to cause estrogen accumulation.

6-D. While they may be associated with loss of libido and erectile disorder, treatment with fluoxetine and other selective serotonin reuptake inhibitors (SSRIs) is most likely to result in delayed or absent orgasm (orgasmic disorder). That is why, although they do not yet have this Food and Drug Administration (FDA) indication, the SSRIs are currently being used to treat premature ejaculation. Dyspareunia is not associated with SSRI treatment.

7-C. The neurotransmitter alteration most likely to be associated with delayed or absent orgasm is increased serotonin resulting from treatment with the SSRI fluoxetine. Increased dopamine tends to increase sexual interest and performance. Decreased dopamine, decreased serotonin, and decreased norepinephrine are less likely to be associated with delayed orgasm than increased serotonin.

8-A. Because tissue tears providing access to the blood supply are more likely to occur in anal intercourse, this is the type of sexual behavior which poses the most risk for transmitting HIV. While theoretically it is possible to transmit HIV by other sexual behaviors (e.g., fellatio, cunnilingus, vaginal intercourse, and kissing), such transmission is much less likely than with anal intercourse.

9-B. Of the listed agents, the one most likely to have caused erectile disorder is propranolol, an antihypertensive medication (β-blocker). Cocaine, amphetamines, and L-dopa tend to increase sexual interest and performance by elevating dopamine availability. Amyl nitrate (a vasodilator) is used to enhance the sensation of orgasm.

10-B. This 65-year-old married couple is most likely to be having sexual problems because of vaginal dryness due to lack of estrogen after menopause. Aging is also characterized by a longer refractory period and delayed ejaculation in men and decreased intensity of orgasm in men and women. Although sexual behavior may decrease with aging because of these problems, sexual interest remains about the same. Vaginismus is not particularly associated with aging.

11-E. This man is describing premature ejaculation, a common sexual dysfunction which can be effectively treated with the squeeze technique (not psychotherapy). Premature ejaculation is associated with an absent plateau phase of the sexual response cycle and is not commonly associated with depression.

12-C. Untreated diabetes is most likely to be associated with erectile dysfunction in a 62-year-old patient. Although the medications used to treat these conditions are associated with erectile dysfunction, untreated cardiac problems, hypertension, and schizophrenia are not associated with erectile dysfunction. Dementia of the Alzheimer type is not associated with erectile dysfunction. In fact, sexual expression may be the last form of communication between a couple in which one partner has dementia of the Alzheimer type.

13-C. This man who masturbates by rubbing against women in crowded buses is exhibiting frotteurism. Exhibitionism involves a sexual preference for revealing one's genitals to unsuspecting persons so that they will be shocked. Fetishism is a sexual preference for inanimate objects. Sexual masochism is a preference for receiving physical pain or humiliation. Voyeurism is a preference for secretly watching people undressing or engaging in sexual activity.

14-A. The tenting effect begins during the excitement phase of the sexual response cycle.

15-D. Resolution shows the greatest difference between men and women. Men have a resting (refractory) period when restimulation is not possible. Women are unlikely to have a refractory period.

16-C. Uterine contractions occur mainly during the orgasm phase of the sexual response cycle.

17-B. The sex flush first appears during the plateau phase of the sexual response cycle in both men and women.

20

Aggression and Abuse

Typical Board Question

A 3-month-old infant is brought to the emergency department unconscious. While no external injuries are seen, physical examination reveals a subdural hematoma and retinal hemorrhages. The parents tell the physician that the child fell off his changing table. After stabilizing the child, the emergency department physician should

(A) contact the state child-protective service agency
(B) question the parents to determine if they have abused the child
(C) inform the parents that he suspects that they have abused the child
(D) obtain the parents' permission to hospitalize the child
(E) obtain the parents' permission to call a pediatric neurologist

(See "Answers and Explanations" at end of Chapter)

I. Aggression

A. Social determinants of aggression

1. Factors associated with increased aggression include poverty, frustration, physical pain, and exposure to aggression in the media (e.g., **violence on television**).

2. Homicide occurs more often in **low socioeconomic populations** and its incidence is increasing. At least half of homicides are accomplished with **guns.**

3. In **African-American** males **15–24 years of age,** homicide is the **leading cause of death;** it is the second leading cause of death (after accidents) in white males in this age group.

4. Children at risk for showing aggressive behavior in adulthood frequently **abuse animals,** have low intelligence, and cannot defer gratification. Their parents frequently display criminal behavior, abuse drugs and alcohol, and have physically or sexually abused them (or both).

B. Biological determinants of aggression

1. **Hormones**
   a. **Androgens** are closely associated with aggression; in most animal species and human societies, males are more aggressive than females; **homicide** involving strangers is **committed** almost exclusively by **men.**

189

   b. **Androgenic** or **anabolic steroids,** often taken by body builders to increase muscle mass, can result in **high levels of aggression** and even psychosis. Severe depression frequently occurs with withdrawal from these hormones.

   c. **Estrogen, progesterone,** and **antiandrogens,** all of which block androgen receptors, decrease sexual interest and behavior and may be useful in treating male sex offenders.

2. **Substances of abuse and their effect on aggression**

   a. Low doses of **alcohol** and **barbiturates** inhibit aggression while high doses facilitate it.

   b. While intoxicated heroin users show little aggression, increased aggression is associated with the use of **cocaine, amphetamines,** and **phencyclidine (PCP).**

3. **Neural bases of aggression**

   a. **Serotonin** and γ-aminobutyric acid (GABA) inhibit aggression, and dopamine and norepinephrine facilitate it; low levels of the serotonin metabolite 5-hydroxyindoleacetic acid (5-HIAA) are associated with impulsive aggression (see Chapter 4).

   b. Drugs used to treat inappropriate aggressiveness include antidepressants, benzodiazepines, antipsychotics, and antimanics (e.g., lithium, used especially in adolescent boys).

   c. **Abnormalities of the brain** (e.g., abnormal activity in the **amygdala** and prepyriform area and psychomotor and temporal lobe epilepsy) and lesions of the temporal lobe, frontal lobe, and hypothalamus are associated with increased aggression.

   d. Violent people often have a history of **head injury** or show abnormal electroencephalogram (EEG) readings.

II. Abuse and Neglect of Children and the Elderly

A. Overview

1. Types of child and elder abuse include **physical abuse** (e.g., the "battered child syndrome"), **emotional** or **physical neglect,** and **sexual abuse.** The elderly may also be exploited for monetary gain.

2. **Abuse-related injuries** must be differentiated from injuries obtained during normal activity. Examples of **non-abuse injuries** in children include bruises and scrapes on the chin, forehead, knees, and elbows; or, in the elderly, excessive skin bruising due to aging.

3. Occurrence of abuse and characteristics and signs which indicate neglect and abuse are shown in **Table 20-1.**

B. Sequelae of child abuse

1. Adults who were abused as children are more likely to suffer from:

   a. **Dissociative disorders, (e.g. dissociative identity disorder)** (see Chapter 14)

   b. **Posttraumatic stress disorder** and other anxiety disorders (see Chapter 13)

   c. **Depression** and substance abuse disorders (see Chapter 12 and Chapter 9)

Table 20-1. Physical Abuse of Children and Elders

Category	Features of child abuse	Features of elder abuse
	Occurrence	
Annual occurrence	• At least 1 million cases are reported • Most cases are not reported • 2000–4000 abuse-related deaths	• At least 1 million cases are reported • Most cases are not reported
Most likely abuser	• The closest family member (e.g., the mother)	• The closest family member (e.g., spouse, daughter, son, or other relative) with whom the person lives (and who is often supported financially by the elder)
	Characteristics of the Abused and the Abuser	
Characteristics of the abused	• Hyperactivity or mild physical handicap; child is perceived as slow or different • Premature, low-birthweight infant • Colicky or "fussy" infant • Physical resemblance to the abuser's absent, rejecting, or abusive partner • In 1/3 of cases, victims are younger than 5 years of age; in 1/4 of cases, victims are 5–9 years of age	• Some degree of worsening cognitive impairment (e.g., dementia of the Alzheimer's type) • Physical dependence on others • Does not report the abuse, but instead says that he fell and injured himself
Characteristics of the abuser	• Substance abuse • Poverty • Social isolation • Personal history of victimization by caretaker or spouse	• Substance abuse • Poverty • Social isolation
	Signs of Abuse	
Neglect	• Poor personal care and hygiene (e.g., diaper rash, dirty hair) • Lack of needed nutrition	• Poor personal care and hygiene (e.g., urine odor in incontinent person), lack of medication or health aids (e.g., eyeglasses, dentures) • Lack of needed nutrition
Bruises	• Particularly in areas not likely to be injured during normal play, such as buttocks or lower back • Belt or belt buckle marks	• Often bilateral and often on the arms from being grabbed
Fractures and burns	• Fractures at different stages of healing • Spiral fractures caused by twisting the limbs • Cigarette burns • Wrist or ankle rope burns caused by tying to a bed or chair • Burns on the feet or buttocks due to immersion in hot water	• Fractures at different stages of healing • Spiral fractures caused by twisting the limbs • Cigarette and other burns • Wrist or ankle rope burns caused by tying to a bed or chair
Other signs	• Internal abdominal injuries (e.g., ruptured spleen) • "Shaken baby" syndrome (i.e., retinal detachment or hemorrhage, and subdural hematoma caused by shaking the infant to stop it from crying)	• Internal abdominal injuries (e.g., ruptured spleen) • Evidence of depleted personal finances (their money was spent by the abuser and other family members) • Head and neck injuries

2. People abused in childhood also are at substantially greater risk for abusing their own children.

C. Sexual abuse of children

1. Signs

   a. Sexually transmitted diseases (STDs) in children are signs of sexual abuse; children do not contract STDs through casual contact with an infected person or with their bedclothes, towels, or toilet seats.

   b. Genital or **anal trauma** also are signs of sexual abuse.

   c. Young children have only a vague knowledge about sexual activities; specific **knowledge about sexual acts** (e.g., fellatio) in a young child often indicates that the child has been sexually abused.

   d. Recurrent **urinary tract infections** and excessive **initiation of sexual activity** with friends also are signs of sexual abuse.

2. Occurrence

   a. Sexual abuse of children is now being reported more frequently than in the past; at least 250,000 cases are reported annually.

   b. Most sexually abused children are **9–12 years of age,** and 25% are younger than 8 years old.

   c. Approximately 25% of all women and 12% of all men report sexual abuse at some time during their childhood and adolescence.

3. Characteristics of the sexual abuser

   a. Most abusers are **male** and **known to the child** (e.g., uncle, father, mother's boyfriend, family acquaintance); fewer than 5% of sexual abusers are strangers to the child.

   b. Alcohol and **drugs** are commonly used by the abuser.

   c. The abuser typically has **marital problems** and **no appropriate alternate sexual partner;** occasionally, he is a pedophile (i.e., he prefers children to appropriate sexual partners) (see Chapter 19).

III. Physical and Sexual Abuse of Domestic Partners

A. Occurrence

1. Domestic abuse is a common reason that women come to a hospital emergency room. The abuser is almost always male.

2. The abused woman **may not report to the police** or **leave the abuser** because she has nowhere to go and because he has **threatened to kill her** if she reports or leaves him. (In fact, she does have a greatly increased risk of being killed by her abusive partner if she leaves.)

B. Physical evidence of domestic abuse

1. The victim commonly has **bruises** (e.g., blackened eyes, bruises on the breasts) and broken bones.

2. In **pregnant women** (who have a higher risk of being abused), the **injuries** are often in the **"baby zone"** (i.e., the breasts and abdomen).

C. The **cycle of abuse** includes three phases:

1. Buildup of tension in the abuser

    2. Abusive behavior (battering)

    3. Apologetic and **loving behavior** by the abuser toward the victim

D. Characteristics of abusers and abused partners

    1. Abusers often use **alcohol or drugs,** are impulsive, have a low tolerance for frustration, and displace their angry feelings onto their partner.

    2. The abused partner is often emotionally or **financially dependent** on the abuser, pregnant, and blames herself for the abuse.

    3. Both the abuser and the abused commonly have **low self-esteem.**

IV. Role of the Physician in Suspected Child, Elder, and Domestic Partner Abuse

A. Child and elder abuse

    1. According to the law in every state, **physicians must report** suspected **physical** or **sexual abuse of a child** or **elderly person** (if the elderly person appears to be physically or mentally impaired) to the appropriate family social service agency (e.g., state child-protective service or state adult-protective service) **before** or **in conjunction with treatment** of the patient.

    2. The physician is **not required to tell the suspected abuser of the child** or **impaired elder** that she suspects abuse.

    3. The physician **does not need family consent** to hospitalize the abused child or elderly person for protection or treatment.

B. Domestic partner abuse

    1. Direct reporting by the physician of domestic partner abuse is not appropriate because the victim is usually a competent adult.

    2. A physician who suspects **domestic partner abuse** should provide emotional support to the abused partner, refer her to an appropriate shelter or program, and encourage her to report the case to law enforcement officials.

V. Sexual Aggression: Rape and Related Crimes

A. Definitions. Rape is a crime of violence, not of passion, and is known legally as **"sexual assault,"** or "aggravated sexual assault."

    1. Rape involves **sexual contact without consent.**

    2. Vaginal penetration by a penis, finger, or other object may occur.

    3. Erection and ejaculation do not have to occur.

    4. Sodomy is defined as the insertion of the penis into the **oral** or **anal orifice.** The victim may be male or female.

B. Legal considerations

    1. Because **rapists may use condoms** to avoid contracting human immunodeficiency virus (HIV), or to avoid DNA identification, or because rapists may have difficulty with erection or ejaculation, semen may not be present in the vagina of a rape victim.

2. A victim is **not required to prove that she resisted the rapist** for him to be convicted. A rapist was convicted recently even though the victim asked him to use a condom.

3. Certain information about the victim (e.g., previous sexual activity, "seductive" clothing worn at the time of the attack) is generally not admissible as evidence in rape trials.

4. In almost every state, **husbands can be prosecuted** for raping their wives. It is illegal to force anyone to engage in sexual activity. Even if a woman consents to go on a date with a man and consents to sexual activity not involving intercourse, a man can be prosecuted for rape (**"date rape"**).

5. Consensual sex may be considered rape (**"statutory rape"**) if the victim is younger than 16 or 18 years old (depending on state law) or is **physically** or **mentally handicapped.**

C. Characteristics of the rapist and victim

1. The rapist
   a. **Rapists** are usually younger than 25 years of age.
   b. They are usually the **same race** as the victim.
   c. They are usually **known to the victim.**
   d. **Alcohol use** by the rapist occurs in at least one third of rape cases.

2. The victim
   a. Rape victims are most typically between **16–24** years of age.
   b. Rape most commonly occurs **inside the victim's home.**
   c. **Vaginal injuries may be absent,** particularly in parous women (those who have had children).

D. The sequelae of rape

1. For a variety of reasons, including shame, fear of retaliation, and the difficulties involved in substantiating rape charges, **only 25% of all rapes are reported to the police.**

2. Others may commonly **blame the victim** in rape cases.

3. The length of the emotional recovery period after rape varies, but is commonly **at least 1 year. Posttraumatic stress disorder** sometimes occurs after rape (see Chapter 14).

4. The most effective type of counseling is group therapy with other rape victims.

E. The Role of the Physician in Rape Cases

1. Immediately after the rape, the physician should
   a. Take the patient's history in a **supportive manner,** and should not question the patient's veracity or judgment.
   b. Perform a general **physical examination** and conduct **laboratory tests** (e.g., cultures for sexually transmitted diseases from the vagina, anus, and pharynx; test for presence of semen).

    c. Prescribe prophylactic **antibiotics** and postcoital **contraceptive measures** (e.g., diethylstilbestrol) if appropriate.

    d. **Encourage** the patient to notify the police. The doctor is not required to notify the police if the woman is a competent adult.

2. Up to 6 weeks after the rape

    a. Discuss with the patient the **emotional** and **physical sequelae** of the rape (e.g., suicidal thoughts, vaginal bleeding) and, if needed, refer her for **long-term counseling** or a **support group.**

    b. Do a **pregnancy test** and repeat other laboratory tests if appropriate.

Review Test

Directions: Each of the numbered items or incomplete statements in this section is followed by answers or by completions of the statement. Select the **one** lettered answer or completion that is **best** in each case.

1. A 4-year-old girl tells the physician that her mother's boyfriend asked her to touch his penis. Physical examination of the child is unremarkable. The next thing that the physician should do is to

(A) contact the state child-protective service agency
(B) contact the child's biological father
(C) speak to the boyfriend about the child's remark
(D) contact a child psychiatrist to determine if the child is telling the truth
(E) question the child at length to determine if she is telling the truth

2. A 33-year-old single woman who has a 4-year-old child comes to the emergency room and reports that she was raped by a man she was on a date with 2 days ago. The physical examination shows no physical evidence of rape (i.e., no injuries, no semen). She appears anxious, disheveled, and "spacey." It is most likely that this woman

(A) is delusional
(B) is malingering
(C) is suffering from hypochondriasis
(D) is suffering from conversion disorder
(E) has been raped and the rapist used a condom

3. A 7-year-old child and her mother both have chlamydia. The child's infection is most likely to be the result of

(A) sleeping in the same bed as the mother
(B) sexual abuse
(C) masturbation
(D) using the mother's towel
(E) bathing in the mother's bathtub

4. Which of the following injuries in a 4-year-old child is most likely to be the result of abuse?

(A) Cut chin
(B) Bilateral bruises on the knees
(C) Scraped forehead
(D) Cut elbow
(E) Ruptured spleen

5. A 93-year-old mildly demented woman who lives with her daughter attends a day care program from 9:00 am–1:00 pm. From 1:00–4:00 pm a neighbor (who has an alcoholic son and an unemployed son) takes care of the elderly woman. The woman is brought to the emergency room by her daughter with injuries that suggest physical abuse. The person most likely to have abused this woman is

(A) a day care program worker
(B) the neighbor's alcoholic son
(C) the neighbor
(D) the woman's own daughter
(E) the neighbor's unemployed son

6. An 18-year-old retarded woman with an IQ of 50 agrees to have sexual intercourse with the 18-year-old president of the high school senior class. Sexual intercourse between these two people is best described as

(A) consensual sex
(B) statutory rape
(C) sodomy
(D) child abuse
(E) sexual abuse

Answers and Explanations

TBQ-A. After stabilizing the infant, the emergency department physician should contact the state child-protective service agency to report suspected child abuse. Subdural hematoma, retinal hemorrhage and retinal detachment are signs of the "shaken baby syndrome," a form of child abuse in which an adult shakes a child to stop its crying. The shaken child may have no external injuries. Parents commonly make up some explanation for the injuries such as "the child fell." The physician must report any suspicion of abuse to the appropriate authority but does not have to question the parents or inform them of his suspicions. Similarly, when a physician suspects child physical or sexual abuse he does not need a parent's permission to examine, hospitalize, or treat the child or to consult with a specialist.

1-A. As in the TBQ, when a child of any age reports inappropriate sexual touching, the physician must call the state child-protective service agency. This example demonstrates that a child may show no physical signs of sexual abuse. The physician must assume that patients (even young ones) are telling the truth. The physician does not need to talk to the child at length, consult a child psychiatrist, or talk to the mother's boyfriend to confirm the story. The state agency will handle these matters. The child's biological father is not relevant to the situation at this time.

2-E. It is most likely that this woman has been raped by the man she went out with ("date rape"). Because there is no semen, the rapist may have used a condom. Parous women like this patient may show no physical signs of rape. Rape victims may appear anxious, disheveled, and "spacey"(i.e., showing dissociation). Patients rarely lie to doctors. There is no indication that this woman is lying for obvious gain (malingering) or is delusional or suffering from hypochondriasis or conversion disorder.

3-B. The child's chlamydia infection is most likely to be the result of sexual abuse. Sleeping in the same bed as the mother, masturbation, using the mother's towel, or bathing in the mother's bathtub are unlikely ways to contract a sexually transmitted disease.

4-E. An internal injury like a ruptured spleen is most likely to be the result of abuse in a 4-year-old child. Chin, knee, forehead, and elbow injuries are more likely to have been obtained during normal play.

5-D. A close relative who cares for the person (i.e., the daughter) is most likely to have abused this elderly demented woman. Although no excuse for abuse, this may be due in part to the stresses associated with caring for a demented elderly person. Unrelated people such as caretakers (even if alcoholic or unemployed) are much less likely than a close relative to abuse an elderly person.

6-B. Even though both are legally of adult age, sexual intercourse between this retarded person and a non-retarded person is best described as statutory rape. Because the woman has impaired mental functioning (i.e., a mental age of 7.5 years, per Chapter 2), she may not fully understand the meaning of her consent in this context. Consensual sex implies that both people have the ability to decide to interact. Sodomy is oral-penile or anal-penile contact. Child abuse and sexual abuse are not the best identifiers for the behavior described here.

21

The Doctor-Patient Relationship

Typical Board Question

When a doctor prescribed fluoxetine [Prozac] for a 35-year-old male patient, she explained the major side effects of the drug. Four months later, the patient asks her whether fluoxetine has any side effects. The doctor's best response is to say

(A) "The side effects are nervousness, insomnia, and sexual dysfunction."
(B) "I will have the nurse go over the side effects with you again."
(C) "Why do you ask?"
(D) "Would you like me to check for possible side effects?"
(E) "The side effects are minor; do not worry."

(See "Answers and Explanations" at end of Chapter)

I. Medical Practice

A. Seeking medical care

1. Patients' behavior when ill and their expectations of doctors are influenced by their **culture** (see Chapter 18), their previous experiences with medical care, their physical and mental condition, and their personality styles (not necessarily personality disorders) (Table 21-1).

2. Only about **one third of individuals with symptoms seek medical care;** most people contend with illnesses at home with over-the-counter medications and home treatment.

B. Seeking psychiatric care

1. In the United States, there is a **stigma** to having a psychiatric illness. Psychiatric symptoms are considered by many Americans to indicate **"moral weakness"** or a **lack of self control.** Because of this stigma, many patients fail to seek help.

2. It is important for patients to seek help since there is a strong **correlation between psychological illness** and **physical illness.** Morbidity rates and mortality rates are much higher in patients who need psychiatric attention.

Table 21-1. Patient Personality Style and Behavioral Characteristics During Illness

Personality style	Behavioral characteristics during illness
Dependent	• Has a need to be cared for by others, resulting in the desire for excessive attention from the physician during an illness
Obsessive-compulsive and Type A	• Fear loss of control and may in turn become controlling during illness • Characterized by time pressure (i.e., feels rushed most of the time) and competitiveness • May also show hostility which is associated specifically with the development of coronary artery disease
Histrionic	• May be dramatic, emotionally changeable, and approach the physician in an inappropriate sexual fashion during illness
Narcissistic	• Has a perfect self-image which is threatened by illness • Often feels superior to others and therefore may request that only the "top" physicians be involved in treatment
Paranoid	• Often blames the physician for the illness • Is overly sensitive to a perceived lack of attention or caring from the physician
Passive-aggressive	• Asks for help but then does not comply with the physician's advice
Schizoid	• Becomes even more withdrawn during illness

C. **"The sick role"**

1. A person assumes a particular role in society and certain behavioral patterns when he is ill (the "sick role," described by T. Parsons). The sick role includes **exemption from usual responsibilities** and expectation of care by others as well as working towards becoming healthy, and cooperating with health care personnel in getting well.

2. Critics of the sick role theory argue that it **applies only to middle-class** patients with acute physical illness, and that it emphasizes the power of the doctor and undervalues the individual's social support network in getting well.

D. **Telling patients the truth**

1. In the United States, adult patients generally are **told the complete truth** about the diagnosis, the treatment and its side effects and the prognosis of their illness. **Falsely reassuring** or **patronizing statements** in response to patient questions, (e.g., "do not worry about anything, we will take good care of you") are not appropriate.

2. Information about the illness must be **given directly to the patient** and **not relayed to the patient through relatives.**

   a. With the patient's permission, the physician can tell relatives this information in conjunction with or after telling the patient.

   b. Relieving the fears of **close relatives** of a seriously ill patient can bolster the support system and thus help the patient.

E. Special situations

1. Patients may be **afraid to ask questions** about issues that are **embarrassing** (e.g., sexual problems) or **fear-provoking** (e.g., laboratory results). A doctor should not try to guess what is troubling a patient; it is the doctor's responsibility to ask about such issues in an open-ended fashion (see III A 2 b) and address them truthfully and fully with the patient.

2. Doctors have the primary responsibility for dealing with **compliance issues** (see II below), as well as with **angry, seductive,** or **complaining behavior** by their patients (Table 21-2). Referrals to other doctors should be reserved only for medical and psychiatric problems outside of the range of the expertise of the treating physician.

Table 21-2. Dr. Fadem's Do's and Do Not's for Answering USMLE Questions Involving Common Problems in the Doctor-Patient Relationship

Problem	Do	Do not
Angry patient	• **Do** acknowledge the patient's anger	• **Do not** take the patient's anger personally (the patient is probably fearful about becoming dependent as well as of being ill)
Seductive patient	• **Do** call in a chaperone when you are with the patient • **Do** gather information using direct rather than open-ended questions • **Do** set limits on the behavior that you will tolerate	• **Do not** refuse to see the patient • **Do not** refer the patient to another doctor
Non-compliant patient	• **Do** examine the patient's willingness to change his health-threatening behavior (e.g., smoking); if he is not willing, you must address that issue • **Do** identify the real reason for the patient's refusal to comply or to consent to a needed intervention and address it	• **Do not** attempt to scare the patient into complying (e.g., showing frightening photographs of untreated illness) • **Do not** refer the patient to another doctor
Suicidal patient	• **Do** assess the seriousness of the threat • **Do** suggest that the patient remain in the hospital voluntarily, if the threat is serious	• **Do not** release a hospitalized patient who is a threat to himself [patients who are a threat to self or others can be held involuntarily (see Chapter 23)]
Complaining patient	• **Do** encourage the patient to speak to the other doctor directly if the patient complains about a relationship with another doctor • **Do** speak to your own office staff if the patient has a complaint about one of them	• **Do not** intervene in the patient's relationship with another doctor unless there is a medical reason to do so • **Do not** blame the patient for problems with office staff

Table 21-3. Compliance with Medical Advice

Factors Associated with Increased Compliance	Factors Associated with Decreased Compliance	Comments
Good physician-patient relationship	Poor physician-patient relationship	• Liking the doctor is the most important factor in compliance; it is even more important than the doctor's technical skill • Physicians perceived as unapproachable have low compliance from patients
Patient feels ill and usual activities are disrupted by the illness	Patient experiences few symptoms and little disruption of usual activities	• In asymptomatic illnesses such as hypertension, only about half of patients initially comply with treatment • Many asymptomatic patients who initially complied have stopped complying within 1 year of diagnosis
Short time spent in the waiting room	Long time spent in the waiting room	• Patients kept waiting get angry and then fail to comply
Belief that the benefits of care outweigh its financial and time costs	Belief that financial and time costs of care outweigh its benefits	• The "Health Belief Model" of health care
Written diagnosis and instructions for treatment	Verbal diagnosis and instructions for treatment	• Patients often forget what is said during a visit to the doctor because they are anxious • Asking the patient to repeat your verbal instructions can improve understanding and thus increase compliance
Acute illness	Chronic illness	• Chronically ill people see doctors more often but are more critical of them than acutely ill people
Recommending only one behavioral change at a time	Recommending multiple behavioral changes at once	• To increase compliance, instruct the patient to make one change (e.g., stop smoking) this month, and make another change (e.g., go on a diet) next month. • Recommending too many changes at once will reduce the likelihood that the patient will make any changes
Simple treatment schedule	Complex treatment schedule	• Compliance is higher with medications that require once daily dosing, preferably with a meal • Patients are more likely to forget to take medications requiring frequent or between meal dosing
Older physician	Younger physician	• Usually young physician age is only an issue for patients in the initial stages of treatment
Peer support	Little peer support	• Membership in a group of people with a similar problem [(e.g., smoking (see Chapter 9)] can increase compliance

II. Compliance

A. Patient characteristics associated with compliance

1. Compliance is the extent to which a patient follows the instructions of the physician such as **taking medications on schedule, having a needed medical test** or surgical procedure and following directions for **changes in life-style** such as diet or exercise.

2. Patients' **unconscious** transference reactions to their doctors, which are

Table 21-4. Aims of the Clinical Interview and Interviewing Techniques

Aim	Technique	Specific use	Example
To establish rapport	Support and empathy	To express the physician's interest, understanding, and concern for the patient	"You must have really been frightened when you realized you were going to fall."
	Validation	To give value and credence to the patient's feelings	"Many people would feel the same way if they had been injured as you were."
To maximize information gathering	Facilitation	To encourage the patient to elaborate on an answer; can be a verbal question or body language such as a quizzical expression	"And then what happened?"
	Reflection	To encourage elaboration of the answer by repeating part of the patient's previous response	"You said that your pain increased after lifting the package?"
	Silence	To increase the patient's responsiveness	Waiting silently for the patient to speak
To clarify information	Confrontation	To call the patient's attention to inconsistencies in his or her responses or body language	"You say that you are not worried about tomorrow's surgery, but you seem really nervous to me."
	Recapitulation	To sum up all of the information obtained during the interview to ensure that the doctor understands the information provided by the patient	"Let's go over what happened. You fell last night and hurt your side. You husband called 911. The paramedics came but the pain got worse until they gave you a shot in the emergency room."

Adapted from Fadem and Simring, *High Yield Psychiatry,* Williams & Wilkins, 1998.

based in childhood parent-child relationships, can increase or decrease compliance (see Chapter 6).

3. Only about **one-third of patients comply with treatment,** one-third comply some of the time, and one-third do not comply with treatment.

B. **Factors that increase and decrease compliance**

1. Compliance is **not related to patient intelligence, education,** sex, religion, race, socioeconomic status, or marital status.

2. Factors associated with compliance are listed in **Table 21-3.**

III. The Clinical Interview

A. **Communication skills**

1. Patient compliance with medical advice, detection of both physical and psychological problems, and patient satisfaction with the physician are improved by good doctor-patient communication.

2. One of the most important skills for a physician to have is how to interview patients. In the interview, the physician must first **establish trust in** and **rapport with the patient** and then gather physical, psychological, and social information to identify the patient's problem.

3. The interview serves to obtain the **patient's psychiatric history** including information about prior mental problems, drug and alcohol use, sexual activity, current living situation, and sources of stress.

B. **Specific interviewing techniques**

1. **Direct questions.** Direct questions are used to elicit specific information quickly from a patient in an emergency situation (e.g., "Have you been shot?") or when the patient is seductive, or overly talkative.

2. **Open-ended questions**

a. Although direct questions can elicit information quickly, open-ended types of questions are more likely to aid in obtaining information about the patient, and not close off potential areas of pertinent information.

b. Using open-ended questions (e.g., "What brings you in today?"), the interviewer gives little structure to the patient and **encourages the patient to speak freely.**

3. **Table 21-4** lists aims of the clinical interview and gives examples of some specific interviewing techniques.

Review Test

Directions: Each of the numbered items or incomplete statements in this section is followed by answers or by completions of the statement. Select the **one** lettered answer or completion that is **best** in each case.

Questions 1–2

A 38-year-old salesman who previously had a myocardial infarction, comes to the doctor's office for a routine visit. On seeing the doctor, he angrily exclaims, "What is the matter with this place? I can never find a parking space around here!" He then insists on making a phone call while the doctor waits to examine him.

1. Most appropriately, the physician should now say

A.   "I cannot examine you until you calm down."
B.   "Are you always this angry?"
C.   "You seem upset."
D.   "Would you like a referral to another doctor?"
E.   "I will reschedule your appointment for another day."

2. The personality type that best describes this patient is

A.   histrionic
B.   narcissistic
C.   obsessive-compulsive
D.   passive-aggressive
E.   dependent

Questions 3–4

A patient comes to the doctor's office wearing a low-cut blouse. She comes up very close to him and begins to ask him questions about his personal life.

3. The doctor's most appropriate behavior is to

A.   refuse to examine her but give her another appointment
B.   call in a chaperone
C.   use only open-ended questions in interviewing her
D.   refer her to another doctor
E.   ask her about her personal life

4. The personality type that best describes this patient is

A.   histrionic
B.   narcissistic
C.   obsessive-compulsive
D.   passive-aggressive
E.   dependent

5. A 46-year-old man comes to the emergency department complaining of chest pain. Which of the following statements will elicit the most information from this patient?

A.   "Point to the area of pain in your chest."
B.   "Tell me about the pain in your chest."
C.   "Tell me about the pain."
D.   "Have you been to a physician within the past 6 months?"
E.   "Is there a history of heart disease in your family?"

6. A 50-year-old woman presents with a complaint of gastric distress. She seems agitated and says that she is afraid she has cirrhosis of the liver but then stops speaking. Which of the following will best encourage her to continue speaking?

A.   "Please go on."
B.   "How much liquor do you drink?"
C.   "Do you drink?"
D.   "Why did you wait so long to come in?"
E.   "I see that the situation upsets you."

7. On the day he is to receive the results of a biopsy, a patient tells the doctor that he feels fine. However, the doctor notices that the patient is pale, sweaty, and shaky. Which of the following is the most appropriate statement for the doctor to make?

A.   "Tell me again about the pain in your back."
B.   "How do you feel?"
C.   "You'll be fine."
D.   "You look frightened."
E.   "How do you feel about being in the hospital?"

8. Patients are most likely to comply with medical advice for which of the following reasons?

A. The illness has few symptoms.
B. The patient likes the doctor.
C. The doctor is young.
D. The illness is chronic.
E. The treatment schedule is complex.

9. A 50-year-old African-American male patient who is well-educated has a herniated disc. The characteristic of this patient most likely to increase his compliance with the treatment plan is his

A. race
B. socioeconomic status
C. back pain
D. education
E. gender

10. The "sick role" as described by Parsons

A. applies mainly to low socioeconomic groups
B. overvalues people's social support networks
C. includes lack of cooperation with health care workers
D. includes exemption from usual responsibilities
E. applies mainly to chronic illness

11. A 34-year-old father of two children smokes two packs of cigarettes a day but believes that smoking does not cause him harm. Instead, he believes that smoking prevents him from getting colds. To get him to smoke less, the physician should first

A. recommend a smoking cessation support group
B. recommend a nicotine patch
C. show him photographs of the lungs of patients with lung cancer
D. determine how willing he is to stop smoking
E. tell him his children will be fatherless if he continues smoking

12. A patient whose father died of prostate cancer says that he cannot take a prostate-specific antigen test because "the needle will leave a mark." The doctor's most appropriate behavior is to

A. speak to his wife and ask her to convince him to have the test
B. reassure him that the needle mark will fade with time
C. show him photographs of patients with untreated prostate cancer
D. reassure him that whatever the outcome of the test, he can be cured
E. discuss his feelings about his father's illness with the patient

13. The parents of a critically ill 6-year-old patient tell the doctor that when the child became ill, his 14-year-old brother started to behave badly in school and at home. The younger child's doctor, should

A. refer the teenager to an adolescent psychologist
B. speak to the teenager as soon as possible
C. speak to the teenager when the younger child is out of danger
D. tell the parents that the patient is the younger child, not the teenager
E. tell the parents to concentrate on the younger child

Answers and Explanations

TBQ-C. The doctor's best response is to say, "Why do you ask?," an open-ended question meant to encourage the patient to speak freely. It is likely that the patient is having sexual side effects, common with fluoxetine, and is uncomfortable about discussing them. It is not appropriate to just repeat the possible side effects, reassure the patient, or have the nurse do the doctor's work by talking to the patient (see also Table 23-1).

1-C. Before examining this patient, the physician should acknowledge his anger by saying "You seem upset." While directed at the doctor via the parking problem, the patient's anger is more likely to be related to his anxiety about having a serious illness. Treating him in a childlike way (i.e., telling him that he cannot be examined until he calms down) will further anger him. The doctor is are responsible for dealing with illness-related emotional needs and problems of patients. There is no reason to refer this patient to another physician.

2-C. The personality type that best describes this patient is obsessive-compulsive. Obsessive-compulsive patients fear loss of control and may in turn become controlling (i.e., having the doctor wait while he makes a phone call) during illness.

3-B. The doctor's most appropriate behavior is to call in a chaperone when dealing with this seductive patient. Refusing to treat her, asking about her personal life, and referring her to another physician are not appropriate. For seductive patients, closed-ended questions which limit responsiveness are often more appropriate than open-ended questions.

4-A. The personality type that best describes this patient is histrionic. Histrionic patients are dramatic and may behave in a sexually inappropriate fashion to get attention during illness. Characteristics of other personality types and disorders can be found in Chapter 14.

5-C. The most open-ended of these questions, "Tell me about the pain," gives little structure to the patient and can therefore elicit the most information.

6-A. The interview technique known as facilitation is used by the interviewer to encourage the patient to elaborate on an answer. The phrase, "Please go on," is a facilitative statement.

7-D. The physician's statement, "You look frightened," demonstrates the interviewing technique of confrontation which calls the patient's attention to the inconsistency in his response and his body language and helps him to express his fears.

8-B. Patients are most likely to comply with medical advice because they like the doctor. Compliance is also associated with symptomatic illnesses, older doctors, acute illnesses, and simple treatment schedules.

9-C. The fact that he is experiencing pain is most likely to increase this patient's compliance with the treatment plan. There is no clear association between compliance and race, socioeconomic status, education, or gender.

10-D. The "sick role" applies mainly to middle-class patients with acute physical illnesses. It includes the expectation of care by others, lack of responsibility for becoming ill, and exemption from one's usual responsibilities. It undervalues social support networks.

11-D. In order to get this patient to smoke less, the physician should first determine how willing he is to stop smoking. A support group or nicotine patch are only useful for motivated patients. This patient is not motivated, in fact, he believes that smoking helps him avoid colds. Scaring patients about the consequences of their behavior is not appropriate or effective in gaining compliance.

12-E. The doctor's most appropriate behavior with this patient who refuses a needed test is to determine the basis of his refusal—probably his feelings about his father's fatal illness. The reason he refuses to have the test probably has little to do with the mark it will leave. Telling him that he can be cured is patronizing, inappropriate, and possibly untrue. Speaking to his wife also is not appropriate; doctors should deal directly with patients whenever possible. Scaring patients about the consequences of their behavior is not appropriate or effective in gaining compliance (see also Table 23-1).

13-B. The younger child's doctor should speak to the teenager as soon as possible to provide information and relieve his fears. This teenager is likely to be frightened about his sibling's illness and the changed behavior of his parents. Adolescents often "act out" when fearful or depressed (see Chapter 6). It is the doctor's role to deal with problems in the patient's support system to reduce stress and thus help in recovery. There is usually no need to refer family members to mental health professionals. Waiting until the younger child is out of danger will needlessly prolong the older child's problem and further stress the family.

22

Psychosomatic Medicine

*Typical **B**oard **Q**uestion*

A 45-year-old man has a routine yearly physical examination. While taking the history, the doctor determines that during the last year, the patient took out a substantial mortgage and moved to a new house. During the move, he fell and sustained a head injury requiring him to be hospitalized. While recuperating, he and his wife of 10 years went on a 2-week vacation. He recovered completely, but after the vacation, the couple separated. According to the Holmes and Rahe scale, which of these social experiences puts this man at the highest risk for physical illness in the present year?

(A) Taking out a large mortgage
(B) Changing residence
(C) Sustaining a serious injury
(D) Going on vacation
(E) Obtaining a marital separation

(See "Answers and Explanations" at end of Chapter)

I. Stress and Health

A. Psychological factors affecting health

—Psychological factors may initiate or **exacerbate symptoms of medical disorders** (psychosomatic symptoms) involving almost all body systems. These factors include:

1. **Poor health behavior** (e.g., smoking, failure to exercise)

2. **Maladaptive personality styles** (e.g., type A personality) (see Chapter 21).

3. **Chronic or acute life stress** due to emotional (e.g., depression), social (e.g., divorce), or economic (e.g., job loss) problems.

B. Mechanisms of the physiologic effects of stress

1. Acute or chronic life stress leads to **activation of the autonomic nervous system,** which in turn affects cardiovascular and respiratory changes.

2. Stress also leads to **altered levels of neurotransmitters** (e.g., serotonin, norepinephrine), which result in changes in mood and behavior.

3. Stress can **increase the release of adrenocorticotropic hormone**

(ACTH), which leads to the release of cortisol, ultimately resulting in depression of the immune system as measured by **decreased lymphocyte response** to mitogens and **impaired function** of natural killer (NK) cells.

C. **Stressful life events**

—High levels of stress in a patient's life may be related to an **increased likelihood of medical** and **psychiatric illness.**

1. The **Social Readjustment Rating Scale** by **Holmes and Rahe** (which also includes "positive" events like holidays) ranks the effects of life events (Table 22-1). Events with the highest scores require people to make the most "social readjustment" in their lives.

2. The need for social readjustment is directly correlated with increased risk of medical and psychiatric illness; in studies by Holmes and Rahe, **80% of patients with a score of 300 points in a given year became ill during the next year.**

II. Psychological Stress in Hospitalized Patients

A. **Overview**

1. Not uncommonly, medical and surgical patients have concurrent psychological problems. These problems cause psychological stress which can exacerbate the patient's physical disorder.

2. Usually, the treating physician handles these problems by **organizing the patient's social support systems** and by using specific psychotropic medications.

3. For severe psychiatric problems (e.g., psychotic symptoms) in hospitalized patients, consultation–liaison **(CL) psychiatrists** may be called.

Table 22-1. Magnitude of Stress Associated With Selected Life Events According to the Holmes and Rahe Social Readjustment Rating Scale

Relative Stressfulness	Life Event (exact point value)
Very high	• Death of a spouse (100) • Divorce (73) • Marital separation (65) • Death of a close family member (63)
High	• Major personal loss of health due to illness or injury (53) • Marriage (50) • Job loss (47) • Retirement (45) • Major loss of health of a close family member (44) • Birth or adoption of a child (39)
Moderate	• Assuming major debt (e.g., taking out a mortgage) (31) • Promotion or demotion at work (29) • Child leaving home (29)
Low	• Changing residence (20) • Vacation (15) • Major holiday (12)

B. Problems of hospitalized patients

1. Common psychological complaints in hospitalized patients include anxiety, sleep disorders, and disorientation, often as a result of **delirium** (see Chapter 14).

2. Patients who are at the **greatest risk** for such problems include those undergoing surgery, those on renal dialysis, and those who are being treated in the intensive care unit (ICU) or coronary care unit (CCU).

C. Surgical patients

1. Patients undergoing surgery who are at greatest psychological and medical risk are those who **believe that they will not survive** surgery as well as those who **do not admit that they are worried** before surgery.

2. To reduce risk, the doctor should **encourage patients to take a positive attitude** and to **talk about their fears** and explain to patients what they can expect during and after the procedure (e.g., mechanical support, pain).

D. Patients undergoing renal dialysis

1. Patients on renal dialysis are at increased risk for psychological problems (e.g., depression, suicide, and sexual dysfunction) in part because their lives **depend on other people** and **on machines.**

2. Psychological and medical risk can be **reduced** through the use of **in-home dialysis units,** which cause less disruption of the patient's life.

E. ICU or CCU patients

1. Patients treated in the ICU or CCU are at increased risk for depression and delirium (**ICU psychosis**).

2. Because these patients have **life-threatening illnesses,** their clinical stability is **particularly vulnerable** to psychological symptoms.

3. Psychological and medical risk can be reduced by **enhancing sensory** and **social input** (e.g., encouraging the patient to talk) and allowing the patient to control the environment (e.g., lighting, pain medication) as much as possible.

III. Patients With Chronic Pain

A. Psychosocial factors

1. Chronic pain (pain lasting >6 months) is a **commonly encountered complaint** of patients. It may be associated with physical factors, psychological factors, or a combination of both.

   a. **Decreased tolerance for pain** is associated with depression, anxiety, and life stress in adulthood and physical and sexual abuse in childhood.

   b. **Pain tolerance** can be increased through biofeedback, physical therapy, hypnosis, psychotherapy, meditation, and relaxation training.

2. Depression may predispose a person to develop chronic pain. More commonly, **chronic pain results in depression.**

3. Religious, cultural, and ethnic factors may influence the patient's expression of pain and the responses of the **patient's support systems** to the pain (see Chapter 18).

4. Psychological "benefits" (**secondary gain**) of chronic pain include attention from others, financial gain, and justification of inability to establish social relationships.

B. Treating pain

1. **Pain relief** in pain caused by physical illness is best achieved by **analgesics** (e.g., opiates) or nerve-blocking surgical procedures.

2. **Antidepressants,** particularly tricyclics, are useful in the management of pain.

   a. Antidepressants are most useful for patients with **arthritis, facial pain,** and **headache.**

   b. Their analgesic effect may be the result of **stimulation of efferent inhibitory pain pathways.**

   c. Although they have direct analgesic effects, antidepressants also may decrease pain indirectly by **improving symptoms of depression.**

3. According to the **gate control theory,** the perception of pain can be blocked by electric stimulation of large-diameter afferent nerves. Some patients are helped by this treatment.

4. Patients with pain caused by physical illness also benefit from **behavioral, cognitive,** and **other psychological therapies** (see Chapter 17), by needing less pain medication, becoming more active, and showing increased attempts to return to a normal lifestyle.

C. Programs of pain treatment

1. **Scheduled administration of an analgesic** before the patient requests it (e.g., every 3 hours) is more effective than medication administered when the patient requests it (on demand). Scheduled administration separates the experience of pain from the receipt of medication.

2. Many **patients with chronic pain are undermedicated** because the physician fears that the patient will become addicted to opiates. However, recent evidence shows that patients with chronic pain **easily discontinue the use of opiates** as the pain remits.

3. Pain patients are at much higher risk for depression than they are for drug addiction.

D. Pain in children

1. Children feel pain and remember pain as much as adults do.

2. Children who experience pain due to a procedure have a higher risk of morbidity and mortality and a slower recovery from the procedure.

3. The most useful ways of administering pain medications to children are **orally** (e.g., a Fentanyl "lollipop"), **transdermally** (e.g., a skin cream to prevent pain from injections or spinal taps) or via patient-controlled analgesia.

IV. Patients with Acquired Immune Deficiency Syndrome (AIDS)

A. Psychological stressors. AIDS and human immunodeficiency virus (HIV)-positive patients must deal with particular psychological stressors not seen together in other disorders.

1. These stressors include having a **fatal illness,** feeling **guilt** about how they contracted the illness (e.g., sex with multiple partners, intravenous drug use) and about possibly infecting others, and being met with **fear of contagion** from medical personnel, family, and friends.

2. HIV-positive **homosexual patients** may be forced to **"come out"** (i.e., reveal their sexual orientation) to others.

3. **Depression** is commonly seen in AIDS patients.

4. Medical and psychological **counseling** can reduce medical and psychological risk for HIV-positive patients.

B. Contagion

1. Only a total of about **50 medical personnel** (mostly laboratory workers, less than 10 doctors) **have contracted HIV** from patients in this country.

2. If they comply with methods of infection control, HIV-positive physicians pose no risk to their patients. In the United States, **no physician-to-patient transmission** of HIV has ever been confirmed.

3. Doctors can identify HIV-positive patients to those they put at imminent risk (e.g., sexual partners)(see Chapter 23).

Review Test

Directions: Each of the numbered items or incomplete statements in this section is followed by answers or by completions of the statement. Select the **one** lettered answer or completion that is **best** in each case.

Questions 1–2

A 35-year-old woman with a herniated disc has been suffering from back pain for the past two years. To help control her pain she takes an opiate-based medication daily.

1. Which of the following is most likely to be true about this patient?

(A) She is at high risk for drug addiction
(B) Psychological therapies will not benefit her
(C) Her expression of pain is related exclusively to the extent of her pain
(D) She is at high risk for depression
(E) She is receiving too much pain medication

2. Psychological stress engendered by this patient's pain is most likely to result in increased

(A) lymphocyte response to mitogens
(B) release of adrenocorticotropic hormone (ACTH)
(C) function of natural killer cells
(D) function of the immune system
(E) cortisol suppression

3. In the United States, the number of physicians who have contracted HIV from patients is

(A) between 0 and 50
(B) between 51 and 100
(C) between 101 and 200
(D) between 201 and 300
(E) more than 300

4. In the United States, the number of patients confirmed to have contracted HIV from physicians is

(A) between 0 and 50
(B) between 51 and 100
(C) between 101 and 200
(D) between 201 and 300
(E) more than 300

Questions 5–6

A 65-year-old male patient is scheduled for cardiac surgery. After the surgery he will be in the intensive care unit (ICU) for about 12 hours and will require a mechanical ventilator.

5. To reduce this patient's likelihood of psychological problems in the ICU, the physician should

(A) severely limit visits from family
(B) reduce exposure to ambient light
(C) explain the need for and function of the mechanical ventilator
(D) discourage communication between patient and staff
(E) have the nurses control the patient's lighting level

6. During his stay in the intensive care unit (ICU) after surgery, this patient is most likely to experience which of the following disorders?

(A) Panic disorder
(B) Obsessive-compulsive disorder
(C) Hypochondriasis
(D) Somatization disorder
(E) Delirium

Answers and Explanations

TBQ-E. According to the Holmes and Rahe scale, marital separation puts this man at the highest risk for physical illness this year. The events in this man's life in decreasing order of stressfulness are: marital separation, serious head injury, large mortgage, changing residence, and going on vacation.

1-D. This chronic pain patient is at high risk for depression but at relatively low risk for drug addiction. Pain patients tend to be undermedicated; it is more likely that this patient is receiving too little rather than too much pain medication. Psychological therapies can be of significant benefit to chronic pain patients. This patient's expression of pain is related not only to the extent of her pain, but also to religious, cultural, and ethnic factors.

2-B. Psychological stress engendered by this patient's pain is likely to result in increased release of adrenocorticotropic hormone (ACTH) and cortisol. This in turn results in decreased function of the immune system as reflected in decreased lymphocyte response to mitogens and function of natural killer cells.

3-A. In the United States, fewer than 10 physicians have contracted HIV from patients.

4-A. In the United States, no physician-to-patient transmission of HIV has been confirmed.

5-C. To reduce this patient's likelihood of psychological problems in the intensive care unit (ICU), the physician should explain the need for and function of the mechanical ventilator and any other mechanical support that he will need. The physician should also encourage visits from family and communication between patient and staff. The patient should also be encouraged to control aspects of his environment (e.g., lighting level). Outside stimuli (e.g., light) should be increased rather than decreased.

6-E. Because of the disorienting nature of the intensive care unit (ICU), delirium is commonly seen in ICU patients. Panic disorder, obsessive-compulsive disorder, hypochondriasis, and somatization disorder are no more common in ICU patients than in the general population.

23

Legal and Ethical Issues in Medicine

Typical Board Question

A legally competent 65-year-old man signs a document that states that he does not want any measures taken to prolong his life should he go into a persistent vegetative state. Five days later he has a stroke. He goes into a coma and requires life support. Extensive evaluation reveals that he will never recover consciousness. The patient's wife urges the physician to keep her husband alive. The physician should

(A) get a court order to start life support
(B) follow the wishes of the wife and start life support
(C) carry out the patient's prior request and not provide life support
(D) ask the patient's adult children for permission to continue life support
(E) turn the case over to the ethics committee of the hospital

(See "Answers and Explanations" at end of Chapter)

I. Legal Competence

A. Definition

1. To be **legally competent** to make health care decisions, a patient must understand the **risks, benefits,** and likely outcome of such decisions.

2. **All adults** (persons 18 years of age and older) are assumed to be legally competent to make health care decisions for themselves.

B. Minors

1. **Minors** (persons younger than 18 years of age) usually are **not** considered legally competent.

2. **"Emancipated minors"** are people under 18 years of age who meet at least one of the criteria below. Emancipated minors are considered competent adults and can give consent for their own medical care.

   a. They are **self-supporting** or in the **military.**

   b. They are **married.**

   c. They **have children** whom they care for.

C. Questions of competence

1. If an adult's competence is in question (e.g., a mentally retarded or demented person), **a judge** (not the patient's family or physician) **makes the determination** of competence. Doctors are often consulted by the judge for information about whether the patient has the capacity to make health care decisions.

2. A person **may meet the legal standard** for competence to accept or refuse medical treatment **even if she is mentally ill** or **retarded** or is incompetent in other areas of her life (e.g., with finances).

II. Informed Consent

A. Overview

—With the exception of life-threatening emergencies, physicians must obtain consent from competent, informed adult patients before proceeding with **any medical or surgical treatment.**

1. Although a signature may not be required for minor medical procedures, patients usually **sign a document** of consent for major medical procedures or for surgery.

2. **Other hospital personnel** (e.g., nurses) usually **cannot** obtain informed consent.

B. Components of informed consent

1. Before patients can give consent to be treated by a doctor, they must be informed of and **understand the health implications of their diagnosis.**

2. Patients must also be informed of the **health risks and benefits** of treatment **and the alternatives** to treatment.

3. Patients must know the likely **outcome if they do not consent** to the treatment.

4. They also must be informed that they can **withdraw consent for treatment at any time** before the procedure (even on the way to the operating room after preanesthetic medication has been administered).

C. Special situations

1. Competent patients have the **right to refuse to consent** to a needed test or procedure for religious or other reasons even if their health will suffer or death will result from such refusal.

2. Although medical or surgical intervention may be necessary to protect the health or life of the fetus, a **competent pregnant woman has the right to refuse** such intervention (e.g., cesarean section) even if the fetus will die or be seriously injured without the treatment.

3. While all of the medical findings are generally provided to a patient, a doctor does not have to relay the findings immediately if the doctor believes such knowledge will **adversely affect the patient's health**

(e.g., a coronary patient). The doctor can **delay** telling the patient the diagnosis until the patient indicates that he is ready to receive the news.

4. The **opinions of family members** as to whether to tell the patient the diagnosis and prognosis **are not relevant.** At the patient's request, family members may be present when the doctor provides the diagnosis.

D. Unexpected findings

—If an **unexpected finding** during surgery necessitates a non-emergency procedure for which the patient has not given consent (e.g., biopsy of an unsuspected ovarian malignancy found during a tubal ligation), the patient must **wake up** and **give informed consent** before the additional procedure can be performed.

E. Treatment of minors [i.e., people younger than 18 years of age, unless emancipated (see I.B.2)]

1. Only the **parent** or **legal guardian** can give consent for surgical or medical treatment of a minor.

2. Parental consent is **not required** in the treatment of minors in the following instances:

   a. **Emergency** situations (i.e., when the parent or guardian cannot be located and a delay in treatment can potentially harm the child)

   b. Treatment of sexually transmitted diseases (**STDs**)

   c. Prescription of **contraceptives**

   d. Medical care during **pregnancy**

   e. Treatment of **drug and alcohol dependence**

3. About 80% of the states require parental consent when a minor seeks an **abortion.**

4. A **court order** can be obtained from a judge (within hours if necessary) if a child has a life-threatening illness or accident and the **parent or guardian refuses to consent to an established** (but not an experimental) medical procedure for religious or other reasons.

III. Confidentiality

A. Although physicians are **expected ethically to maintain patient confidentiality,** they are **not required** to do so if:

1. Their patient is suspected of **child or elder abuse**

2. Their patient has a significant **risk of suicide**

3. Their patient poses a serious **threat to another person.**

B. **Intervention by the physician if the patient poses a threat**

1. The physician must first ascertain the **credibility** of the threat or danger.

2. If the threat or danger is credible, the doctor must **notify** the appropri-

ate law enforcement officials or social service agency and **warn** the intended victim (the **Tarasoff** decision).

IV. Reportable Illnesses

A. Most states require physicians to report certain infectious illnesses to their state health departments (reportable illnesses). State health departments report these illnesses to the federal Centers for Disease Control and Prevention (**CDC**) for statistical purposes.

B. Requirements as to which specific illnesses are reportable may vary from state to state:

1. In all states, **varicella, hepatitis, measles, mumps, rubella, salmonellosis, shigellosis,** and **tuberculosis** are reportable.

2. Sexually transmitted diseases (**STDs**) which are reportable in all states include acquired immune deficiency syndrome (**AIDS**) (but not HIV-positive status in all states), **syphilis,** and **gonorrhea.**

3. Chlamydia and genital herpes are not reportable in most states.

V. Ethical Issues Involving HIV Infection

A. **HIV-positive colleagues**

—Doctors are **not required to inform** either patients or the medical establishment about another doctor's HIV-positive status since, if the doctor follows procedures for infection control, he poses no risk to his patients (see Chapter 22).

B. **HIV-positive patients**

1. Ethically, a doctor **cannot refuse** to treat HIV-positive patients because of fear of infection. There is no legal requirement for a doctor to treat any patient.

2. **A pregnant patient** at high risk for HIV infection **cannot be tested** for the virus or treated [(e.g., with zidovudine (AZT)] against her will even if the fetus could be adversely affected by such refusal.

3. Doctors are not required to maintain confidentiality when an HIV-positive patient habitually puts another person at risk by engaging in unprotected sex (see III, B above).

VI. Involuntary and Voluntary Psychiatric Hospitalization

—Under certain circumstances that vary according to state law, patients with psychiatric disorders who are a **danger to themselves or others** may be hospitalized against their will (involuntary hospitalization).

A. In psychiatric **emergency situations,** patients who will not or cannot agree to be hospitalized may be hospitalized against their will or without consent with the certification of **one or two physicians,** for up to 60 days (depending on state law) before a court hearing.

B. Even if a psychiatric patient **chooses voluntarily to be hospitalized,** he may be required to wait 24–48 hours before he is permitted to sign out against medical advice.

C. Patients who are confined to mental health facilities, whether voluntarily or involuntarily, have the **right to receive treatment** and **to refuse treatment** (e.g., medication, electroconvulsive therapy).

VII. Advance Directives

A. Overview

1. Advance directives are instructions given by patients **in anticipation of the need for a medical decision.** A durable power of attorney and a living will are examples of advance directives.

   a. A **durable power of attorney** is a document in which a competent person **designates another person** (e.g., spouse, friend) as her legal representative (i.e., health care proxy) to make decisions about her health care when she can no longer do so.

   b. A **living will** is a document in which a competent person gives directions for his future health care if he becomes incompetent to make decisions when he needs care.

2. Health care facilities that receive Medicare payments (most hospitals and nursing homes) **are required to ask patients** whether they have advance directives and, if necessary, **help patients** to write them. They must also inform patients of their **right to refuse** treatment or resuscitation.

B. Surrogates

1. If an incompetent patient does not have an **advance directive,** health care providers or family members (**surrogates**) must determine **what the patient would have done if she were competent** (the substituted judgment standard). The **personal wishes of surrogates are irrelevant** to the medical decision.

2. Even if a health care proxy or surrogate has been making decisions for an incompetent patient, if the patient **regains function** (competence) even briefly or intermittently, she regains the right during those periods to make decisions about her health care.

VIII. Death and Euthanasia

A. Legal standard of death

1. In the United States, the legal standard of death (when cardiorespiratory criteria are not met) is **irreversible cessation of all functions of the entire brain,** including the brain stem.

2. If the patient is dead according to the legal standard, the physician is authorized to **remove life support.** A court order or relative's permission is not necessary.

3. Physicians certify the **cause of death** (e.g., natural, suicide, accident) and sign the death certificate.

B. Euthanasia

According to medical codes of ethics (e.g., those of the American Medical Association and medical specialty organizations), **euthanasia (mercy killing) is a criminal act** and is **never appropriate.**

1. **Physician-assisted suicide** is not strictly legal in any state, but is not generally an indictable offense as long as the physician does not actually perform the killing (i.e., the patient injects himself).

—Dr. Jack Kevorkian recently challenged the law in Michigan regarding physician-assisted suicide by actually administering a lethal injection to a patient himself and was convicted of murder.

2. Under some circumstances, food, water, and medical care can be withheld from a terminally ill patient who has **no reasonable prospect of recovery** but is not legally dead.

3. If a competent patient **requests cessation of artificial life support,** it is both legal and ethical for a physician to comply with this request. Such action by the physician is not considered euthanasia.

IX. Medical Malpractice

A. Overview

1. Medical malpractice occurs when harm comes to a patient as a result of actions or inactions of a physician. The elements of malpractice (**the 4 "D"s**) are:
   a. **Dereliction,** or negligence (i.e., deviation from normal standards of care), of a
   b. **Duty** (i.e., there is an established physician-patient relationship) that causes
   c. **Damages** (i.e., injury)
   d. **Directly** to the patient (i.e., the damages were caused by the negligence, not by another factor).

2. **Surgeons** (including obstetricians) and **anesthesiologists** are the specialists most likely to be sued for malpractice. Psychiatrists and family practitioners are the least likely to be sued.

3. Malpractice is a **tort,** or **civil wrong,** not a crime. A finding for the plaintiff (the patient) results in a financial award to the patient from the defendant physician or his insurance carrier, not a jail term or loss of license.

4. Recently there has been an increase in the number of malpractice claims. This increase is due mainly to a **breakdown** of the traditional **physician-patient relationship** because of:
   a. **Technological advances** in medicine, which reduce personal contact with the doctor.

     b. Limits on time for personal interaction and physician autonomy, partly as a result of the growth of managed care.

  B. Damages. The patient may be awarded compensatory damages only, or both compensatory and punitive damages.

    1. Compensatory damages are given to **reimburse** the patient for medical bills or lost salary and to compensate the patient for pain and suffering.

    2. Punitive damages are awarded to the patient to **punish the physician** and set an example for the medical community. Punitive damages are rare and are awarded only in cases of wanton carelessness or gross negligence (e.g., a drunk doctor who cuts a vital nerve).

  C. Sexual relationships with patients

    1. Sexual relationships with current or former patients are **inappropriate** and are **prohibited** by the ethical standards of most specialty boards.

    2. Patients who claim that they had a sexual relationship with a physician may **file an ethics complaint or a medical malpractice complaint,** or both.

X. Impaired Physicians

  A. Causes of impairment in physicians include

    1. Drug or alcohol abuse

    2. Physical or mental illness

    3. Impairment in functioning associated with old age

  B. Reporting of an impaired colleague, medical student, or resident is an ethical requirement because patients must be protected and the impaired colleague must be helped. The legal requirement for reporting impaired colleagues varies among states.

    1. An **impaired medical student** should be reported to the **dean** of the medical school or the dean of students.

    2. An **impaired resident** or **attending physician** should be reported to the person directly in charge of him, (e.g., the residency training director or the chief of the medical staff, respectively).

    3. A licensed physician should report an **impaired colleague** to the state licensing board or the impaired physicians program, usually part of the state medical society.

XI. Answering USMLE Legal and Ethical Issues Questions

  —Table 23–1 provides "Do's" and "Do Not's" for answering questions on the USMLE involving legal and ethical issues.

Table 23-1. Dr. Fadem's "Do's" and "Do Not's" for Answering USMLE Ethical and Legal Questions

Do	Do Not
• **Do** tell patients the complete truth about their illness and prognosis	• **Do not** "cover up" the truth about a patient's condition
• **Do** tell patients the truth about your qualifications (e.g., "I am a third-year medical student")	• **Do not** "cover up" the true status of medical students or residents (e.g., "I am a member of the doctor's team")
• **Do** speak to competent adult patients directly	• **Do not** discuss issues concerning patients with their relatives (e.g., spouse, adult children) or anyone else (e.g., insurance companies) without the patient's permission
• **Do** ask patients to consent to their own treatment	• **Do not** ask a relative for consent to treat a patient unless the relative has a durable power of attorney or is the legal guardian
• **Do** encourage competent patients to make their own health care choices (i.e., be autonomous)	• **Do not** try to "scare" patients into consenting to any medical test (e.g., mammogram) or surgical procedure (e.g., coronary bypass)
• **Do** take care of your patient yourself	• **Do not** refer your patient (no matter how difficult or offensive) to another student, resident, or doctor
• **Do** spend time with your patient	• **Do not** delegate your responsibilities (e.g., giving patients lengthy medical instructions) to office staff (e.g., nurses)
• **Do** make health care decisions based on what is best for the health of the patient	• **Do not** make health care decisions based on expense in time or money
• **Do** discuss with a pregnant patient the practical issues of having and caring for the child	• **Do not** advise a patient to have an abortion (unless she is at medical risk) no matter what the age of the mother (e.g., teenage) or the condition of the fetus (e.g., Down syndrome)
• **Do** encourage a pregnant patient to make her own decision about whether or not to have an abortion	• **Do not** accede to the demand of the pregnant woman's own parents to perform an abortion (even if the patient is mentally retarded)
• **Do** provide medically needed analgesia to a terminally ill patient even if it coincidentally may shorten the patient's life	• **Do not** administer an analgesia overdose with the purpose of shortening a terminally ill patient's life.

Review Test

Directions: Each of the numbered items or incomplete statements in this section is followed by answers or by completions of the statement. Select the **one** lettered answer or completion that is **best** in each case.

1. A competent 30-year-old patient who is 38 weeks' pregnant refuses to have a cesarean delivery despite the fact that without the surgery the fetus will probably die. Both her physician and a consultation-liaison psychiatrist have failed to convince her to have the surgery. The most appropriate action for her physician to take at this time is to

(A) get permission from the patient's husband to do the surgery
(B) ask a judge to issue a court order to do the surgery
(C) tell the patient that she can be criminally prosecuted if the child dies
(D) deliver the child vaginally
(E) refer the patient to another doctor

2. A 19-year-old man who is HIV-positive tells his physician that he is regularly having unprotected sex with his 18-year-old girlfriend. The girlfriend does not know the patient's HIV status. At this time his physician should

(A) inform state health authorities about the patient's HIV status
(B) keep the information about the patient's HIV status confidential
(C) inform the girlfriend of the patient's HIV status
(D) inform the girlfriend's parents of the patient's HIV status
(E) advise the girlfriend not to have unprotected sex with the patient

3. A 15-year-old patient who has contracted chlamydia consults her family physician. Prior to treating her infection, the physician should

(A) notify her parents
(B) notify her sexual partner
(C) get written permission from her parents
(D) counsel her on safe sex practices
(E) report the case to state health authorities

4. A clearly competent 50-year-old woman who has religious beliefs that preclude blood transfusion is scheduled for major surgery. Prior to the surgery, she states that the physician is not to give her a blood transfusion, although she may need it during surgery. If a transfusion becomes necessary during surgery, the physician should

(A) replace lost body fluids but not give the woman the transfusion
(B) get a court order to do the transfusion
(C) get permission from the woman's family to do the transfusion
(D) give the woman the transfusion but not tell her about it
(E) give the woman the transfusion and inform her of it when she recovers from the anesthetic

5. A 30-year-old man and his 10-year-old son are injured in a train crash. Both of them need surgery within the next 12 hours. The father is clearly mentally competent but refuses the surgery for both himself and his son. The physician should

(A) get a court order for the surgery on the child but do not operate on the father
(B) get a court order for the surgery for both the father and child
(C) get permission for the surgery for both the father and child from the mother
(D) have the father moved to another hospital
(E) follow the father's wishes and do not operate on either the father or the son

6. A 60-year-old man has a suspicious mass biopsied. He is clearly mentally competent but has been very depressed over his wife's recent death. His daughter asks the doctor not to tell the patient the diagnosis if the results show a malignancy because she fears that he will kill himself. If the mass proves to be malignant, the doctor should

(A) follow the daughter's wishes and not tell the patient the diagnosis
(B) tell the patient the diagnosis immediately
(C) tell the patient not to worry and that he will be well cared for
(D) ask the patient when he would like to receive the diagnosis
(E) have the daughter tell the patient the diagnosis

7. A 10-year-old boy who was injured during gym class is brought to the emergency department. He has a severe laceration that requires immediate suturing. His parents are on vacation and cannot be located and an aunt is babysitting for the child. The most appropriate action for the physician to take is to

(A) obtain consent from the aunt
(B) obtain consent from the gym teacher
(C) suture the laceration without obtaining consent
(D) keep the patient comfortable until you reach the parents
(E) obtain consent from the child himself

8. On his surgery rotation, medical student X frequently smells alcohol on the breath of medical student Y. The most appropriate action for medical student X to take is to

(A) talk to medical student Y about his drinking on the floor
(B) warn medical student Y that he will be reported if he continues to drink on the floor
(C) report medical student Y to the dean of students
(D) report medical student Y to the police
(E) ask that medical student Y be transferred to another rotation site

9. A surgeon to whom an internist has regularly referred patients tells the internist in confidence that he (the surgeon) is HIV positive. The most appropriate action for the internist to take is to

(A) stop referring patients to the surgeon
(B) report the surgeon to the state health authorities
(C) report the surgeon to the hospital administration
(D) continue to refer patients to the surgeon

(E) continue to refer patients to the surgeon but first tell them about his HIV status

10. A 25-year-old man who is HIV-positive comes to a doctor's office for treatment of a skin lesion. Because she is afraid of infection, the doctor refuses to treat him. This doctor's refusal to treat the patient is best described as

(A) unethical and illegal
(B) ethical and legal
(C) unethical but legal
(D) ethical but illegal

11. A legally competent, terminally ill 70-year-old patient on life support asks her physician to turn off the machines and let her die. The doctor follows the patient's wishes and discontinues life support. The physician's action is best described as

(A) unethical and illegal
(B) ethical and legal
(C) unethical but legal
(D) ethical but illegal

12. A clearly competent, pregnant 25-year-old woman tells her obstetrician that over the past year she has abused intravenous drugs and has had at least 10 sexual partners. The doctor suggests that she be tested for HIV but she refuses. The most appropriate action for the doctor to take is to

(A) perform the test without the patient's knowledge
(B) give her a prescription for zidovudine (AZT)
(C) refer her to another obstetrician
(D) note in her chart that she has refused to be tested and continue caring for her
(E) ask the father of the child for permission to test the patient

13. A married 17-year-old woman sustains brain damage after an unsuccessful suicide attempt. She is in a coma and requires life support. Clinical examination and electroencephalogram (EEG) reveal irreversible cessation of brain function. Her father insists that the physician not withdraw life support. The most appropriate action for the doctor to take is to

(A) withdraw life support
(B) do nothing
(C) get a court order to withdraw life support
(D) get the patient's husband to authorize withdrawal of life support
(E) get the patient's mother to authorize withdrawal of life support

14. A 55-year-old woman undergoes surgery to repair a torn knee ligament. After the surgery, she has partial paralysis of the affected leg and sues the surgeon for malpractice. The lawsuit will be successful if the patient can prove that

(A) the physician did not follow the usual standards of professional care
(B) the paralysis is permanent
(C) the physician was not board-certified in orthopedic surgery
(D) her sexual function is negatively affected by the paralysis
(E) she will lose a significant amount of time from work because of the paralysis

15. A 35-year-old man who has paranoid type schizophrenia and lives in a subway station is brought to the emergency department. This patient can be hospitalized against his will if he

(A) is dirty and disheveled
(B) is malnourished
(C) has attempted to push a passenger onto the train tracks
(D) is hearing voices
(E) believes the FBI is listening to his conversations

Answers and Explanations

TBQ-C. Because the patient is in a persistent vegetative state, the physician should carry out the patient's request and not provide life support. This decision is based on the patient's prior instructions as put forth in his living will. The wife's or adult children's wishes are not relevant to this decision. Under these circumstances, the patient's wishes are clear, and there is no need to approach the court or the ethics committee of the hospital.

1-D. The most appropriate action for the physician to take is to deliver the child vaginally. Competent pregnant women, like all competent adults, can refuse medical treatment, even if the fetus will die as a result. Neither the patient's husband (even if he is the father) nor the court has the right to alter this decision. Trying to frighten the patient by telling her that she can be criminally prosecuted if the child dies or referring her to another doctor are not appropriate actions.

2-C. The physician should inform the patient's girlfriend (but not her parents) about his infection. The usual standards of doctor-patient confidentiality do not apply here since the patient's failure to use condoms poses a significant threat to his girlfriend's life (Tarasoff decision). If the patient is using condoms, the doctor does not have to inform his partner of his HIV-positive status. However, even if he is using condoms, the doctor should encourage the patient to disclose his medical condition to his sexual partner. Not all states require reporting of HIV-positive patients.

3-D. Prior to treating the patient, the physician should counsel her on safe sexual practices. There is no need to break doctor-patient confidentiality by telling the sexual partner since chlamydia is not life-threatening. Parental consent is not required for treating minors in cases of sexually transmitted disease, pregnancy, and substance abuse. Chlamydia is not generally "reportable" to state health authorities.

4-A. The physician can use alternative means of replacing lost body fluids but should not give the patient a blood transfusion. Legally competent patients may refuse treatment even if death will result. Getting a court order or obtaining permission from the woman's family to do the transfusion are not appropriate or ethical actions. Failing to tell a patient the truth, (i.e., giving the woman the transfusion but not telling her about it), or going against a competent patient's expressed wishes (i.e., informing her of the transfusion when she recovers from the anesthetic), are never appropriate.

5-A. As noted above, a patient who is legally competent can refuse lifesaving treatment for himself for religious or other reasons, even if death will be the outcome. However, a parent (or guardian) cannot refuse lifesaving treatment for his child for any reason. When there is time, a court order should be obtained before treatment is started. In an emergency, the physician can proceed without a court order. Competent patients (i.e., the father) can refuse treatment for themselves even if death or injury will result.

6-D. Before this patient's cancer can be treated, he must be informed of the diagnosis. Since there is some question about his emotional state, asking the patient when he would like to receive the diagnosis is the best choice. Only the doctor (not a family member) should tell the patient the results of a medical test. If the doctor believes that the patient's health will be adversely affected by the news of a malignancy, she can delay telling the patient the diagnosis until he is ready to receive the biopsy report. The opinions of family members as to whether to tell the patient the diagnosis and prognosis are not relevant.

7-C. Only the parent can give consent for surgical or medical treatment of a minor. In an emergency such as this, if the parent or guardian cannot be located, treatment may proceed without consent. The babysitting aunt and gym teacher have no legal standing to make health care decisions for this child. Waiting to act until the parents are reached could be harmful to the child.

8-C. The most appropriate action for medical student X to take is to report medical student Y to the dean of students. Reporting of an impaired colleague is required ethically because patients must be protected and the impaired colleague must be helped. Even if medical student X talks to or warns medical student Y about his drinking, there is no guarantee that Y will listen and that the patients will be protected. Reporting Y to the police is not appropriate.

9-D. The most appropriate action for the internist to take is to continue to refer patients to the surgeon without mentioning his HIV status, provided that the surgeon is physically and mentally competent to treat patients and he complies with precautions for infection control. Physician-to-patient transmission of HIV has never been confirmed in the United States. Doctors are not required to inform either patients or the medical establishment about another doctor's HIV-positive status.

10-C. It is unethical but not illegal for doctors to refuse to treat patients because of fear of infection.

11-B. If a competent patient requests cessation of artificial life support, it is both legal and ethical for a physician to comply with this request.

12-D. The most appropriate action for the doctor to take is to note in the patient's chart that she has refused to be tested and continue to care for her. Although providing zidovudine (AZT) to an HIV-positive woman during pregnancy can significantly reduce the danger of HIV transmission to the unborn child (see Table 19-6), a pregnant woman has the right to refuse medical tests or treatment even if the fetus will die or be seriously injured as a result.

13-A. The most appropriate action for the doctor to take is to withdraw life support. If a patient is legally dead ("brain dead"), the physician is authorized to remove life support without a court order or consent from family.

14-A. The lawsuit will be successful if the patient can prove that the physician did not follow the usual standards of professional care. An unfavorable outcome alone (e.g., paralysis of the leg as an unavoidable complication of the surgical procedure) or negative effects on functioning because of the injury do not constitute malpractice. Licensed physicians are legally allowed to perform any medical or surgical procedure; they do not have to be boarded in a specialty.

15-C. This patient can be hospitalized involuntarily if he poses a significant danger to himself or to others. Trying to push a passenger onto the tracks is such a danger. Self-neglect (e.g., poor grooming, malnutrition) or psychotic symptoms (e.g., hearing voices or having delusions—see Chapter 11) are not grounds for involuntary hospitalization unless they constitute a significant, imminent danger to this patient's life.

24

Health Care In the United States

Typical ***Board*** *Question*

A first-year resident who has recently starting working in a hospital emergency department sees 4 patients during his first hour on the service. Which of these patients is likely to be the most ill when first seen by the resident?

(A) A 45-year-old man from a low socioeconomic group
(B) A 45-year-old woman from a low socioeconomic group
(C) A 45-year-old man from a high socioeconomic group
(D) A 45-year-old woman from a high socioeconomic group

(See "Answers and Explanations" at end of Chapter)

I. Health Care Delivery Systems

A. Hospitals

1. The United States has **too many hospitals** (over 6,000) and too many hospital beds (about 1,000,000). Currently, approximately 33% of hospital beds (especially in city hospitals) are unoccupied.

2. Most stays in general hospitals average **6–7 days. Length of stay is decreasing** because of the increase in managed care. Types of hospitals and their ownership are listed in Table 24-1.

B. Nursing homes and other health care facilities

1. There are currently about 25,000 **nursing homes** with a capacity of 1.5 million beds. Because of the aging of the population, these numbers are increasing.

2. Rehabilitation centers, visiting nurses associations, and hospices provide alternatives to hospital and nursing home care (Table 24-2).

C. Physicians

1. Currently, there are **126 medical schools** and **16 colleges of osteopathic medicine** in the United States, graduating annually over 15,000 medical doctors (M.D.s) and 1800 doctors of osteopathy (D.O.s). Both M.D.s and D.O.s are correctly called "physicians."

Table 24-1. Types of Hospitals in the United States

Hospital type	Ownership	Comments
Voluntary (not-for-profit)	Private owners, churches, universities	• Most hospitals are in this category
For-profit	Investors	• Oriented toward general or to specialty care • About 12% of all hospitals are in this category
Municipal	City governments	• Often are teaching hospitals affiliated with medical schools
Psychiatric (long-term)	State governments	• Numbers are decreasing due to the success of psychoactive medication leading to deinstitutionalization
Veterans Administration (VA) and military	Federal government	• Reserved for those who have served (veterans) or are currently serving in the military

Table 24-2. Other Health Care Facilities

Type of care or facility	Services provided	Comments
Nursing home (skilled care facility, intermediate care facility, or residential facility—these types vary in the level of nursing care provided)	• Long-term care • Room and board • Assistance with self care • Nursing care	• Cost ranges from about $35,000–$75,000 per year depending on geographical area and level of nursing care provided
Rehabilitation centers and halfway houses	• Short-term care • Room and board	• Goal is to help hospitalized patients reenter society.
Visiting nurse associations	• Nursing care, physical and occupational therapy, and social work services • Care given in a patient's own home	• Funded by Medicare • Serves as a less expensive alternative to hospitalization or nursing home placement
Hospice organizations	• Supportive care to terminally ill patients (i.e., those expected to live less than 6 months) and their families using physicians, nurses, social workers, and volunteers • Care usually given in a patient's own home	• Funded by Medicare • Goal is to allow patient to die at home to be with their families and preserve their dignity • Pain medication is used liberally

    a. Training and practice are essentially the same for **D.O.s** as for M.D.s; however, the philosophy of osteopathic medicine stresses the **interrelatedness of body systems** and the use of **musculoskeletal manipulation** in the diagnosis and treatment of physical illness.

    b. There are currently about **650,000 physicians** in the United States; about 35,000 of these are D.O.s and 140,000 are foreign medical school graduates.

    c. Overall, physicians earn an average salary of **$200,000 annually.** Psychiatrists, pediatricians, and family practitioners typically earn less than this average figure and surgeons typically earn more.

2. **Primary care** physicians, including family practitioners, internists, and pediatricians, provide initial care to patients and account for at least one third of all physicians. This **number is increasing** and is expected to reach one half of all physicians. The number of **specialists is decreasing.**

3. The **ratio of physicians to patients** is higher in the Northeastern states and in California than in the Southern and Mountain states.

4. People in the United States average **about 5 visits** to physicians per year. This is significantly **fewer yearly visits** than people in developed countries with systems of government-funded medical care.

    a. **High-income patients are more likely to seek treatment** and to visit private doctor's offices than are low-income patients.

    b. **Low-income patients** are more likely to seek treatment in hospital emergency departments and to **delay** seeking treatment, in part because of the cost. Illnesses often become more severe when patients delay seeking treatment.

    c. **Women are more likely to seek treatment** than men.

    d. Children and the elderly are more likely to seek treatment than people of other ages.

5. Seventy-five percent of people visit physicians in a given year. In all age groups, the **most common medical conditions** for which treatment is sought are upper respiratory ailments and injuries.

II. Costs of Health Care

A. Health Care Expenditures

1. Health care expenditures in the United States will soon make up **over 15% of the gross domestic product (GDP), more than in any other industrialized society.**

2. Health care expenditures have increased because of the **increasing age of the population,** advances in medical technology, and the availability of health care to the poor and elderly through Medicaid and Medicare, respectively.

B. Allocation of health care funds

—The origins of health care expenses and the sources of payment for health care are listed in Table 24-3.

Table 24-3. Health Care Expenses and Payment

Origin of health care expenses (in decreasing order of magnitude)	Sources of payment for health care expenses (in decreasing order of magnitude)
Hospitals	Federal government
Doctor's fees	State governments
Nursing homes	Private health insurance
Medications and medical supplies	Individuals
Mental health services	Other
Dental and other care	

III. Health Care Insurance

A. Overview

1. The United States is the only industrialized country that **does not have publicly mandated health care insurance coverage funded by the government** for all citizens. This is one reason that the United States has **higher infant mortality** rates and **lower life expectancies** than many other developed countries.

2. Most Americans must **obtain health insurance** through their employer or on their own. About 15% of Americans have **no health insurance** and must pay the costs of health care themselves. The percentage of uninsured people is increasing.

3. Certain citizens (e.g., the **elderly** and the **poor**) have government-funded health care insurance through **Medicare** and **Medicaid,** respectively (see III. E).

B. Private health insurers

1. **Blue Cross/Blue Shield (BC/BS),** a nonprofit private insurance carrier, is regulated by insurance agencies in each state and pays for hospital costs (Blue Cross) and physician fees and diagnostic tests (Blue Shield) for 30%–50% of working people in the United States.

2. Individuals can also contract with one of approximately 1000 other **private insurance carriers,** such as Aetna or Prudential.

C. Fee-for-service care versus managed care

1. Whichever the insurance carrier, patients usually can choose either a traditional fee-for-service indemnity plan or a managed care plan.

   a. A traditional **fee-for-service** indemnity plan has no restrictions on provider choice or referrals. It also commonly has higher premiums.

   b. A **managed care** plan has restrictions on provider choice and referrals and lower premiums. Approximately 50% of BC/BS subscribers are enrolled in a managed care plan.

2. Many insurance plans have a **deductible** (e.g., the amount the patient must pay out-of-pocket before the insurance company begins to cover ex-

penses), or a co-payment (i.e., a percentage, typically 20%, of the total bill that the patient must pay), or both.

D. Managed care

1. **Managed care** describes a health care delivery system in which all aspects of an individual's health care are coordinated or managed by a group of providers to enhance cost effectiveness.

2. Although cost is controlled in managed care, **patients are restricted** in their choice of a doctor. Thus, while the number of managed care plans is increasing, **managed care is more popular with the government** than with the public.

3. Because fewer patient visits result in lower costs, the philosophy of managed care stresses **primary, secondary,** and **tertiary prevention** (Table 24-4) rather than acute treatment.

4. Types of managed care plans including health maintenance organizations **(HMOs),** independent practice associations **(IPAs),** preferred provider organizations **(PPOs)** and point of service **(POS)** plans are described in Table 24-5.

E. Federal and state-funded insurance coverage

1. Medicare and Medicaid are government-funded programs that provide medical insurance to certain groups of people. Eligibility requirements and coverage provided by these programs are outlined in Table 24-6.

2. **Diagnosis-related groups (DRGs)** are used by Medicare to pay hospital bills. The amount paid is based on an estimate of the cost of hospitalization for each illness rather than the actual charges incurred.

Table 24-4. Primary, Secondary, and Tertiary Prevention in Health Care

Types of prevention	Goal	Examples
Primary	To reduce the incidence of a disorder by reducing its associated risk factors	• Immunization of infants to prevent infectious illnesses • Improved obstetrical care to avoid premature birth and its associated problems
Secondary	To reduce the prevalence of an existing disorder by decreasing its severity	• Early identification and treatment of otitis media in children to prevent hearing loss • Mammography for the early identification and treatment of breast cancer
Tertiary	To reduce the prevalence of problems caused by an existing disorder	• Physical therapy for stroke patients so that they can care for themselves • Occupational training for mentally retarded persons so that they can gain the skills needed to join the work force

Table 24-5. Managed Care Plans

Type of plan	Definition	Comments
Health Maintenance Organization (HMO) (staff model or closed panel)	• Physicians and other health care personnel are paid a salary to provide medical services to a group of people who are enrolled voluntarily and who pay an annual premium • HMOs may operate their own hospitals and clinics • Services include hospitalization, physician services, preventive medicine services, and often dental, eye, and podiatric care	• These plans are the most restrictive for the patient in terms of choice of doctor • Patient is assigned a "gatekeeper" (a primary care doctor from within the network who decides if and when a patient needs to see a specialist)
HMO [Independent Practice Association (IPA) model]	• Physicians in private practice are hired by an HMO to provide services to HMO patients • About 65% of HMOs have IPA components	• Private practice physicians receive a fee, or capitation, for each HMO patient they see
Preferred Provider Organization (PPO)	• A third-party payor (e.g., a union trust fund, insurance company, or corporation) contracts with physicians in private practice and with hospitals to provide medical care to its subscribers • Participants choose physicians from a listing of member practitioners (the network) • Physicians in the network receive capitation for each patient they see	• These plans guarantee doctors in private practice a certain volume of patients • By paying a larger share of the cost, patients can choose a doctor who is not in the network • There is no "gatekeeper" physician
Point of Service Plan (POS)	• Variant of a PPO in which a third party payor contracts with physicians in private practice to provide medical care to its subscribers • Physicians in the network receive capitation for each patient they see	• As with a PPO, patients can choose a doctor who is not in the network by paying an extra fee • As with an HMO, there is a "gatekeeper" physician

Table 24-6. Medicare and Medicaid

Source of Funding	Eligibility	Coverage
Medicare		
The federal government (through the social security system)	• People eligible for social security benefits (e.g., those ≥ 65 years of age regardless of income) • People of any age with chronic disabilities or debilitating illness • Covers about 34 million people	• **Part A:** Inpatient hospital costs, home health care, medically necessary nursing home care for a limited time after hospitalization, hospice care • **Part B:** Dialysis, physical therapy, laboratory tests, out-patient hospital care, physician bills, ambulance service, medical equipment (Part B is optional and has a 20% co-payment and a $100 deductible) • **Neither Part A nor Part B** covers outpatient prescription drugs or long-term nursing home care
Medicaid (MediCal in California)		
Both federal and state governments (the state contribution is determined by average per capita income of the state)	• Indigent (very low income) people • One third of all monies are allocated for nursing home care for indigent elderly people • Covers about 25 million people	• Inpatient and outpatient hospital costs • Physician services • Home health care, hospice care • Laboratory tests, dialysis, therapy • Ambulance service, medical equipment • Prescription drugs • Long-term nursing home care

IV. Demographics of Health

A. Lifestyle, habits, and attitudes

1. Lifestyle and poor dietary and other habits, particularly smoking and drinking alcohol, are responsible for about **70% of physical and mental illness.** For example, alcohol abuse is related to liver dysfunction and to increased suicide risk.

2. **Social attitudes** involving health care issues also affect health care delivery. For example, although organ transplants can save many lives, fewer transplant procedures are done than are needed. This is primarily because there are not enough people willing to donate their organs at death.

B. Socioeconomic status and health

1. Socioeconomic status is determined primarily by **occupation,** with secondary emphasis on **educational level;** it is also associated with place of residence and with income.

2. People in low socioeconomic groups typically have decreased life expectancy and **poorer mental** and **physical health.**

3. Approximately 85% of people in low socioeconomic groups are African-American or Hispanic American (see also Chapter 18).

C. Gender and health

1. **Men** have shorter life expectancies and are more likely to have heart disease than women.

Table 24-7. Leading Causes of Death by Age Group (across sex and ethnic group)

Age group	Causes of death (in decreasing order of frequency)
Infants (< 1 year of age)	Congenital anomalies Prematurity, low birth weight Sudden infant death syndrome (SIDS)
Children (1–4 years of age)	Accidents Congenital anomalies Cancer (primarily leukemia and CNS malignancies)
Children (5–14 years of age)	Accidents (most by failure to use seat belts) Cancer (primarily leukemia and CNS malignancies) Homicide and legal intervention Suicide
Adolescents and young adults (15–24 years of age)	Accidents (most in motor vehicles) Homicide and legal intervention Suicide
Adults (25–44 years of age)	Accidents HIV infection Cancer
Adults (45–64 years of age)	Cancer Heart disease Accidents
Elderly (65 years of age and over)	Heart disease Cancer Stroke
All ages combined	Heart disease Cancer (lung, breast and prostate, and colorectal, in decreasing order) Stroke

CNS=central nervous system; *HIV*=human immunodeficiency virus

2. While they have less heart disease overall, **women** are more likely than men to **die during their first heart attack.**

3. Women are also at higher risk than men for developing
   a. **Autoimmune diseases** (75% percent of victims),
   b. **Smoking-related illnesses** like lung cancer
   c. **AIDS (when they are already HIV positive** and have the same viral load as a man).

D. **Age and health**
   1. The likelihood of physical and mental illness and hospitalization increases with age.
   2. Although the **elderly** comprise only 12% of the population, they currently incur over **30% of all health care costs;** this figure is expected to rise to 50% by the year 2020.

E. **Causes of death**
   ––The death rate for adults is lower now than in previous years. The leading causes of death differ by age group (Table 24-7).

Review Test

Directions: Each of the numbered items or incomplete statements in this section is followed by answers or by completions of the statement. Select the **one** lettered answer or completion that is **best** in each case.

1. Of the following patients, the one likely to use the least Medicare services and funds during his or her lifetime is a(n)

(A) African-American man
(B) African-American woman
(C) white man
(D) white woman
(E) Native-American man

Questions 2–3

A 45-year-old stockbroker with three children must choose a health insurance plan at work.

2. In which of the following plans will she have the most choice in choosing a doctor?

(A) A health maintenance organization (HMO)
(B) A preferred provider organization (PPO)
(C) A point of service (POS) plan
(D) A fee-for-service plan

3. In which of the following plans will she have the least choice in choosing a doctor?

(A) A health maintenance organization (HMO)
(B) A preferred provider organization (PPO)
(C) A point of service (POS) plan
(D) A fee-for-service plan

4. Parents bring their 8-year-old child in for a school physical. Both of the parents smoke cigarettes. The child plays soccer, swims, and bicycles. In order to protect the child's life and health, which is the most important suggestion the doctor can give the parents?

(A) Stop smoking to reduce the child's exposure to secondhand smoke
(B) Put smoke alarms in the home
(C) Have the child wear a helmet while bicycling
(D) Learn cardiopulmonary resuscitation
(E) Be sure the child wears a seatbelt in the car

5. A first-year resident who has recently starting working in a hospital emergency department sees 4 patients during his first hour on the service. Which of these patients is likely to be healthiest when first seen by the resident?

(A) A 45-year-old man from a low socioeconomic group
(B) A 45-year-old woman from a low socioeconomic group
(C) A 45-year-old man from a high socioeconomic group
(D) A 45-year-old woman from a high socioeconomic group

6. Parents bring their 2-year old to a well-child clinic. In order to protect the child's life and health, the most important suggestion the doctor can give is to tell the parents to

(A) keep ipecac in the medicine cabinet
(B) put smoke alarms in the home
(C) observe safety measures in (i.e., "safe proof") the home
(D) learn cardiopulmonary resuscitation
(E) have the child immunized against measles, mumps, and rubella

7. In the United States, the percentage of the gross domestic product spent on health care is about

(A) 1%
(B) 8%
(C) 15%
(D) 30%
(E) 50%

8. In the United States, the largest percentage of personal health care expenses is paid by which of the following sources?

(A) The federal government
(B) State governments
(C) Municipal governments
(D) Private health insurance
(E) Personal funds

9. In the United States, the largest percentage of health care expenditures is for

(A) physician fees
(B) nursing home care
(C) medications
(D) hospital care
(E) dental services

10. A mother brings her infant daughter to the doctor for a checkup. The most common cause of death in infants between birth and 1 year of age is

(A) leukemia
(B) sudden infant death syndrome (SIDS)
(C) congenital anomalies
(D) accidents
(E) respiratory distress syndrome

Questions 11–12

A 70-year-old female patient is hospitalized for a fractured hip. The patient, who has $100,000 in savings, was brought to the hospital by ambulance. She stayed in the hospital for 5 days and required physical therapy and a "walker" for help with mobility for the next 6 weeks.

11. This patient can expect that Medicare Part A will cover which of the following costs related to this injury?

(A) Inpatient hospital care
(B) The "walker"
(C) Ambulance service
(D) Physician bills
(E) Physical therapy

12. After 6 months at home it is determined that this patient is unable to care for herself and requires care in a nursing home, probably for the rest of her life. Which of the following will pay for the first few years of this care?

(A) Medicare Part A
(B) Medicare Part B
(C) Blue Cross
(D) Blue Shield
(E) The patient's savings

13. Which of the following are the three leading causes of death in the United States in order of magnitude (higher to lower)?

(A) AIDS, heart disease, cancer
(B) Heart disease, cancer, stroke
(C) Cancer, heart disease, AIDS
(D) Heart disease, cancer, AIDS
(E) Stroke, heart disease, cancer

14. In women in the United States, which is the most common cause of cancer death?

(A) Cervical cancer
(B) Colorectal cancer
(C) Breast cancer
(D) Lung cancer
(E) Uterine cancer

15. Most patients in the United States can expect to receive care in which of the following types of hospital?

(A) For-profit
(B) Voluntary
(C) Federal
(D) Municipal
(E) State

16. An educational program is developed to teach mentally ill adults skills necessary to get them into the employment force. This program is an example of

(A) primary prevention
(B) secondary prevention
(C) tertiary prevention
(D) managed care

Answers and Explanations

TBQ-A. A man from a low socioeconomic group is likely to be most ill when the resident first sees him. This is because low-income patients and male patients are more likely to delay seeking treatment due to costs and attitudes, respectively. Delay in seeking treatment commonly results in more severe illness.

1-A. Medicare pays for health care services for persons 65 years of age and older and others who are eligible to receive Social Security benefits. Because statistically he is likely to have a shorter life than a white or Native-American man, an African-American woman, or a white woman, an African-American man is likely to use the least Medicare services over the course of his lifetime (see Table 3-1).

2-D, 3-A. Patients have the most choice in choosing a doctor in a traditional fee-for-service indemnity plan. In this type of plan there are no restrictions on provider choice or referrals. Managed care plans [e.g., health maintenance organizations (HMOs), preferred provider organizations (PPOs), and point of service (POS) plans] have restrictions on doctor choice. Patients have the least choice in choosing a doctor in a health maintenance organization (HMO). HMOs are the most restrictive of managed care plans for the patient in terms of choice of doctor. Rather than choosing a doctor from the network as in the PPO and POS, in HMOs the patient is assigned a doctor.

4-E. While house fires, bicycling accidents, and drowning are causes of death in children, failure to wear seatbelts is the major cause of accidental death in children 4–14 years of age. Secondhand smoke has not been shown statistically to be of significant danger to life.

5-D. A woman from a high socioeconomic group is likely to be healthiest when the resident first sees her. Women and people from higher socioeconomic groups are more likely to seek treatment and therefore to be less ill when first seen by a doctor than men and people from low socioeconomic groups (see also Explanation to TBQ).

6-C. While accidental poisoning, house fires, and drowning are causes of death in children, accidents in the home are a more important cause of accidental death in children 1–4 years of age. Infectious illnesses due to lack of immunization are not common causes of death in American children.

7-C. The percentage of the gross domestic product (GDP) spent on health care is about 15%, a percentage that is larger than that of any other developed country.

8-A. The largest percentage of personal health care expenses are paid by the federal government. In decreasing order, other sources of payment for health care expenses are state governments, private health insurance and personal funds. Municipal governments pay a relatively small percentage of these expenses.

9-D. In the United States, most health care expenditures are for hospital care. In decreasing order, other sources of health care expenses are physician fees, nursing home care, medications, mental health services, and dental services.

10-C. The most common cause of death in infants up to 1 year of age is congenital anomalies. Prematurity and low birth weight, sudden infant death syndrome (SIDS), and respiratory distress syndrome are the second, third, and fourth leading causes of death in this age group.

11-A, 12-E. Medicare Part A will cover inpatient hospital costs. Part B covers ambulance services, physician fees, medical equipment (the "walker"), and therapy. The patient herself is responsible for long-term nursing home costs. Neither Part A nor Part B of Medicare nor Blue Cross/Blue Shield will cover long term nursing home costs. After the patient's $100,000 is exhausted (proba-

239

bly within 3 years at \$35,000–\$75,000 per year), she will be poor and therefore eligible for Medicaid. Medicaid pays for nursing home care and all other health care for poor people.

13-B. The leading cause of death in the United States is heart disease, followed by cancer and stroke.

14-D. In women, as in men, the most common cause of cancer death in the United States is cancer of the lung. In women, this is followed by breast cancer and colorectal cancer. The number of women getting lung cancer is increasing with increased smoking rates in women.

15-B. Most hospital care in the United States is provided by voluntary (not-for-profit) hospitals.

16-C. This educational program for mentally ill adults is an example of tertiary prevention. Tertiary prevention is aimed at reducing the prevalence of problems caused by an existing disorder, mental illness in this case. Primary prevention is aimed at reducing the occurrence or incidence of disorder by reducing its associated risk factors (e.g., immunization against measles). Secondary prevention is aimed at reducing the prevalence of an existing disorder by reducing its severity, (e.g., early identification and treatment of breast cancer using mammography). Managed care is a system of health care in which all aspects of health care are coordinated by providers to control costs.

25

Epidemiology

Typical Board Question

A study is designed to compare a new medication for Crohn's disease with a standard medication. Each of 50 Crohn's disease patients is allowed to decide which of these two treatment groups to join. The major reason that the results of this study may not be valid is because of

(A) selection bias
(B) recall bias
(C) sampling bias
(D) differences in the sizes of the two groups
(E) the small number of patients in the study

(See "Answers and Explanations" at end of Chapter)

I. Epidemiology—Incidence and Prevalence

—Epidemiology is the study of the factors determining the occurrence and distribution of diseases in human populations.

A. Incidence

—**Incidence rate** is the number of individuals who **develop an illness in a given time period (commonly 1 year)** divided by the total number of individuals at risk for the illness during that time period [e.g., the number of intravenous (IV) drug abusers newly diagnosed as HIV-positive in 2001divided by the number of IV drug abusers in the population during 2001].

B. Prevalence

—**Prevalence ratio** is the number of individuals in the population who have an illness (e.g., are HIV-positive) divided by the total population.

1. **Point prevalence** is the number of individuals who have an illness at a specific point in time (e.g., the number of people who are HIV-positive on August 31, 2001 divided by the total population on that date).

2. **Period prevalence** is the number of individuals who have an illness during a specific time period (e.g., the number of people who are HIV-positive in 2001 divided by the total population mid-year in 2001).

C. Relationship between incidence and prevalence

1. Prevalence is equal to incidence rate multiplied by the average duration of the disease process (if incidence and duration are stable).

2. Prevalence is greater than incidence if the disease is long term. For example, because diabetes lasts a lifetime its prevalence is much higher than its incidence. In contrast, the prevalence of influenza, an acute illness, is approximately equal to the incidence.

II. Research Study Design

A. Cohort studies

1. Cohort studies begin with the identification of specific populations (cohorts), who are free of the illness under investigation at the start of the study.

2. Following assessment of exposure to a risk factor [a variable linked to the cause of an illness (e.g., smoking)], incidence rates of illness between exposed and nonexposed members of a cohort are compared.

    —An example of a cohort study would be one that followed healthy adults from early adulthood through middle age to compare the health of those who smoke versus those who do not smoke.

3. Cohort studies can be **prospective** (taking place in the present time) or **historical** (some activities have taken place in the past).

4. **A clinical treatment trial** is a special type of cohort study in which members of a cohort with a specific illness are given one treatment and other members of the cohort are given another treatment or a placebo. The results of the two treatments are then compared.

    —An example of a clinical treatment trial would be one in which the differences in survival rates between men with lung cancer who receive a new drug and men with lung cancer who receive a standard drug are compared.

B. Case–control studies

1. Case–control studies begin with the identification of subjects who have a specific disorder (cases) and subjects who do not have that disorder (controls).

2. Information on the prior exposure of cases and controls to risk factors is then obtained.

    —An example of a case–control study would be one in which the smoking histories of women with and without breast cancer are compared.

C. Cross-sectional studies

1. Cross-sectional studies begin when information is collected from a group of individuals who provide a "snapshot" in time of disease activity.

2. Such studies can provide information on the relationship between risk factors and health status of a group of individuals at one specific point in time (e.g., a random telephone sample is done to determine if men who smoke have more back pain than men who do not smoke). They can also be used to calculate the prevalence of a disease in a population.

III. Quantifying Risk

—Relative risk, attributable risk, and the odds (or odds risk) ratio are measures used to quantify risk in population studies. **Relative risk** and **attributable risk** are calculated for **cohort** studies, while the **odds ratio** is calculated for **case-control** studies.

A. **Relative risk.** Relative risk compares the incidence rate of a disorder among individuals exposed to a risk factor (e.g., smoking) with the incidence rate of the disorder in nonexposed individuals.

1. For example, the incidence rate of lung cancer among smokers in New Jersey is 20/1000, while the incidence rate of lung cancer among non-smokers in New Jersey is 2/1000. Therefore, the chance of getting lung cancer (the relative risk) for this New Jersey population is 20/1000 divided by 2/1000, or 10.

2. A relative risk of 10 means that in New Jersey, if an individual smokes, his or her risk of getting lung cancer is 10 times that of a non-smoker.

B. **Attributable risk**

1. Attributable risk is useful for determining what would happen in a study population if the risk factor was removed (e.g., determining how common lung cancer would be in a study if people did not smoke).

2. To calculate attributable risk, the incidence rate of the illness in nonexposed individuals is subtracted from the incidence rate of the illness in those who have been exposed to a risk factor.

3. For the example above, the risk of lung cancer attributable to smoking (the attributable risk) in this New Jersey population is 20/1000 minus 2/1000 or 18/1000.

C. **Odds ratio**

—Since incidence data are not available in a case-control study, the **odds ratio** can be used as an estimate of relative risk when a disease is uncommon (Example 25-1).

Example 25-1. Calculating the Odds Ratio

Of 200 patients in the hospital, 50 have lung cancer. Of these 50 patients, 45 are smokers. Of the remaining 150 hospitalized patients who do not have lung cancer, 60 are smokers. Use this information to calculate the odds ratio for smoking and the risk of lung cancer.

	Smokers	Nonsmokers
People with lung cancer	A = 45	B = 5
People without lung cancer	C = 60	D = 90

$$\text{Odds Ratio} = \frac{(A)(D)}{(B)(C)} = \frac{(45)(90)}{(5)(60)} = 13.5$$

An odds ratio of 13.5 means that the risk of lung cancer is 13.5 times higher in people who smoke than in those who do not smoke.

IV. Bias, Reliability, and Validity

—To be useful, testing instruments must be bias-free, reliable, and valid (i.e., sensitive and specific).

A. Bias

1. A biased test or study is one constructed so that **one outcome is more likely to occur than another.** Selection, recall, or sampling bias can flaw all types of research studies.

2. **Selection bias**

   a. Selection bias can occur if subjects are permitted to choose whether to go into a drug or a placebo group rather than being assigned randomly.

   —For example, if in a study on the effectiveness of estrogen replacement therapy on menopausal symptoms, menopausal women who have many hot flashes are more likely to choose the estrogen group rather than the placebo group because they want relief. Thus, women with more symptoms end up in the estrogen group, making it more difficult to show a positive effect of estrogen.

   b. Selection bias can also occur if, rather than making random assignments, the investigator purposely chooses which patients go into the drug group and which patients go into the placebo group.

   —For example, a physician investigator, believing that a new drug for relief of menopausal symptoms being tested in clinical trials will be effective, will put all of her most serious cases into the new drug group. Thus, women with more symptoms end up in the new drug group, making it more difficult to show a positive effect of the new drug.

3. **Recall bias.** In recall bias, knowledge of the presence of a disorder alters the way the subject remembers his or her history.

   —For example, if mothers of children with cleft palate overestimate how much medication they took during pregnancy, the overestimation can make it appear (erroneously) that certain medications are related to formation of cleft palate deformities.

4. **Sampling bias.** In sampling bias, subjects who volunteer to be in a study may not be representative of the population being studied. Factors unrelated to the subject of the study may have led them to volunteer, but could also distinguish the subjects from the rest of the population. Because of these factors, the results of the study may not be generalizable to the entire population.

   —For example, if college students who volunteer for an experiment on the physiological bases of sexual response are more sexually active than students who do not volunteer, the students who volunteered may not be representative of the entire population of college students; thus the data are not generalizable.

B. Reducing bias

Blind studies, placebos, crossover studies, and randomized studies are used to reduce bias.

1. **Blind studies.** The expectations of patients can influence the effectiveness of treatment. Blind studies attempt to reduce this influence.
    a. In a single-blind study, the subject does not know what treatment he or she is receiving.
    b. In a double-blind study, neither the subject nor the clinician-evaluator knows what treatment the subject is receiving.

2. **Placebo responses**
    a. In a blind drug study, a patient may receive a placebo (an inactive substance) rather than the active drug.
    b. People receiving the **placebo** are the **control group;** those receiving the **active drug** are the **experimental group.**
    c. At least one-third of patients respond to treatment with placebos (the placebo effect); in psychiatric illnesses, the placebo effect is even greater (see also Chapter 4).

3. **Crossover studies**
    a. In a crossover study, subjects in Group 1 first receive the drug and subjects in Group 2 first receive the placebo.
    b. Later in the crossover study, the groups switch—those in Group 1 receive the placebo, and those in Group 2 receive the drug.
    c. Because subjects in both groups receive both drug and placebo, **each subject acts as his or her own control.**

4. **Randomization**
    —In order to ensure that the proportion of sicker and healthier people is the same in the treatment and control (placebo) groups, patients are randomly assigned to the groups. The number of patients in each group does not have to be equal.

C. **Reliability and validity**
    1. Reliability refers to the reproducibility of results.
        a. **Interrater reliability** is a measure of whether the results of the test are similar when the test is administered by a different rater or examiner.
        b. **Test–retest reliability** is a measure of whether the results of the test are similar when the person is tested a second or third time.
    2. **Validity** is a measure of whether the test assesses what it was designed to assess (e.g., does a new IQ test really measure IQ or does it instead measure educational level) (see Chapter 8). Sensitivity and specificity are components of validity.

D. **Sensitivity and specificity** (Example 25-2)
    1. **Sensitivity** measures how well a test identifies truly ill people.
        a. **True positives** are ill people whom a test has correctly identified as being ill.
        b. **False negatives** are ill people whom a test has incorrectly identified as being well.
        c. **Sensitivity** is calculated by dividing the number of true positives by the sum of the number of true positives and false negatives.

Example 25-2. Sensitivity, Specificity, Predictive Value, and Prevalence

A new blood test to detect the presence of HIV was given to 1000 patients. Although 200 of the patients were actually infected with the virus, the test was positive in only 160 patients (true +); the other 40 infected patients had negative tests (false −) and thus were not identified by this new test. Of the 800 patients who were not infected, the test was negative in 720 patients (true −) and positive in 80 patients (false +).

Use the following information to calculate sensitivity, specificity, positive predicitive value, and negative predicitive value of this new blood test and the prevalence of HIV in this population.

	Patients infected with HIV	Patients not infected with HIV	Total patients
Positive HIV blood test	160 (true +)	80 (false +)	240 (those with + test)
Negative HIV blood test	40 (false −)	720 (true −)	760 (those with − test)
Total patients	200	800	1000

$$\text{Sensitivity} = \frac{160\ (\text{true +})}{160\ (\text{true +}) + 40\ (\text{false −})} = \frac{160}{200} = 80.0\%$$

$$\text{Specificity} = \frac{720\ (\text{true −})}{720\ (\text{true −}) + 80\ (\text{false +})} = \frac{720}{800} = 90.0\%$$

$$\text{Positive predictive value} = \frac{160\ (\text{true +})}{160\ (\text{true +}) + 80\ (\text{false +})} = \frac{160}{240} = 66.67\%$$

$$\text{Negative predictive value} = \frac{720\ (\text{true −})}{720\ (\text{true−}) + 40\ (\text{false−})} = \frac{720}{760} = 94.7\%$$

$$\text{Prevalence} = \frac{200\ (\text{total of those infected})}{1000\ (\text{total patients})} = 20.0\%$$

2. **Specificity** measures how well a test identifies truly well people.
   a. **True negatives** are well people whom a test has correctly identified as being well.
   b. **False positives** are well people whom a test has incorrectly identified as being ill.
   c. **Specificity** is calculated by dividing the number of true negatives by the sum of the number of true negatives and false positives.

E. **Predictive value** (see Example 25-2)
   1. **The predictive value** of a test is a measure of the percentage of test results that match the actual diagnosis.
      a. **Positive predictive value** is the probability that someone with a positive test actually has the illness. It is calculated by dividing the number of true positives by the sum of the number of true positives and false positives.
      b. **Negative predictive value** is the probability that a person with a

---

Example 25-3.   Clinical Probability

After 3 years of clinical trials of a new medication to treat erectile dysfunction, it is determined that 20% of patients taking the new medication develop hypertension. If two patients (patients A and B) take the drug, calculate the following probabilities.

1. The probability that both patient A and patient B will develop hypertension:

This is calculated by multiplying the probability of A developing hypertension by the probability of patient B developing hypertension (the multiplication rule for independent events)

The probability of A developing hypertension = 0.20.

The probability of B developing hypertension = 0.20.

The probability of both A and B developing hypertension = $0.20 \times 0.20 = 0.04$

2. The probability that at least one of the two patients (either A or B or both A and B) will develop hypertension.

This is calculated by adding the probability of A developing hypertension to the probability of B developing hypertension and then subtracting the probability of both A and B developing hypertension (see 1. above) (the addition rule).

$= 0.20 + 0.20 - 0.04 = 0.36.$

3. The probability that neither patient A nor patient B will develop hypertension:

This is calculated by multiplying the probability of patient A being normotensive by the probability of patient B being normotensive: probability (normotensive) = probability (hypertensive): $= 0.80 \times 0.80 = 0.64.$

---

negative test is actually well. It is calculated by dividing the number of true negatives by the sum of the number of true negatives and false negatives.

2. If the prevalence of a disease in the population is low, even tests with very high sensitivity and specificity will have low positive predictive value.

V. Clinical Probability and Attack Rate

A. Clinical probability is the number of times an **event actually occurs** divided by the number of times the **event can occur** (Example 25-3).

B. Attack rate is a type of incidence rate used to describe disease outbreaks. It is calculated by dividing the number of people who become ill during a study period by the number of people at risk during the study period.

—For example, if 20 out of 40 people who drank apple juice and 10 out of 50 people who drank orange juice become ill after a picnic, the attack rate is 50% for apple juice and 20% for orange juice.

Review Test

Directions: Each of the numbered items or incomplete statements in this section is followed by answers or by completions of the statement. Select the **one** lettered answer or completion that is **best** in each case.

Questions 1–2

A town in the western United States has a population of 1200. In 1998, 200 residents of the town are diagnosed with a disease. In 1999, 100 residents of the town are discovered to have the same disease. The disease is lifelong and chronic but not fatal.

1. The incidence rate of this disease in 1999 among this town's population is

(A) 100/1200
(B) 200/1200
(C) 300/1200
(D) 100/1000
(E) 300/1000

2. The prevalence rate of this disease in 1999 among the town's population is

(A) 100/1200
(B) 200/1200
(C) 300/1200
(D) 100/1000
(E) 300/1000

3. In which of the following infectious illnesses is prevalence most likely to exceed incidence?

(A) Measles
(B) Influenza
(C) Leprosy
(D) Rubella
(E) Rabies

4. A study is designed to determine the relationship between emotional stress and ulcers. To do this, the researchers used hospital records of patients diagnosed with peptic ulcer disease and patients diagnosed with other disorders over the period from July 1988–July 1998. The amount of emotional stress each patient was exposed to was determined from these records. This study is best described as a

(A) cohort study
(B) cross-sectionals study
(C) case–control study
(D) historical cohort study
(E) clinical treatment trial

5. A study is done to determine the effectiveness of a new antihistamine. To do this, 25 allergic patients are assigned to one of two groups, the new drug (13 patients) or a placebo (12 patients). The patients are then followed over a 6-month period. This study is best described as a

(A) cohort study
(B) cross-sectional study
(C) case–control study
(D) historical cohort study
(E) clinical treatment trial

6. After a new antidepressant has been on the market for 5 years, it is determined that of 2,400 people who have taken the drug, 360 complained of persistent nausea. If a physician has 2 patients on this antidepressant, the probability that both of them will experience persistent nausea is approximately

(A) .02
(B) .09
(C) .24
(D) .30
(E) .64

7. An intelligence quotient (IQ) test has high interrater reliability. This means that

(A) the test involves structured interviews
(B) a new assessment strategy is being used
(C) the test actually measures IQ and not educational level
(D) the results are very similar when the test is administered a second time
(E) the results are very similar when the test is administered by a different examiner

8. There are 100,000 people in Hobart, Tasmania. On January 1, 2000, 50 of these people have stomach cancer. Fifty divided by 100,000 on that date gives the

(A) point prevalence
(B) period prevalence
(C) incidence rate
(D) odds ratio
(E) relative risk

9. A patient has a new test for tuberculosis. Although the patient is infected, the test does not detect the presence of the bacillus. This is known as

(A) a false positive result
(B) a false negative result
(C) a true positive result
(D) a true negative result
(E) a predictive result

Questions 10–12

A study is undertaken to determine if prenatal exposure to marijuana is associated with low birth weight in infants. Mothers of 50 infants weighing less than 5 lbs (low birth weight) and 50 infants weighing more than 7 lbs (normal birth weight) were questioned about their use of marijuana during pregnancy. The study found that 20 mothers of low birth weight infants and 2 mothers of normal birth weight infants used the drug during pregnancy.

10. In this study, the odds ratio associated with smoking marijuana during pregnancy is

(A) 2
(B) 16
(C) 20
(D) 30
(E) 48

11. An odds ratio of X, calculated in the preceding question, means that

(A) the incidence of low birth weight in infants whose mothers smoke marijuana is X
(B) an infant whose mother uses marijuana during pregnancy is X times as likely to be of low birth weight as an infant whose mother does not use the drug
(C) a child has a 1/X chance of being born of low birth weight if its mother uses marijuana
(D) the risk of low birth weight in infants whose mothers use marijuana is no different from that of infants whose mothers do not use the drug
(E) the prevalence of low birth weight in infants whose mothers smoke marijuana is X

12. This study is best described as a

(A) cohort study
(B) cross-sectional study
(C) case–control study
(D) historical cohort study
(E) clinical treatment trial

13. A case–control study is done to determine if elderly demented patients are more likely to be injured at home than elderly patients who are not demented. The results of the study show an odds ratio of 3. This figure means that when compared to nondemented elderly patients, demented elderly patients

(A) should be institutionalized
(B) have one-third the risk of injury
(C) have the same risk of injury
(D) should be kept at home
(E) have three times the risk of injury

Questions 14–15

14. A blood test to detect prostate cancer was given to 1000 male members of a large HMO. Although 50 of the men actually had prostate cancer, the test was positive in only 15; the other 35 patients with prostate cancer had negative tests. Of the 950 men without prostate cancer, the test was positive in 200 men and negative in 750. The specificity of this test is approximately

(A) 15%
(B) 30%
(C) 48%
(D) 79%
(E) 86%

15. The positive predictive value of this blood test is

(A) 7%
(B) 14%
(C) 21%
(D) 35%
(E) 93%

Answers and Explanations

TBQ-A. The major reason that the results of this study are not valid is because of selection bias (i.e., the subjects were able to choose which group to go into). If very ill people were more likely to choose the standard treatment, people in the experimental treatment group (who were healthier to begin with) would have had a better outcome. In recall bias, knowledge of the presence of a disorder alters the way subjects remember their histories. In sampling bias, subjects choose to be in a study because of factors which may be unrelated to the subject of the study but which distinguish them from the rest of the population. A study can be valid even though two groups may be of different sizes or there is a small number of patients in a study.

1-D, 2-C. The incidence rate of the disease in 1999 is 100/1000, the number who were diagnosed with the illness divided by the number of people at risk for the illness. Because the 200 people who got the disease in 1998 are no longer at risk for getting the illness in 1999, the denominator in the equation (number of people at risk) is 1000 (rather than 1200). The prevalence rate of this disease in 1999 is 300/1200. This figure represented the people who were diagnosed in 1999 (100) plus the people who were diagnosed in 1998 and still have the disease. (200) divided by the total population at risk (1200).

3-C. In leprosy, a long-lasting infectious illness, the number of people in the population who have the illness (prevalence) is likely to exceed the number newly developing the illness in a given year (incidence). Measles, influenza, rubella, and rabies are shorter-lasting illnesses than leprosy.

4-C. Case-control studies begin with the identification of subjects who have a specific disorder (cases—i.e., ulcer patients) and subjects who do not have that disorder (controls—i.e., those diagnosed with other disorders). Information on the prior exposure of cases and controls to risk factors is then obtained. In this case-control study, the investigators used cases (ulcer patients) and controls (patients with other disorders) and looked into their histories (hospital records), to determine the occurrence of the risk factor (i.e., emotional stress) in each group. Cohort studies begin with the identification of specific populations (cohorts), who are free of illness at the start of the study and can be prospective (taking place in the present time) or historical (some activities have taken place in the past). Clinical treatment trials are cohort studies in which members of a cohort with a specific illness are given one treatment and other members of the cohort are given another treatment or a placebo. The results of the two treatments are then compared. Cross-sectional studies involve the collection of information on a disease and risk factors in a population at one point in time.

5-E. This study is best described as a clinical treatment trial—a study in which a cohort receiving a new antihistamine is compared with a cohort receiving a placebo (see also the explanation for Question 4).

6-A. The probability of both patients (A and B) on this antidepressant experiencing nausea equals the probability of A experiencing nausea ($360/2400 = 0.15$) times the probability of B experiencing nausea ($360/2400 = 0.15$) = $0.15 \times 0.15 = .0225$.

7-E. Interrater reliability is a measure of how similar test findings are when used by two different examiners.

8-A. Point prevalence is the number of people who have an illness at a specific point in time (i.e., January 1, 2000) divided by the total population at that time. Incidence rate is the number of individuals who develop an illness in a given time period (commonly 1 year) divided by the total number of individuals at risk for the illness during that time period. Period prevalence is the number of individuals who have an illness during a specific time period. Relative risk compares the incidence rate of a disorder among individuals exposed to a risk factor (e.g., smoking) with the incidence rate of the disorder in nonexposed individuals. The odds ratio is an estimate of the relative risk in case–control studies.

250

9-B. A false negative result occurs if a test does not detect tuberculosis in someone who truly is infected. True positives are ill people whom a test has correctly identified as being ill. True negatives are well people whom a test has correctly identified as being well. False positives are well people whom a test has incorrectly identified as being ill.

10-B, 11-B, 12-C. The odds ratio is 16 and is calculated as follows:

	Mother smoked marijuana	**Mother did not smoke marijuana**
Low birth weight babies	A = 20	B = 30
Normal birth weight babies	C = 2	D = 48

$$\textbf{Odds ratio} = (A)(D)/(B)(C) \text{ or } (20)(48)/(30)(2) = 960/60 = 16$$

The odds ratio of 16 means that an infant whose mother uses marijuana during pregnancy is 16 times as likely to be of low birth weight as an infant whose mother does not use the drug. This study is best described as a case-control study; the risk factor here is fetal exposure to marijuana (see also the explanation for Question 4).

13-E. An odds ratio of 3 means that when compared to nondemented elderly persons, demented elderly persons have three times the risk of injury. This number does not indicate whether or not certain people should be institutionalized.

14-D, 15-A. Calculations shown below indicate that the specificity of this blood test is 79%.

	Those who have prostate cancer	**Those who do not have prostate cancer**	**Total**
Positive blood test	15 (true +)	200 (false +)	215
Negative blood test	35 (false −)	750 (true −)	785
Total patients	50	950	1000

Specificity: 750 (true −)/[750 (true −) + 200 (false +)] = 0.789 or 78.9%

The calculations shown below indicate that the positive predictive value of this test is 7%.

Positive predictive value: 15 (true +)/(15 + 200) (those with + test) = 0.07 or 7.0%.

26

Statistical Analyses

Typical Board Question

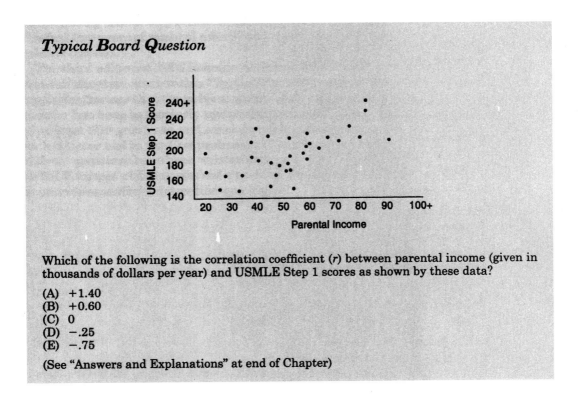

Which of the following is the correlation coefficient (*r*) between parental income (given in thousands of dollars per year) and USMLE Step 1 scores as shown by these data?

(A) +1.40
(B) +0.60
(C) 0
(D) −.25
(E) −.75

(See "Answers and Explanations" at end of Chapter)

I. Elements of Statistical Analyses

A. Variables

—A **variable** is a quantity that can change under different experimental situations; variables may be independent or dependent.

1. An **independent variable** is a predictive factor which has an impact on a dependent variable (e.g., the amount of fat in the diet).

2. A **dependent variable** is the outcome that reflects the effects of changing the independent variable (e.g., body weight under different dietary fat regimens).

B. Measures of dispersion

1. **Standard deviation** (σ) is the average distance of observations from their mean. Standard deviation is calculated by squaring each variation, or deviation from the mean in a group of scores, then adding the squared deviations; this sum is then divided by the number of scores in the group minus 1, and the square root of the result is determined.

2. A standard normal value, or **z score,** is the difference between an individual variable and the population mean in units of standard deviation.

Example: $$z = \frac{\text{A score in the distribution} - \text{The mean score of the distribution}}{\text{The standard deviation of the distribution}}$$

3. **Standard error** is the standard deviation divided by the square root of the number of scores in a sample.

C. Measures of central tendency

1. The **mean** is the average and is obtained by adding a group of numbers and then dividing by the quantity of numbers in the group.

2. The **median,** or the 50th percentile value, is the middle value in a **sequentially ordered** group of numbers (i.e., the value which divides the data set into two equal groups).

3. The **mode** is the value that appears most often in a group of numbers.

D. Normal distribution

—A **normal** distribution, also referred to as a **gaussian** or **bell-shaped** distribution, is a theoretical distribution of scores in which the mean, median, and mode are equal.

1. The highest point in the distribution of scores is the **modal peak.** In a **bimodal distribution,** there are two modal peaks (e.g., two distinct populations).

2. In a normal distribution, approximately 68% of the population scores fall within one standard deviation of the mean; approximately 95% of scores fall within two, and 99.7% of scores fall within three standard deviations of the mean (Figure 26-1).

E. Skewed distributions

—In a skewed distribution, the modal peak shifts to one side (Figure 26-2).

1. In a **positively skewed** distribution (skewed to the right), the tail is toward the right and the modal peak is toward the left side (i.e., scores cluster toward the low end).

2. In a **negatively skewed** distribution (skewed to the left), the tail is toward the left and the modal peak is toward the right side (i.e., scores cluster toward the high end).

II. Hypothesis Testing

A. A **hypothesis** is a statement based on inference, existing literature, or preliminary studies that postulates a difference existing between two groups.

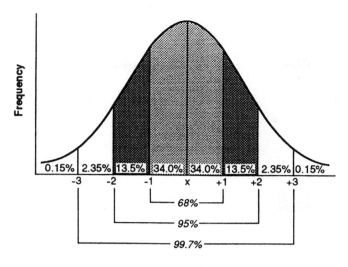

Area under the curve

Figure 26-1. The normal (gaussian) distribution. The number of standard deviations (-3 to $+3$) from the mean is shown on the x-axis. The percentage of the population that falls under the curve within each standard deviation is shown. (From Fadem B, *High-Yield Behavioral Science,* Baltimore, Williams & Wilkins, 1996, p 101)

The possibility that this difference occurred by chance is tested using statistical procedures.

B. The **null hypothesis,** which postulates that no difference exists between two groups, can either be rejected or not rejected following statistical analysis.

—Example of the null hypothesis:

1. A group of 20 patients who have similar systolic blood pressures at the beginning of a study (Time 1) is divided into two groups of 10 patients each. One group is given daily doses of an experimental drug meant to lower blood pressure (experimental group); the other group is given daily doses of a placebo (placebo group). Blood pressure is measured 2 weeks later (Time 2).

2. The null hypothesis assumes that there are no significant differences in blood pressure between the two groups at Time 2.

3. If, at Time 2, patients in the experimental group show systolic blood pressures similar to those in the placebo group, the null hypothesis (i.e., there is no significant difference between the groups) is **not** rejected.

4. If, at Time 2, patients in the experimental group have significantly lower or higher blood pressures than those in the placebo group, the null hypothesis is rejected.

C. **Alpha (α) and beta (β)**

1. α is a preset level of significance, usually set at **0.05** by convention.

2. Power (1 minus β) is the ability to detect a difference between groups if it is truly there. The larger the sample size, the more power a researcher has to detect this difference.

D. **Type I (α) and type II (β) error**

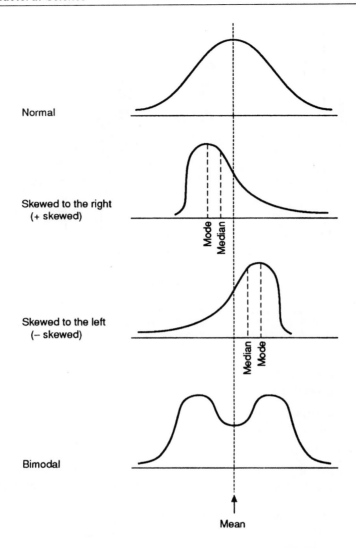

Figure 26-2. Frequency distributions. (From Fadem B, *High-Yield Behavioral Science,* Baltimore, Williams & Wilkins, 1996, p 102)

1. A **type I error** occurs when the null hypothesis is rejected although it is true (e.g., the drug really does not lower blood pressure).

2. A **type II error** occurs when the null hypothesis is not rejected although it is false (e.g., the drug really does lower blood pressure) but there may not have been enough power to detect this difference.

E. **Statistical probability**

1. The p (probability) value is the chance of a type I error occurring. If a p value is equal to or less than 0.05, the preset α level, it is unlikely that a type I error has been made (i.e., a type I error is made 5 or fewer times out of 100 attempts).

2. A p value equal to or less than 0.05 (e.g., $p < 0.01$) is generally considered to be statistically significant.

III. Specific Statistical Tests

—Statistical tests are used to analyze data from medical studies. The results of statistical tests tell whether to reject or not reject the null hypothesis. Statistical tests can be parametric or nonparametric.

A. Parametric statistical tests for continuous data

1. Parametric tests are commonly used to evaluate the presence of statistically significant differences between groups when the distribution of scores in a population is normal and when the sample size is large.

2. Commonly used parametric statistical tests include *t*-**tests and analysis of variance (ANOVA),** and **linear correlation** (Example 26-1).

3. **Linear correlation** is the degree of relationship between two continuous variables which can be assessed using linear correlation coefficients (*r*) that range between **−1 and +1.**

Example 26-1. Commonly Used Statistical Tests

A consumer group would like to evaluate the success of three different commercial weight loss programs. To do this, subjects are assigned to one of three programs (group A, group B, and group C). The average weight of the subjects is not significantly different at the start of the study (Time 1). Each group follows a different diet regimen. At Time 1 and at the end of the 6-week study (Time 2), the subjects are weighed and their blood pressure meansurements are obtained. Examples of how statistical tests can be used to analyze the results of this study are given below.

t-**test: Difference between the means of two samples**

Independent (nonpaired) test: Tests the mean difference in body weights of subjects in group A and subjects in group B at Time 1 (i.e., two groups of subjects are sampled on one occasion).

Dependent (paired) test: Tests the mean difference in body weights of people in group A at Time 1 and Time 2 (i.e., the same people are sampled on two occasions).

Analysis of variance: Differences between the means of more than two samples.

One-way analysis: Tests the mean differences in body weights of subjects in group A, group B, and group C at Time 2 (i.e., one variable: group).

Two-way analysis: Tests the mean differences in body weights of men and women and in body weights of group A, group B, and group C at Time 2 (i.e., two variables: sex and group)

Correlation: The mutual relation between two continuous variables

Tests the relation between blood pressure and body weight in all subjects at Time 2.

Chi-square test: Differences between frequencies in a sample

Tests the difference among the percentage of subjects with body weight of 140 lbs or less in group A, B, and C at Time 2.

    a. If the two variables move in the same direction, ρ is **positive** (e.g., as height increases, body weight increases, or, as calorie intake decreases, body weight decreases).

    b. If the two variables move in opposite directions, ρ is **negative** (e.g., as time spent exercising increases, body weight decreases).

B. Nonparametric statistical tests

    1. If the distribution of scores in a population is not normal or if the sample size is small, nonparametric statistical tests are used to evaluate the presence of statistically significant differences between groups.

    2. Commonly used nonparametric statistical tests include Wilcoxon's (rank sum and signed-rank), Mann-Whitney or Kruschal-Wallis tests.

C. Categorical tests

    —To analyze categorical data or compare proportions, the **chi-square** (see Example 26-1) or **Fisher's Exact tests** are used.

Review Test

1. Analysis of the data from a large research study reveals a p value of 0.001. These results indicate that the researcher

(A) has committed a type I error
(B) has committed a type II error
(C) can reject the null hypothesis
(D) cannot reject the null hypothesis
(E) has biased the study

Questions 2–3

On a gross anatomy quiz, test scores of 10, 10, 10, 70, 40, 20, and 90 are obtained by seven students in a laboratory group.

2. Which of the following correctly describes these quiz scores?

(A) Positively skewed
(B) A normal distribution
(C) Negatively skewed
(D) The mode is higher than the mean
(E) The mode is equal to the mean

3. The median of these quiz scores is

(A) 10
(B) 20
(C) 40
(D) 70
(E) 90

Questions 4–5

Systolic blood pressure is normally distributed with a mean of 120 mm Hg and a standard deviation of 10.

4. What percentage of people would be expected to have systolic blood pressure at or above 140 mm Hg?

(A) 1.9%
(B) 2.5%
(C) 13.5%
(D) 34.0%
(E) 64.2%

5. In a population of 500 people, how many would be expected to have systolic blood pressure between 110 mm Hg and 120 mm Hg?

(A) 80
(B) 100
(C) 125
(D) 170
(E) 250

6. Which of the following statistical tests is most appropriately used to evaluate the difference in the percentage of women who lose weight on a protein-sparing diet versus the percentage who lose weight on a high-protein diet?

(A) Paired t-test
(B) Analysis of variance
(C) Chi-square test
(D) Correlation
(E) Independent t-test

7. Which of the following statistical tests is most appropriately used to evaluate differences between initial body weight and final body weight for each woman on a protein-sparing diet?

(A) Paired t-test
(B) Analysis of variance
(C) Chi-square test
(D) Correlation
(E) Independent t-test

8. Which of the following statistical tests is most appropriately used to evaluate the relationship between body weight and systolic blood pressure in a group of 25-year-old women?

(A) Paired t-test
(B) Analysis of variance
(C) Chi-square test
(D) Correlation
(E) Independent t-test

9. In a study to determine the usefulness of a new antihypertensive medication, 12 hypertensive patients are given the new drug and 10 hypertensive patients are given a placebo. The dependent variable in this study is

(A) the experimenter's bias
(B) giving the patients the drug
(C) giving the patients a placebo
(D) the patients' blood pressure following treatment with the drug or placebo
(E) the daily variability in the patients' blood pressure before the drug treatment

Answers and Explanations

TBQ-B. The correlation between parental income and USMLE Step 1 scores as shown by these data is positive (+) (i.e., as parental income increases, scores increase). Since a correlation coefficient (r) cannot be more than +1 the only possible answer is + 0.60.

1-C. With a p value of 0.001 (which is smaller than the preset α level of 0.05), the findings are statistically significant and the researcher can reject the null hypothesis. A type I error occurs when the null hypothesis is rejected although it is true. A type II error occurs when the null hypothesis is not rejected although it is false. There is no evidence of a type I or type II error or that the researcher has biased the study (see Chapter 25).

2-A, 3-B. Because of all the low scores, the distribution of these test scores is skewed to the right (positively skewed). Also, the mode (10) of these scores is lower than the mean 35.7, a characteristic of a positively skewed distribution. In a negatively skewed distribution (skewed to the left), the tail is toward the left (i.e., scores cluster toward the high end). In a normal distribution, the mean, median, and mode are equal. When they are sequentially ordered, the median (middle value) of these scores is 20.

4-B, 5-D. Systolic blood pressure of 140 mmHg is 2 standard deviations above the mean (120 mmHg). The area under the curve between 2 and 3 standard deviations above the mean is about 2.35% plus about 0.15% (everything above 3 standard deviations). Thus, a total of about 2.50% of the people will have blood pressure of 140 mmHg and above. Systolic blood pressure between 110–120 mmHg is one standard deviation below the mean. The percentage of people in this area on a normal curve is 34%. Thus, 34% of 500 people, or 170 people, will have systolic blood pressure in the range of 110–120 mmHg.

6-C. The chi-square test is used to examine differences between frequencies in a sample—in this case, the percentage of women who lose weight on a protein-sparing diet versus the percentage of women who lose weight on a high-protein diet.

7-A. The t-test is used to examine differences between means of two samples. This is an example of a paired t-test because the same women are examined on two different occasions.

8-D. Correlation is used to examine the relationship between two continuous variables—in this case, systolic blood pressure and body weight.

9-D. The dependent variable is a measure of the outcome of an experiment. In this case, blood pressure following treatment with the drug or placebo is the dependent variable. The independent variable is a characteristic that an experimenter examines to see if it changes the outcome. In this case, giving the patient a drug or placebo is the independent variable.

Comprehensive Examination

Directions: Each of the numbered items or incomplete statements in this section is followed by answers or by completions of the statement. Select the **one** lettered answer or completion that is **best** in each case.

1. A mother brings her 3-year-old son to the pediatrician for a well-child checkup. The doctor observes that the child relates well to her and is able to speak in complete sentences. In speaking to the mother, the doctor determines that the child cannot ride a tricycle, nor does he play cooperatively with other children. Select the best description of this child's development in language, motor, and social skills, respectively.

(A) Normal, normal, delayed
(B) Normal, delayed, normal
(C) Delayed, normal, normal
(D) Delayed, delayed, normal
(E) Normal, normal, normal
(F) Delayed, delayed, delayed
(G) Normal, delayed, delayed

2. The parents of a 17-year-old young woman with Down syndrome and an intelligence quotient (IQ) of 70 bring her in for a school physical. The physical is required for admission to a highly recommended special education co-ed boarding school. The parents are worried about sending her to the school because they are afraid that she will get pregnant. Although she has been on oral contraceptives for the past year, her mother must often remind her to take them. The parents ask for the physician's advice. The doctor's most appropriate recommendation is

(A) to do a tubal ligation
(B) to do an oophorectomy
(C) to enroll her in a local day school so that she can live at home
(D) to prescribe a long-acting contraceptive
(E) to send her to the boarding school and take no further action

3. A 6-year-old child with an intelligence quotient (IQ) of 50 is most likely to be able to do which of the following?

(A) Read a sentence
(B) Identify colors
(C) Copy a triangle
(D) Ride a 2-wheeled bicycle
(E) Understand the moral difference between right and wrong

4. A physician diagnoses genital herpes in a 16-year-old male high school student. Prior to treating him, the physician should

(A) notify his parents
(B) get permission from his parents
(C) notify his sexual partner(s)
(D) recommend that he tell his sexual partners
(E) notify the appropriate state agency

5. A 14-year-old boy tells his physician that he masturbates every day. He is doing well in school and is the captain of the school basketball team. The doctor's next move should be to

(A) notify his parents
(B) refer him to an adolescent psychologist
(C) reassure him that his behavior is normal
(D) tell him to become more involved in school sports
(E) measure his level of circulating testosterone

6. A 49-year-old sexually active woman tells her physician that she is experiencing hot flashes and has not menstruated in 4 months. She asks the doctor when she can discontinue use of birth control. The physician's most correct response is

(A) 6 months after the last menstrual period
(B) 1 year after the last menstrual period
(C) after age 55
(D) immediately
(E) when the hot flashes subside

7. "Head Start," an early-intervention enrichment program for normal but disadvantaged preschoolers, is aimed at reducing the likelihood of school failure in grade school. "Head Start" is an example of

(A) primary prevention
(B) secondary prevention
(C) tertiary prevention
(D) systematic desensitization
(E) behavior modification

8. Of the following people, which one is likely to use the most Medicare services and funds during his or her lifetime?

(A) African-American male smoker
(B) African-American female smoker
(C) African-American male nonsmoker
(D) African-American female nonsmoker
(E) White male smoker
(F) White female smoker
(G) White male nonsmoker
(H) White female nonsmoker

9. A child uses about 10 individual words, climbs stairs using one foot at a time, can stack 3 blocks and runs from but quickly returns to his mother. This child's age is most likely to be

A. 8 months
B. 12 months
C. 18 months
D. 36 months
E. 48 months

10. Of the following, the most likely reason for a physician to be sued for malpractice is that the physician

(A) prescribed a medication incorrectly
(B) had poor rapport with a patient
(C) did an unsuccessful surgery
(D) canceled an appointment with a patient
(E) made a poor medical decision

11. A 65-year-old woman signs a document that gives her husband durable power of attorney. Five days later she has a stroke, goes into a coma, and enters a persistent vegetative state. The most appropriate action for the physician to take is to

(A) get a court order to start life support
(B) follow the wishes of the husband
(C) not provide life support
(D) contact the women's adult children
(E) turn the case over to the ethics committee of the hospital

12. The majority of elderly Americans spend most of the last 5 years of their lives

(A) in a nursing home
(B) with family
(C) on their own
(D) in a hospice
(E) in a hospital

13. The husband of an 85-year-old patient with dementia of the Alzheimer's type tells the doctor that he is worried because the patient keeps wandering out the front door of the house. Of the following, the most appropriate recommendation for the doctor to make is to

(A) use restraints
(B) label all the doors
(C) prescribe diazepam
(D) prescribe donepezil [Aricept]
(E) place the patient in a nursing home

14. An 8-year-old child with normal intelligence reads, communicates well, and gets along well with the other children in school. However, he often argues with the teacher. His parents tell the doctor that he often seems angry toward them and rarely follows their rules. The best description for this child's behavior is

(A) normal
(B) attention-deficit hyperactivity disorder (ADHD)
(C) autistic disorder
(D) oppositional defiant disorder
(E) conduct disorder

15. Which of the following agents is most useful to treat a 28-year-old male patient who experiences cataplexy, hypnagogic hallucinations, and a very short rapid eye movement (REM) latency?

(A) A benzodiazepine
(B) A barbiturate
(C) An amphetamine
(D) An antipsychotic
(E) An antidepressant

16. A woman who had a normal delivery 2 days ago tells her doctor that she feels sad and cries for no reason. She appears well-groomed and is taking congratulatory calls and visits from friends and family. Her physician should

(A) tell her to stop worrying
(B) have her call his office daily over the next two weeks to report how she is feeling
(C) recommend a consultation with a psychiatrist
(D) prescribe an antidepressant
(E) prescribe a benzodiazepine

17. Although transplants can save many lives, there are fewer transplants done than are needed. Of the following, the primary reason for this is because

(A) there are not enough donors
(B) patients are usually too ill to withstand surgery
(C) transplants are too expensive
(D) transplants have a high chance of rejection
(E) the drugs used to prevent rejection are too toxic

18. A 22-year-old medical student has a parotid gland abscess and an excessive number of dental caries. She is of normal weight for her height, but seems distressed when the doctor questions her about her eating habits. This young woman is most likely to be suffering from

(A) bulimia nervosa
(B) anorexia nervosa
(C) conversion disorder
(D) avoidant personality disorder
(E) passive-aggressive personality disorder

19. After a 20-year-old woman ingests wine and cheese she is brought to the emergency department in a hypertensive crisis. The prescription drug most likely to have caused this problem is

(A) an antidepressant agent
(B) an antipsychotic agent
(C) an antimanic agent
(D) a benzodiazepine
(E) a barbiturate

20. Which of the following patients is at highest risk for suicide?

(A) A 55-year-old divorced woman
(B) A 55-year-old divorced man
(C) A 55-year-old married woman
(D) A 55-year-old married man
(E) A 55-year-old widowed woman

21. Which of the following is most likely to be seen in 50-year-old women in all cultures?

(A) The "empty-nest" syndrome
(B) Depression
(C) Anxiety
(D) Insomnia
(E) Hot flashes

22. Patients commonly prefer selective serotonin reuptake inhibitors (SSRIs) to tricyclic antidepressants because SSRIs are more likely to

(A) elevate mood
(B) work quickly
(C) lower blood pressure
(D) enhance sleep
(E) be well tolerated

23. A 28-year-old man who is afraid to drive a car is taught relaxation techniques and is then shown a photograph of a car. Later in treatment, he is exposed to toy cars, then to real cars. Finally, he drives a car. This treatment technique is best described as

(A) implosion
(B) biofeedback
(C) aversive conditioning
(D) token economy
(E) flooding
(F) systematic desensitization

(G) cognitive therapy

24. A 59-year-old male patient has just recovered from a myocardial infarction. During a follow-up examination he asks the physician what is the best position for sexual intercourse with his wife. The physician's best recommendation is

(A) face to face, lying on their sides
(B) face to face, female superior
(C) face to face, male superior
(D) male behind female, lying on their sides
(E) avoid sexual activity for at least 1 year

25. A mildly demented 83-year-old man is brought to the emergency department by his daughter with whom he lives. He smells of urine, is undernourished, and has bruises on both of his arms and abrasions on one wrist. He denies that anyone has harmed him. The most appropriate first action for the doctor to take after treating the patient is to

(A) speak to the daughter about the possibility that the man has been abused
(B) send him home with his daughter
(C) contact the appropriate state social service agency
(D) order a neurological evaluation
(E) release the patient into the care of another relative

26. Of the following, the ethnic group with the longest life expectancy is

(A) Asian Americans
(B) African Americans
(C) White Americans
(D) Native Americans

27. In the United States, which of the following is the most common belief concerning mental illness?

(A) It is therapeutic to discuss your internal emotional problems with others
(B) Mental illness signifies personal weakness
(C) Unconscious conflicts can be manifested as physical illness
(D) Mentally ill people have good self control
(E) Mentally ill people usually seek help

28. A 30-year-old man presents with a severe headache. During the interview, he states that he believes that his headache started when his neighbors came into his home and harassed him while he was sleeping the previous night, as they have done many times in the past. The patient has no history of psychiatric illness. He has good social and work relationships. Except for his comments about the neighbors, his thoughts seem clear, logical, and appropriate. The most likely diagnosis for this man is

(A) schizophrenia
(B) bipolar disorder
(C) delusional disorder
(D) schizoaffective disorder
(E) schizoid personality disorder

29. A 26-year-old woman tells her friends and family that she is pregnant with Michael Jackson's child. She has never met the singer and 2 pregnancy tests are negative. There is no other evidence of a thought disorder. This woman is most likely to be suffering from

(A) schizophrenia
(B) bipolar disorder
(C) delusional disorder
(D) somatization disorder
(E) schizoid personality disorder

30. A 40-year-old woman goes to her gynecologist for a yearly checkup. Which of the following is most likely to cause death in a woman of this age?

(A) Pregnancy
(B) An intrauterine device
(C) Oral contraceptives
(D) Barrier contraceptives
(E) A progesterone implant

31. A 29-year-old male patient with psoriasis on his hands and arms asks his doctor how to deal with the reaction of people when they see the rash. The doctor's best response is

(A) "Act like nothing is wrong"
(B) "Wear long-sleeved shirts"
(C) "Tell people that it is not contagious"
(D) "Stay at home as much as possible"
(E) "Tell people that it is not their business"

32. The usual standards of doctor–patient confidentiality would apply to which of the following patients?

(A) A man who tells his physician that he plans to shoot his partner
(B) A bereaved woman who tells her physician that she has had thoughts of suicide
(C) A man who tells his physician that he has been sexually abusing his 10-year-old stepdaughter
(D) An HIV-positive man who is engaging in sexual intercourse without condoms
(E) A depressed woman who tells her physician that she has saved up 50 secobarbital tablets and wants to die

33. Doctor A is aware that doctor B has made a serious mistake in treating a very ill hospitalized patient. Most appropriately, Doctor A should

(A) talk to Doctor B about his lapse
(B) warn Doctor B that he will be reported if he continues to make mistakes
(C) report Doctor B's action to Dr. B's superior at the hospital
(D) report Doctor B's action to the police
(E) recommend that Doctor B be transferred to another hospital

34. To evaluate unconscious conflicts in a 20-year-old man using drawings depicting ambiguous social situations, which is the most appropriate test?

(A) Thematic Apperception Test (TAT)
(B) Minnesota Multiphasic Personality Inventory (MMPI)
(C) Wechsler Intelligence Scale for Children-Revised (WISC-R)
(D) Rorschach Test
(E) Vineland Social Maturity Scale
(F) Wide Range Achievement Test (WRAT)
(G) Folstein Mini-Mental State Examination
(H) Glasgow Coma Scale

35. The basic defense mechanism on which all others are based, and which is used to prevent unacceptable emotions from reaching awareness, is known as

(A) repression
(B) sublimation
(C) dissociation
(D) regression
(E) intellectualization

36. An infant's ability to roll over from belly to back usually begins at what age?

(A) 0–3 months
(B) 5–6 months
(C) 7–10 months
(D) 11–15 months
(E) 16–30 months

37. A patient in the emergency department has just been involved in a car accident. The doctor suspects that she has been drinking. For the patient to be declared legally intoxicated, her blood alcohol concentration (BAC) must fall into which of the following ranges?

(A) 0.05%–0.09%
(B) 0.08%–0.15%
(C) 0.40%–0.50%
(D) 1.5%–2.0%
(E) 2.5%–3.0%

38. Of the following agents, which is the most appropriate heterocyclic antidepressant for a 45-year-old air traffic controller who must stay alert on the job?

(A) Isocarboxazid
(B) Tranylcypromine
(C) Trazodone
(D) Doxepin
(E) Amoxapine
(F) Fluoxetine
(G) Desipramine
(H) Nortriptyline
(I) Amitriptyline
(J) Imipramine

39. A 70-year-old woman reports that she has difficulty sleeping through the night because of persistent muscular contractions in her legs. Which of the following sleep disorders best matches this picture?

(A) Kleine-Levin syndrome
(B) Nightmare disorder
(C) Sleep terror disorder
(D) Sleep drunkenness
(E) Circadian rhythm sleep disorder
(F) Nocturnal myoclonus
(G) Restless leg syndrome

40. A pilot whose plane is about to crash explains the technical details of the engine malfunction to his copilot. The defense mechanism that the pilot is using is

(A) repression
(B) sublimation
(C) dissociation
(D) regression
(E) intellectualization

41. Most children begin to walk without assistance at what age?

(A) 0–3 months
(B) 5–6 months
(C) 7–10 months
(D) 11–15 months
(E) 16–30 months

42. A 40-year-old woman with tension headaches has the tension in the frontalis muscle measured regularly. The readings are projected to her on a computer screen. She is then taught to use mental techniques to decrease muscle tension. Which of the following treatment techniques does this example illustrate?

(A) Implosion
(B) Biofeedback
(C) Aversive conditioning
(D) Token economy
(E) Flooding
(F) Systemic desensitization
(G) Cognitive therapy

43. A patient reports that despite the fact that he goes to sleep at 11:00 pm and wakes up at 7:00 am, he does not feel fully awake until about noon each day. His wife states that he appears to be sleeping soundly at night. The patient denies substance abuse. Which of the following sleep disorders best matches this picture?

(A) Kleine-Levin syndrome
(B) Nightmare disorder
(C) Sleep terror disorder
(D) Sleep drunkenness
(E) Circadian rhythm sleep disorder
(F) Nocturnal myoclonus
(G) Restless leg syndrome

44. A 33-year-old patient tells you that he drinks at least 10 cups of coffee per day. Of the following effects, which is most likely in this patient?

(A) Blood pressure reduction
(B) Lethargy
(C) Tachycardia
(D) Decreased gastric acid secretion
(E) Depressed mood

45. The social smile commonly first appears at what age?

(A) 0–3 months
(B) 5–6 months
(C) 7–10 months
(D) 11–15 months
(E) 16–30 months

46. To evaluate reading and arithmetic skills in a 30-year-old hospitalized male patient, which is the most appropriate test?

(A) Thematic Apperception Test (TAT)
(B) Minnesota Multiphasic Personality Inventory (MMPI)
(C) Wechsler Intelligence Scale for Children-Revised (WISC-R)
(D) Rorschach Test
(E) Vineland Social Maturity Scale
(F) Wide Range Achievement Test (WRAT)
(G) Folstein Mini-Mental State Examination
(H) Glasgow Coma Scale

47. Slow-waves are characteristic of what sleep stage?

(A) Stage 1
(B) Stage 2
(C) Stages 3 and 4 (delta)
(D) REM sleep

48. Normal infants begin visually following faces and objects with their eyes (tracking) at what age?

(A) 0–3 months
(B) 5–6 months
(C) 7–10 months
(D) 11–15 months
(E) 16–30 months

49. A 65-year-old physician who has been given a diagnosis of terminal pancreatic cancer repeatedly discusses the technical aspects of his case with other physicians in the hospital. The defense mechanism this physician is using is

(A) acting out
(B) sublimation
(C) denial
(D) regression
(E) intellectualization
(F) reaction formation

50. An anxious, depressed teenager steals a car. The defense mechanism that this teenager is using is

(A) acting out
(B) sublimation
(C) denial
(D) regression
(E) intellectualization
(F) reaction formation

51. A 50-year-old hospitalized patient has just received a diagnosis of breast cancer. She states that the biopsy was in error and checks out of the hospital against the advice of her physician. The defense mechanism that this patient is using is

(A) acting out
(B) sublimation
(C) denial
(D) regression
(E) intellectualization
(F) reaction formation

52. A patient, although she is angry at her doctor because he canceled her previous appointment at the last minute, tells him at her next appointment that she really likes his tie. The defense mechanism that this patient is using is

(A) acting out
(B) sublimation
(C) denial
(D) regression
(E) intellectualization
(F) reaction formation

53. A 28-year-old woman who works as an animal caretaker lives with her elderly aunt and rarely socializes. She reports that, although she would like to have friends, when coworkers ask her to join them for breaks, she refuses because she is afraid that they will not like her. This behavior is most closely associated with which of the following personality disorders?

(A) Passive-aggressive personality disorder
(B) Schizotypal personality disorder
(C) Antisocial personality disorder
(D) Paranoid personality disorder
(E) Schizoid personality disorder
(F) Obsessive-compulsive personality disorder
(G) Avoidant personality disorder
(H) Histrionic personality disorder

54. A 35-year-old man comes to the physician's office dressed all in bright yellow. He reports that his mild earache felt like "a knife in his ear" and says that he feels so hot that he "must be dying." This behavior is most closely associated with which of the following personality disorders?

(A) Passive-aggressive personality disorder
(B) Schizotypal personality disorder
(C) Antisocial personality disorder
(D) Paranoid personality disorder
(E) Schizoid personality disorder
(F) Obsessive-compulsive personality disorder
(G) Avoidant personality disorder
(H) Histrionic personality disorder

55. A 24-year-old patient is experiencing intense hunger as well as tiredness and headache. This patient is most likely to be withdrawing from which of the following agents?

(A) Alcohol
(B) Secobarbital
(C) Phencyclidine (PCP)
(D) Amphetamine
(E) Lysergic acid diethylamide (LSD)
(F) Diazepam
(G) Heroin
(H) Marijuana

56. A 40-year-old man with a history of depression and insomnia is brought to the emergency department with signs of severe respiratory depression. The drug most likely to be responsible for these symptoms is

(A) Alcohol
(B) Secobarbital
(C) Phencyclidine (PCP)
(D) Amphetamine
(E) Lysergic acid diethylamide (LSD)
(F) Diazepam
(G) Heroin
(H) Marijuana

57. The police bring a 25-year-old man to the hospital in a coma. His girlfriend tells the physician that prior to having a convulsion and fainting, he became combative, showed strange darting eye movements, and said that he felt his body expanding and floating up to the ceiling. Of the following, the drug most likely to be responsible for these symptoms is

(A) alcohol
(B) secobarbital
(C) phencyclidine (PCP)
(D) amphetamine
(E) lysergic acid diethylamide (LSD)
(F) diazepam
(G) heroin
(H) marijuana

58. A patient who has been a heavy coffee drinker is hospitalized and not permitted to take anything by mouth. Which of the following is the patient most likely to demonstrate the day after hospitalization?

(A) Excitement
(B) Euphoria
(C) Headache
(D) Decreased appetite
(E) Pupil dilation

59. To evaluate level of consciousness and attention in a 50-year-old female stroke patient, which of the following is the most appropriate test?

(A) Thematic Apperception Test (TAT)
(B) Minnesota Multiphasic Personality Inventory (MMPI)
(C) Wechsler Intelligence Scale for Children-Revised (WISC-R)
(D) Rorschach Test
(E) Vineland Social Maturity Scale
(F) Wide Range Achievement Test (WRAT)
(G) Glasgow Coma Scale

60. The electroencephalogram of a 28-year-old patient shows mainly alpha waves. This patient is most likely to be

(A) awake and concentrating
(B) awake, relaxed, with eyes closed
(C) in Stage 1 sleep
(D) in Stage 4 sleep
(E) in REM sleep

61. A 24-year-old woman experiences pelvic pain when she and her boyfriend attempt to have sexual intercourse. No abnormalities are found during pelvic examination. This woman is most likely to be suffering from

(A) fetishism
(B) functional vaginismus
(C) sexual aversion disorder
(D) orgasmic disorder
(E) functional dyspareunia
(F) female sexual arousal disorder
(G) hypoactive sexual desire

62. A 65-year-old woman whose husband died 3 weeks before cries much of the time and sleeps poorly. Also, she states that she thinks that she saw her husband walking down the street the day before. The most appropriate first action by her physician is to

(A) recommend a vacation
(B) provide support and reassurance
(C) prescribe antipsychotic medication
(D) prescribe antidepressant medication
(E) recommend a psychiatric evaluation

63. Which of the following individuals has the highest risk for developing schizophrenia?

(A) The dizygotic twin of a schizophrenic person
(B) The child of two schizophrenic parents
(C) The monozygotic twin of a schizophrenic person
(D) The child of one schizophrenic parent
(E) A child raised in an institutional setting when neither biological parent was schizophrenic

64. Which of the following statements is most likely to be evidence of psychotic features in a severely depressed 49-year-old man?

(A) "I am an inadequate person"
(B) "I am a worthless human being"
(C) "I will never get better"
(D) "I am a failure in my profession"
(E) "I am personally responsible for the crash of Pan Am Flight 800"

65. A 7-year-old child requires a blood transfusion within 24 hours for a life-threatening injury. If, for religious reasons, the parents refuse to allow the transfusion, the physician should

(A) give the child the transfusion immediately
(B) obtain a court order and then give the child the transfusion
(C) obtain permission from another family member
(D) have the child moved to another hospital
(E) follow the parents' instructions and do not give the child the transfusion

66. A patient who has suffered a major psychological stress is examined because of severe hearing loss. No medical cause can be found. Which of the following is likely to be true about this patient?

(A) The patient is old
(B) The patient is male
(C) The patient is well educated
(D) The patient's hearing loss appeared suddenly
(E) The patient is very upset about the hearing loss

67. Long-term psychiatric hospitals in the United States are owned and operated primarily by

(A) universities
(B) private investors
(C) state governments
(D) municipal governments
(E) the federal government

68. A 60-year-old janitor from New York whose wife died recently is found in Akron, Ohio, working as a salesman. He does not know how he arrived there. This man is probably suffering from

(A) dissociative amnesia
(B) dissociative fugue
(C) somatization disorder
(D) conversion disorder
(E) depersonalization disorder

69. Which of the following conditions commonly becomes apparent in the fourth or fifth decade of life?

(A) Dementia of the Alzheimer's type
(B) Klinefelter's syndrome
(C) Turner's syndrome
(D) Tourette's disorder
(E) Huntington's disease

70. During an ophthalmologic examination, a 30-year-old schizophrenic female patient is found to have retinal pigmentation. This patient is most likely to be taking which one of the following antipsychotic agents?

(A) Chlorpromazine
(B) Haloperidol
(C) Perphenazine
(D) Trifluoperazine
(E) Thioridazine

71. A normal 24-year-old woman in non-REM sleep is likely to show which of the following?

(A) Dreaming
(B) Increased pulse
(C) Clitoral erection
(D) Skeletal muscle relaxation
(E) Delta waves on the electroencephalogram

72. Of the following disorders, the one to show the largest sex difference is

(A) cyclothymic disorder
(B) major depressive disorder
(C) bipolar disorder
(D) hypochondriasis
(E) schizophrenia

73. Negative predictive value is the probability that a person with a

(A) negative test is actually well
(B) positive test is actually well
(C) negative test is actually ill
(D) positive test is actually ill
(E) positive test will eventually show signs of the illness

74. In a laboratory study, it is shown that the uterus rises in the pelvic cavity during sexual activity. In which stage of the sexual response cycle does this phenomenon first occur?

(A) Excitement
(B) Plateau
(C) Orgasm
(D) Emission
(E) Resolution

75. A married couple tells the physician that their sex life has been poor because the husband ejaculates too quickly. The doctor tells them that the "squeeze technique" would be helpful. In this technique the person who applies the "squeeze" is

(A) the husband
(B) the wife
(C) the physician
(D) a sex therapist
(E) a sex surrogate

76. Which of the following statistical tests is most appropriately used to evaluate differences among mean body weights of women in three different age groups?

(A) Dependent (paired) *t*-test
(B) Chi-square test
(C) Analysis of variance
(D) Independent (unpaired) *t*-test
(E) Fisher's exact test

77. A 39-year-old man (who has never before had problems with erections) begins to have difficulty achieving an erection during sexual activity with his wife. The very first time he had trouble maintaining an erection was at a beach party when he had "too much to drink." This man is suffering from which of the following sexual dysfunctions?

(A) Primary erectile dysfunction
(B) Secondary erectile dysfunction
(C) Sexual aversion disorder
(D) Orgasmic disorder
(E) Dyspareunia
(F) Hypoactive sexual desire

78. A study was carried out to determine whether exposure to liquid crystal display (LCD) computer screens in the first trimester of pregnancy results in miscarriage. To do this, 50 women who had miscarriages and 100 women who carried to term were questioned the day after miscarriage or delivery, respectively, about their exposure to LCDs during pregnancy. If 10 women who had miscarriages and 8 women who carried to term used LCDs during their pregnancies, the odds-risk ratio associated with LCDs in pregnancy is approximately

(A) 1.9
(B) 2.9
(C) 10.0
(D) 20.4
(E) 46

79. In a cohort study, the ratio of the incidence rate of miscarriage among women who use liquid crystal display (LCD) computer screens to the incidence rate of miscarriage among women who do not use LCD computer screens is the

(A) attributable risk
(B) odds-risk ratio
(C) incidence rate
(D) prevalence ratio
(E) relative risk

Questions 80 and 81

In a study, the incidence rate of tuberculosis in people who have someone living in their home with tuberculosis is 5 per 1000. The incidence rate of tuberculosis in people who have no one living in their home with tuberculosis is 0.5 per 1000.

80. What is the risk for getting tuberculosis attributable to living with someone who has tuberculosis (attributable risk)?

(A) 1.5
(B) 4.5
(C) 7.5
(D) 9.5
(E) 10.0

81. How many times higher is the risk of getting tuberculosis for people who live with a patient with tuberculosis than for people who do not live with a tuberculosis patient (the relative risk)?

(A) 1.5
(B) 4.5
(C) 7.5
(D) 9.5
(E) 10.0

82. To estimate the relative risk in a case-control study, which of the following is calculated?

(A) Attributable risk
(B) Odds-risk ratio
(C) Incidence rate
(D) Prevalence ratio
(E) Sensitivity

83. A 50-year-old female high school teacher reports that she has been "feeling very low" for the past 3 months. She often misses work because she feels tired and hopeless and has trouble sleeping. When the doctor questions her she says "Doctor, the Lord calls all his children home." This patient is most likely to be suffering from

(A) cyclothymic disorder
(B) major depressive disorder
(C) bipolar disorder
(D) hypochondriasis
(E) schizophrenia

84. A 32-year-old man survives a plane crash in which four passengers died. Two weeks after the crash he has difficulty remembering aspects of the event. He also feels isolated and distant from others. This patient is most likely to be suffering from which of the following disorders?

(A) Post-traumatic stress disorder (PTSD)
(B) Generalized anxiety disorder
(C) Obsessive-compulsive disorder (OCD)
(D) Panic disorder
(E) Acute stress disorder

85. One year after she was robbed at knifepoint in the street, a 28-year-old woman jumps at every loud noise, has nightmares about the robbery, and is anxious much of the time. Of the following, the best diagnosis for this patient is

(A) post-traumatic stress disorder (PTSD)
(B) generalized anxiety disorder
(C) obsessive-compulsive disorder (OCD)
(D) panic disorder
(E) acute stress disorder

86. At the close of a long interview with an elderly male patient, the physician says, "Let's see if I have taken all of the information correctly," and then sums up the information that the patient has given. This interviewing technique is known as

(A) confrontation
(B) validation
(C) recapitulation
(D) facilitation
(E) reflection
(F) direct question
(G) support

87. "Many people feel the way you do when they first need hospitalization" is an example of the interview technique known as

(A) empathy
(B) validation
(C) recapitulation
(D) facilitation
(E) reflection
(F) direct question
(G) support

88. After a patient has described his symptoms and the time of day that they intensify, the interviewer says, "You say that you felt the pain more in the evening?" This question is an example of the interview technique known as

(A) confrontation
(B) validation
(C) recapitulation
(D) facilitation
(E) reflection
(F) direct question
(G) support

89. "You say that you are not nervous, but you are sweating and shaking and seem very upset to me" is an example of the interviewing technique known as

(A) confrontation
(B) validation
(C) recapitulation
(D) facilitation
(E) reflection
(F) direct question
(G) support

90. A patient relates to the doctor, "If I am seated at a table in the center of a restaurant rather than against the wall, I suddenly get dizzy and feel like I cannot breathe." This patient is describing a(n)

(A) hallucination
(B) delusion
(C) illusion
(D) panic attack

91. A patient relates to the doctor, "Last week, I thought I saw my father who died last year go around the corner." This patient is describing a(n)

(A) hallucination
(B) delusion
(C) illusion
(D) panic attack

92. The most appropriate method to determine in what part of the brain oxygen is used during the translation of a written passage from French to English is

(A) computed tomography (CT)
(B) dexamethasone suppression test (DST)
(C) evoked potentials
(D) electroencephalogram (EEG)
(E) galvanic skin response
(F) positron emission tomography (PET)

93. The most appropriate diagnostic technique to evaluate hearing loss in a 3-month-old infant is

(A) computed tomography (CT)
(B) dexamethasone suppression test (DST)
(C) evoked potentials
(D) electroencephalogram (EEG)
(E) galvanic skin response
(F) positron emission tomography (PET)

94. A 42-year-old woman pretends that she is paralyzed following an automobile accident in order to collect money from the insurance company. This woman is demonstrating

(A) psychogenic fugue
(B) derealization
(C) factitious disorder
(D) malingering
(E) conversion disorder
(F) multiple personality disorder
(G) depersonalization disorder
(H) body dysmorphic disorder

95. A 42-year-old woman pretends that she is paralyzed following an automobile accident in order to gain attention from her doctor. This patient is demonstrating

(A) psychogenic fugue
(B) derealization
(C) factitious disorder
(D) malingering
(E) conversion disorder
(F) multiple personality disorder
(G) depersonalization disorder
(H) body dysmorphic disorder

96. A 54-year-old woman who is depressed awakens at 4:00 am every morning and cannot fall back asleep. She is then tired all day. This woman which of the following sleep disorders

(A) narcolepsy
(B) Kleine-Levin syndrome
(C) insomnia
(D) obstructive sleep apnea
(E) sleep terror disorder

97. A 40-year-old man who is overweight reports that he feels tired all day despite having 8 hours of sleep each night. This man's problem indicates that he is suffering from

(A) narcolepsy
(B) Kleine-Levin syndrome
(C) insomnia
(D) obstructive sleep apnea
(E) sleep terror disorder

98. A patient reports, in a dispassionate way, that she has no sensation in her left arm. Physical examination fails to reveal evidence of a physiological problem. This patient is most likely to be suffering from

(A) hypochondriasis
(B) body dysmorphic disorder
(C) conversion disorder
(D) somatization disorder
(E) somatoform pain disorder

99. Despite the doctor's reassurances and negative biopsies of 5 different moles, a 45-year-old patient appears very worried and tells the doctor that he believes that his remaining moles should be biopsied because they are "probably melanomas." Of the following, this patient is most likely to be suffering from

(A) hypochondriasis
(B) body dysmorphic disorder
(C) conversion disorder
(D) somatization disorder
(E) somatoform pain disorder

100. A dog learns to turn a doorknob with its teeth because this behavior has been rewarded with a treat. This is an example of the type of learning best described as

(A) operant conditioning
(B) aversive conditioning
(C) spontaneous recovery
(D) modeling
(E) stimulus generalization

101. Each time a 35-year-old man receives physical therapy for a shoulder injury, his pain lessens. This makes him return for more physical therapy sessions. This is an example of which of the following?

(A) Implosion
(B) Stimulus generalization
(C) Systematic desensitization
(D) Flooding
(E) Intermittent reinforcement
(F) Fixed ratio reinforcement
(G) Negative reinforcement

102. A 75-year-old woman who lives alone develops a high fever and is brought to the hospital by a neighbor. Although the woman can state her name, she is not oriented to place or time and mistakes the orderly for her nephew. This woman is most likely to be suffering from

(A) depression (pseudodementia)
(B) Tourette's disorder
(C) dementia of the Alzheimer's type
(D) delirium
(E) amnestic disorder (Korsakoff's syndrome)

103. A 19-year-old man is brought to the hospital by the police. The policeman states that when stopped for a minor traffic violation, the man cursed at him and showed bizarre grimacing. This young man is most likely to be suffering from

(A) depression (pseudodementia)
(B) Tourette's disorder
(C) dementia of the Alzheimer's type
(D) delirium
(E) amnestic disorder (Korsakoff's syndrome)

104. A 63-year-old female patient cannot identify the man sitting next to her (her husband). Physical examination is unremarkable and there is no history of drug or alcohol abuse. The patient is alert and seems to be paying attention to the doctor. This patient is most likely to be suffering from

(A) depression (pseudodementia)
(B) Tourette's disorder
(C) dementia of the Alzheimer's type
(D) delirium
(E) amnestic disorder (Korsakoff's syndrome)

105. "I will go to church every day if only I can get rid of this illness" is an example of which of the following stages of dying?

(A) Denial
(B) Anger
(C) Bargaining
(D) Depression
(E) Acceptance

106. A mother puts a bitter substance on her 9-year-old son's fingernails in order to break his nail-biting habit. This is an example of the type of learning best described as

(A) operant conditioning
(B) aversive conditioning
(C) spontaneous recovery
(D) modeling
(E) stimulus generalization

107. A 29-year-old woman comes to the physician with symptoms of anxiety which have been present for over 2 years and have no obvious precipitating event. The patient has never previously taken an antianxiety agent. Of the following psychoactive agents, the best choice for this woman is

(A) diazepam (Valium)
(B) haloperidol (Haldol)
(C) fluoxetine (Prozac)
(D) buspirone (BuSpar)
(E) lithium

Answers and Explanations

1-B. Most normal 3-year-old children can ride a tricycle, can speak in complete but short sentences, and can play in parallel with (next to) other children. They generally do not play cooperatively with other children until about 4 years of age. Thus, this child may be delayed in motor skills but is normal in language and social skills.

2-D. The parent's concerns are real. Therefore, to take no further action is not an acceptable choice for the doctor. The doctor's most appropriate recommendation is to recommend a long-acting contraceptive for this young woman. Permanent forms of birth control such as tubal ligation or oophorectomy are not appropriate. Preventing her from going to the school for fear of pregnancy could limit the social, academic, and employment potential of this young woman.

3-B. Using the intelligence quotient (IQ) formula [i.e., mental age (MA)/chronological age (CA) $\times$ 100 = IQ] the MA of this child is 3 years (MA/6 $\times$ 100 = 50). Like a normal 3-year-old child, someone with a mental age of 3 years can identify colors but cannot read, copy a triangle, ride a 2-wheeled bicycle, or understand the moral difference between right and wrong.

4-D. Prior to treating the 16-year-old patient, the physician should recommend that he tell his sexual partner(s). There is no need to break doctor-patient confidentiality by telling the sexual partner(s) since the illness is not life-threatening. Parents do not have to be told or to give permission to treat sexually transmitted diseases in minors. Herpes is not generally reportable to state or federal health authorities.

5-C. The doctor should reassure this 14-year-old boy that masturbation is normal. Any amount of masturbation is normal, provided it does not prevent a person from having an active, successful life. There is no dysfunction in this boy and it is not appropriate to notify his parents, refer him to a psychologist, or to measure his testosterone level.

6-B. One year after the last menstrual period signals the end of menopause, when the use of birth control can be discontinued. The age of menopause and the occurrence of hot flashes vary considerably among women and thus cannot be used to predict the end of fertility.

7-A. "Head Start" and educational programs like it are examples of primary prevention, mechanisms to reduce the incidence of a problem (e.g., school failure) by reducing its associated risk factors (e.g., lack of educational enrichment).

8-H. Because Medicare coverage lasts for life and because she has the longest life expectancy, a white female nonsmoker is likely to use more Medicare services and funds than men, African-Americans and smokers during her lifetime.

9-C. This child is most likely to be 18 months of age. At this age, children can use about 10 words, climb stairs one foot at a time and stack 3 blocks. They also show "rapprochement," the tendency to run away from but then to rapidly return to their primary caregiver.

10-B. The most likely reason for a physician to be sued for malpractice is that the physician had poor rapport with a patient. The doctor-patient relationship is the most important factor in whether or not a patient will sue a doctor. The doctor's medical or surgical skills have relatively little to do with whether or not the doctor will be sued by a patient.

11-B. The most appropriate action for the physician is to follow the wishes of the husband. In this example, the husband can decide whether or not to continue life support since he has assumed the power to speak for the patient by virtue of the "durable power of attorney."

12-C. Most elderly Americans spend the last 5 years of their lives living on their own in their own residences. Approximately 5% end up in nursing homes and 20% live with family. Hospice care is aimed at people expected to die within 6 months. Hospital stays average only 6–7 days.

13-B. The most effective intervention for this 85-year-old patient with dementia of the Alzheimer's type who wanders out of the house is to label all the doors. She may wander out because she no longer knows where each door leads. Medications can be helpful for associated symptoms (i.e., diazepam for anxiety) and to delay further decline (donepezil) but cannot replace lost function. Nursing home placement should only be considered if the patient cannot be kept at home. Long-term use of restraints is never appropriate.

14-D. Since this child's major problem is with authority figures like his parents and teachers, the best description for this child's behavior is oppositional defiant disorder. He reads and communicates well and there is no evidence for attention-deficit hyperactivity disorder (ADHD) or autistic disorder. He relates well to the other children in school so there is no clear evidence for conduct disorder.

15-C. Cataplexy, hypnagogic hallucinations and a very short rapid eye movement (REM) latency indicate that this patient is suffering from narcolepsy. Amphetamines (but not benzodiazepines, barbiturates, antipsychotics, or antidepressants) are indicated in the treatment of narcolepsy.

16-B. The doctor's most appropriate action is to have this patient call the doctor's office daily over the next few weeks to report how she is feeling. This woman is currently suffering from the "baby blues" (i.e., sadness for no obvious reason after a normal delivery). There is no specific treatment for baby blues and the symptoms usually disappear within one week. However, because some women with the baby blues go on to develop a major depressive episode requiring treatment, the doctor should speak to this patient daily until her symptoms remit.

17-A. Fewer transplants are done than are needed primarily because there are not enough people willing to donate their organs at death.

18-A. This young woman is most likely to be suffering from bulimia nervosa, an eating disorder characterized by binge eating and purging but normal body weight. Parotid gland enlargement and abscesses and dental caries are seen in bulimia as a result of the forced vomiting.

19-A. The prescription drug most likely to have caused this problem is an antidepressant agent, namely a monoamine oxidase inhibitor (MAOI). These agents block the breakdown of tyramine (a pressor) in the gastrointestinal tract, resulting in elevated blood pressure and other life-threatening symptoms following ingestion of tyramine-rich foods (e.g. cheese and red wine).

20-B. Being divorced and being male are high risk factors for suicide.

21-E. Because the cause is physiological, hot flashes are the symptom of menopause most likely to be seen in 50-year-old women in all cultures.

22-E. Patients commonly prefer selective serotonin reuptake inhibitors (SSRIs) to tricyclic anti-depressants because SSRIs have fewer side effects and thus are more likely to be well tolerated. Both groups of antidepressants have similar action on mood and sleep. All take 3–4 weeks to work and neither group is particularly effective at lowering blood pressure.

23-F. This treatment technique in which a phobic patient is taught relaxation techniques and is then exposed to increased "doses" of the feared object is best described as systemic desensitization.

24-B. Because it is likely to cause the least exertion for the patient, the physician's best recommendation is face to face, female superior (woman on the top). To enhance the patient's recovery, the couple should be encouraged to return to their normal activities (including sex) as soon as possible. Avoiding sexual activity can delay the patient's recovery.

25-C. Poor physical care, bruises, and abrasions in this demented elderly patient indicate that he has been neglected and abused. Even though he denies that anyone has harmed him, the most likely abuser is his daughter. Therefore, the most appropriate action for the doctor to take after treating this patient is to contact the appropriate state social service agency. As in cases of child abuse, speaking to the likely abuser about the doctor's concerns is not necessary. The doctor also cannot send the patient home with the likely abuser or with another relative. The social service agency will deal with the patient's ultimate placement. If necessary, a neurological evaluation can be done at a later date.

26-A. Asian Americans have a longer life expectancy (82 years for men; 86 years for women) than African Americans (66 years for men; 74 years for women), White Americans (74 years for men; 80 years for women), or Native Americans (71 years for men; 79 years for women).

27-B. While some Americans may understand that it is therapeutic to discuss your internal emotional problems with others or that unconscious conflicts can be manifested as physical illness, much of the population of the United States believes that mental illness is a sign of personal weakness or failure. Many also believe that mentally ill people have poor self control. For these and other reasons, many mentally ill people do not seek help.

28-C. In persons with delusional disorder (paranoid type), delusions are present without abnormal thought processes. Absence of affective symptoms makes the diagnosis of bipolar disorder and schizoaffective disorder unlikely. Social withdrawal but no frank delusions characterize schizoid personality disorder.

29-C. This woman who believes that she is pregnant with the child of a celebrity is probably suffering from delusional disorder (erotomanic type).

30-A. Pregnancy is more likely to cause death in this 40-year-old woman than any contraceptive technique.

31-C. The doctor's best response is "Tell people that it is not contagious." It is better to face the problem than to act like nothing is wrong or to put people off by telling them it is not their business. The patient should be encouraged to get into the world and deal with the problem openly rather than to avoid questions by wearing long-sleeved shirts or by staying at home.

32-B. The usual standards of doctor–patient confidentiality apply to the bereaved woman who has not expressed a plan and is currently not at high risk to kill herself. In contrast, the depressed woman who tells her physician that she has saved up 50 secobarbital tablets (has a suicidal plan) and wants to die is at high risk to kill herself. Other exceptions to confidentiality include patients who commit child abuse, put their sexual partners at risk for HIV infection, or indicate that they plan to harm someone.

33-C. The most appropriate action for Doctor A to take is to report Dr. B to his or her superior at the hospital. Reporting of a lapse by a colleague is required ethically because patients must be protected. Talking to Doctor B about his lapse, warning him, reporting to the police, or recommending a transfer may not accomplish the goal of protecting patients.

34-A. The Thematic Apperception Test (TAT) utilizes drawings depicting ambiguous social situations to evaluate unconscious conflicts in patients.

35-A. Repression, the defense mechanism in use when unacceptable emotions are prevented from reaching awareness, is the defense mechanism on which all others are based.

36-B. Infants begin to roll over from back to belly and belly to back at about 5 months of age.

37-B. Legal intoxication is defined by blood alcohol concentrations of 0.08–0.15%, depending on individual state law.

38-G. Desipramine is non-sedating and thus is the most appropriate heterocyclic antidepressant for someone who must stay alert on the job. While fluoxetine is also non-sedating, it is a selective serotonin reuptake inhibitor (SSRI), not a heterocyclic agent.

39-F. This elderly woman who reports that she has difficulty sleeping through the night because of muscular contractions in her legs is probably suffering from nocturnal myoclonus.

40-E. Intellectualization, using the mind's higher functions to avoid experiencing emotion associated with the likelihood of crashing, is the defense mechanism used by this pilot.

41-D. Children usually begin to walk unassisted between 11 and 15 months of age.

42-B. The treatment technique described here is biofeedback. In this treatment, the patient is given ongoing physiologic information about the tension in the frontalis muscle and learns to use mental techniques to control this tension.

43-D. This patient who has a full night's sleep but does not feel fully awake until hours after he first wakes up is suffering from sleep drunkenness. This condition is rare and the diagnosis can only be made in the absence of other more common problems during sleep (i.e., sleep apnea) or substance abuse.

44-C. Tachycardia (increased heart rate) is seen with the use of all of the stimulant drugs, including caffeine. Stimulant drugs also tend to increase energy, blood pressure and gastric acid secretion, and to improve mood.

45-A. The social smile commonly first appears at 5–7 weeks of age in normal infants.

46-F. The Wide Range Achievement Test (WRAT) is used clinically to evaluate reading, arithmetic and other school-related skills in patients.

47-C. Slow waves are characteristic of delta sleep (stages 3 and 4).

48-A. Infants can visually track a human face and objects starting at birth.

49-E. Like the pilot in questions 40, this physician, who has been given a diagnosis of terminal pancreatic cancer, is using the defense mechanism of intellectualization (i.e., he is using his intellect to avoid experiencing the frightening emotions associated with his illness).

50-A. By acting out, the teenager's unacceptable anxious and depressed feelings are expressed in actions (stealing a car).

51-C. By using denial, this woman unconsciously refuses to believe what to her is the intolerable fact that she has breast cancer.

52-F. This patient is using the defense mechanism of reaction formation, which involves adopting behavior (i.e., complimenting the doctor) that is the opposite of the way she really feels (i.e., anger towards the doctor).

53-G. This woman is most likely to be suffering from an avoidant personality disorder. Because she is overly sensitive to rejection, she has become socially withdrawn. In contrast to the schizoid patient who prefers being alone, this patient is interested in meeting people but is unable to do so because of her shyness, inferiority complex, and timidity.

54-H. This behavior is most closely associated with the histrionic personality disorder. Persons with this disorder are dramatic and call attention to themselves with dress and behavior.

55-D. Intense hunger, tiredness, and headache are all signs of withdrawal from amphetamine.

56-B. The history of insomnia indicates that this patient may have been given a prescription for secobarbital [Seconal]. His history of depression indicates that he may have taken an overdose of the drug in a suicide attempt.

57-C. Phencyclidine (PCP) use, like other hallucinogens, results in feelings of altered body state. In contrast to use of lysergic acid diethylamide (LSD), increased aggressivity is seen with PCP use. Use of PCP also results in nystagmus (i.e., abnormal horizontal or vertical eye movements).

58-C. Withdrawal from caffeine and other stimulant drugs is associated with headache, lethargy, depression, and increased appetite. Pupil dilation is associated with use of, rather than withdrawal from, stimulants.

59-G. The Glasgow Coma Scale is used to evaluate level of consciousness and attention in patients.

60-B. Alpha waves are associated with the awake relaxed state with eyes closed.

61-E. This woman is probably suffering from functional dyspareunia (i.e., physically unexplainable pain with sexual intercourse).

62-B. Within the first 2 months of an important loss, people may respond intensely (e.g. they may even have the illusion that they see the dead person). The physician should provide support and reassurance since this patient probably is experiencing a normal grief reaction. While limited use of benzodiazepines for sleep is appropriate, antipsychotic or antidepressant medications are not indicated as treatment for normal grief.

63-C. The monozygotic twin of a schizophrenic person has about a 50% chance of developing the disorder. The child of one schizophrenic parent or the dizygotic twin of a schizophrenic patient has about a 12% chance; and the child of two schizophrenic parents has about a 40% chance. Being raised in an institutional setting has not been shown to be a risk factor for schizophrenia.

64-E. Feeling that one is personally responsible for a major disaster when one had nothing to do with it is a delusion in this depressed 49-year-old man. His other statements, while indicating feelings of inadequacy and hopelessness, are commonly seen symptoms of depression but not of psychosis.

65-B. Parents cannot refuse life saving treatment for their child for any reason. Because there is some time before the child must have the transfusion, there is time for a court order to be obtained (a court order can be obtained from a judge within a few hours). If there is no time to obtain a court order, treatment can proceed on an emergency basis.

66-D. This patient is probably suffering from conversion disorder, which involves neurological symptoms with no physical cause. Sensory loss in patients with conversion disorder appears suddenly. Patients with this disorder are more likely to be young, female, and less educated. They frequently show "la belle indifference," a curious lack of concern about the dramatic symptom.

67-C. Long-term psychiatric hospitals are owned and operated primarily by state governments.

68-B. Patients with dissociative fugue, a dissociative disorder, wander away from their homes and do not know how they got to another destination. This memory loss and wandering often occur following a very stressful life event, in this case the loss of his wife.

69-E. Huntington's disease commonly first appears between the ages of 35 and 45 years. Klinefelter's syndrome and Turner's syndrome are apparent by puberty; schizophrenia usually appears in adolescence or early adulthood; dementia of the Alzheimer's type most commonly appears in old age.

70-E. Retinal pigmentation is associated primarily with the use of thioridazine.

71-E. Delta waves are seen in non-REM sleep stages 3 and 4. Penile and clitoral erection, increased pulse, increased respiration, elevated blood pressure, dreaming, and complete relaxation of skeletal muscles are all seen in REM sleep.

72-B. Of the disorders listed, the largest sex difference in occurrence of a disorder is seen in major depressive disorder. Two times more women than men have this disorder. There is no significant sex difference in the occurrence of schizophrenia, cyclothymic disorder, hypochondriasis, or bipolar disorder.

73-A. Negative predictive value is the probability that a person with a negative test is actually well.

74-A. Rising of the uterus in the pelvic cavity with sexual activity (i.e., "the tenting effect") first occurs during the excitement phase of the sexual response cycle.

75-B. The wife applies the squeeze in the squeeze technique, a method used to delay ejaculation in men who ejaculate prematurely. In this technique, the man identifies a point at which ejaculation can still be prevented. He then instructs his partner to apply gentle pressure to the corona of the penis. The erection then subsides and ejaculation is delayed.

76-C. Analysis of variance is used to examine differences among means of more than 2 samples or groups. In this example there are 3 samples (i.e., age groups).

77-B. This man is suffering from secondary erectile dysfunction, problems with erection occurring after a period of normal functioning. Alcohol use is commonly associated with secondary erectile dysfunction.

78-B. The odds-risk ratio (odds ratio) is 2.9 and is calculated as follows:

	Liquid crystal display (LCD) exposure	**No LCD exposure**
Women who miscarried	A = 10	B = 40
Women who carried to term	C = 8	D = 92

Odds ratio = (A)(D)/(B)(C) = (10)(92)/(40)(8) = 2.9

79-E. In a cohort study, the ratio of the incidence rate of a condition (e.g., miscarriage) in exposed people to the incidence rate in nonexposed people is the relative risk.

80-B, 81-E. The attributable risk is the incidence rate in exposed people (5.0) minus the incidence rate in unexposed people (0.5) = 4.5. Therefore, 4.5 is the additional risk of getting tuberculosis associated with living with someone with tuberculosis. The relative risk is the incidence rate in exposed people (5.0) divided by the incidence rate in unexposed people (0.5) = 10.0. Therefore, the chances of getting tuberculosis are 10 times greater when living with someone who has tuberculosis than when living in a household in which no one has tuberculosis.

82-B. The odds-risk ratio is used to estimate the relative risk in a case-control study.

83-B. This patient is most likely to be suffering from major depressive disorder. Evidence for this is missing work, feeling hopeless and tired, and having trouble sleeping. Suicidal ideation is shown by her reference to death (i.e., "Doctor, the Lord calls all his children home").

84-E. Since it is only 2 weeks since the traumatic event occurred, this patient is most likely to be suffering from acute stress disorder. Post-traumatic stress disorder (PTSD) cannot be diagnosed until at least one month has passed. Obsessive-compulsive disorder (OCD) is an anxiety disorder characterized by obsessions and compulsions and panic disorder is characterized by sudden attacks of intense anxiety and a feeling that one is about to die. In OCD, generalized anxiety disorder, and panic disorder there is no obvious precipitating event.

85-A. Hypervigilance (i.e., jumping at every loud noise), nightmares, and persistent anxiety after a life-threatening event is post-traumatic stress disorder (PTSD). Acute stress disorder can only be diagnosed within one month of the traumatic event (see also explanation to Question 84).

86-C. Using recapitulation, the interviewer sums up all of the information given by the patient to ensure that it has been correctly recorded.

87-B. "Many people feel the way you do when they first need hospitalization" is an example of the interview technique known as validation. In validation, the interviewer gives credence to the patient's feelings and fears.

88-E. "You say that you felt the pain more in the evening?" is an example of the interview technique known as reflection.

89-A. Commenting on body language indicating anxiety and noting inconsistencies between verbal responses and body language demonstrate the interviewing technique known as confrontation.

90-D. Suddenly feeling anxious, becoming dizzy, and feeling like one cannot breathe when exposed to an open area are manifestations of a panic attack with agoraphobia.

91-C. In an illusion, an individual misperceives a real external stimulus. In this case, the individual has seen someone but has interpreted the person as being her father. Illusions are not uncommon in a normal grief reaction.

92-F. Positron emission tomography (PET) scans, which are used mainly as research tools, can localize metabolically active brain areas in persons who are performing specific tasks.

93-C. Auditory evoked potentials, the response of the brain to sound as measured by electrical activity, are used to evaluate loss of hearing in infants.

94-D. In malingering, the patient pretends that she is ill in order to realize an obvious (i.e., financial) gain.

95-C. In factitious disorder (formerly Munchausen's syndrome), the patient simulates illness for medical attention. The gain to this patient, attention from a doctor, is not as obvious as it is in the malingering patient (see explanation to Question 94).

96-C. Early morning awakening is a type of insomnia that is commonly seen in people with major depressive disorder.

97-D. Patients with obstructive sleep apnea are frequently unaware that they have awakened often during the night because they cannot breathe. They may become chronically tired.

98-C. Conversion disorder involves a dramatic loss of motor or sensory function with no medical cause. There is often a curious lack of concern ("la belle indifference") about the symptoms. Hypochondriasis is an exaggerated concern with illness or normal bodily functions. People with body dysmorphic disorder feel that there is something seriously wrong with their appearance. In somatization disorder, patients have many different physical symptoms over many years which have no biological cause. In somatoform pain disorder, a patient has long-lasting, unexplainable pain.

99-A. This patient is most likely to be suffering from hypochondriasis, an exaggerated concern with illness (and see Explanation to question 98).

100-A. In operant conditioning, a nonreflexive behavior, such as a dog turning a doorknob, is learned by using reinforcement, such as a treat.

101-G. In this example of negative reinforcement, a patient increases his behavior (e.g., going to physical therapy sessions) in order to reduce an aversive stimulus (e.g., his shoulder pain).

102-D. This woman is most likely to be suffering from delirium caused by the high fever.

103-B. Facial tics, cursing, and grimacing seen in this young man are symptoms of Tourette's disorder.

104-C. This patient is most likely to be suffering from dementia of the Alzheimer's type. Because her level of attention is normal, this is not delirium. There is no evidence of depression (pseudo-dementia) and this patient has no history of alcohol abuse to suggest amnestic disorder.

105-C. This statement is an example of the Kübler-Ross stage of dying known as bargaining.

106-B. In aversive conditioning, an unwanted behavior (nail biting) is paired with an unpleasant stimulus (noxious-tasting substance).

107-D. Because it is less likely than the benzodiazepines (e.g., diazepam) to cause dependence, the best medication for this chronically anxious patient is buspirone. Lithium is used to treat bipolar disorder and fluoxetine is used to treat depression and other anxiety disorders, such as panic disorder and obsessive-compulsive disorder.

Index

Page numbers set in *italics* denote figures; those followed by a t denote tables

Children
abuse of
features, 191t
incidence of, 191t
physical, 190–192, 191t,
196–197
review questions re-
garding, 189, 196–197
sequelae, 190
sexual, 192
aggressive behavior signs,
189
costs of raising, 168
custody of, 169
demographics of, 167–168
disorders in, (*see* Childhood disorders)
leading causes of death,
236t, 237, 239
mental retardation of,
16–17
neglect of, 191t
pain in, 212
parents' refusal to treat,
268, 276
preschool age, (*see*
Preschool child)
reactions to illness or
death, 16, 19, 206,
208
school age, (*see* School age
child)
in single-parent families,
168, 173–174
Chi-square test, 257, 257t,
259–260
Chlorazepate, 152t
Chlordiazepoxide, 152t
Chlorpromazine, 146
Cholecystokinin, 35–36, 38
Cholinergic neurons, 34, 36
Chronic pain
definition of, 211
depression and, 211
psychosocial factors,
211–212
review questions regard-
ing, 214–215
treatment for, 212
Circadian rhythm sleep disorder, 90t
Classical conditioning,
55–56, 60
Climacterium, 18
Clinical interview
aims of, 203t
communication skills, 204
interviewing techniques,
204–205, 207
open-ended question use,
199, 205, 207

review questions regard-
ing, 205, 207, 270,
278
Clomipramine, 148t
Clonazepam, 152t
Clonidine, 81t
Clozapine (Clozaril), 41,
44–45, 146, 154, 156
Cocaine
laboratory findings, 80t
neurotransmitter effects,
83, 85
population use of, 74t
pregnancy use, 75
priapism and, 183
review questions regard-
ing, 83–85
sexuality and, 183
smokable forms of, 75
Cognex, (*see* Tacrine)
Cognitive disorders
characteristics of, 127,
128t
dementia, (*see* Dementia)
etiology of, 128t
Cognitive function
age-related declines, 22
development of, 9
of infant, 4–5, 5t
of preschool child, 7t
of toddler, 7t
mental status examina-
tion of, 67t
Cognitive therapy
characteristics of, 161t
description of, 160
review questions regard-
ing, 164–165
Cohort studies, 242, 248,
250, 269, 277
Coma
alcohol-induced, 77
definition of, 68t
Competence, (*see* Legal competence)
Compliance, of patients with
medical advice
characteristics associated
with, 203–204
factors associated with,
202t, 204
review questions regard-
ing, 206–207
Computed tomography, psy-
chiatric patient evalu-
ations using, 43t,
44–45
Conditioned response, 56,
60, 62
Conditioned stimulus, 56,
59–60, 62

Conduct disorder, 140–141,
142t, 143–144
Confidentiality
description of, 219–220
review questions regard-
ing, 225, 227, 261,
264, 272, 274
Confrontation, 203t, 270, 278
Conscious mind, 48, 48t
Consciousness, 68t
Consent, (*see* Informed consent)
Continuous positive airway
pressure, 92t
Continuous reinforcement,
58t
Contraceptives, 15
Conversion disorder, 120t,
123, 125, 268, 271,
276, 278
Correlation, 253, 257,
259–260
Countertransference, 41, 50,
52
CPAP, (*see* Continuous posi-
tive airway pressure)
"Crack," 75
Crossover studies, 245
Cross-sectional studies, 242
Cross-tolerance, 73
Cubans, infant mortality
rate among, 2t
Culture, (*see also specific
culture or race group*)
characteristics of, 169
illness and, 167, 169–170,
174
in United States, 169
Culture shock, 170, 173–174
Custody, of children, 169
Cyclothymic disorder,
111–112, 114–116
Cylert, (*see* Pemoline)

Dalmane, (*see* Flurazepam)
Death, (*see also* Infant mortality rate)
leading causes of, by age
group, 236t, 237–240
legal standard of,
221–222, 226, 228
physician's response to,
24, 26–27
reactions of adolescents
and children to, 16,
19–20
stages of, 23
Defense mechanisms, (*see
also specific defense
mechanism*)
definition of, 48